AF676452

Primary Care Psychiatry and Behavioral Medicine

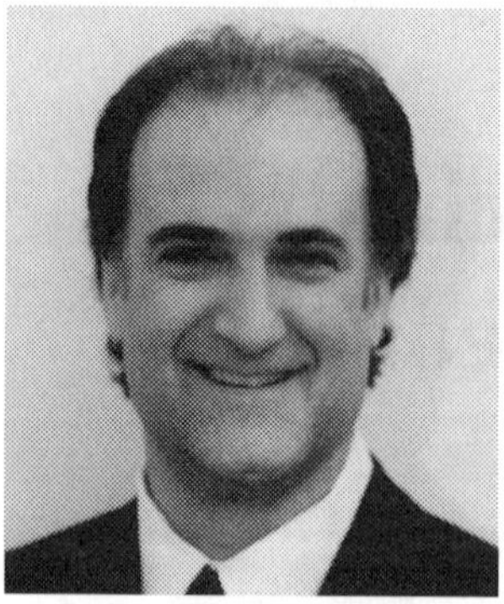

Robert E. Feinstein, M.D. Dr. Feinstein is an Associate Clinical Professor of Psychiatry, Director of Behavioral Science at Stamford Hospital/Columbia University College of Physicians & Surgeons, Program in Family Practice in Stamford, CT. He is also Medical Director of Fairfield County Mental Health Associates, Inc., and is in private psychiatric practice. Dr. Feinstein graduated from the University of Michigan, New York University Medical School, and did his psychiatric residency training at Albert Einstein College of Medicine. He completed his advanced training in psychoanalysis at the Center for Psychoanalytic Training & Research at Columbia University College of Physicians & Surgeons. Dr. Feinstein sees patients, teaches, writes, and does research while living in Stamford, CT with his wife, Marilyn.

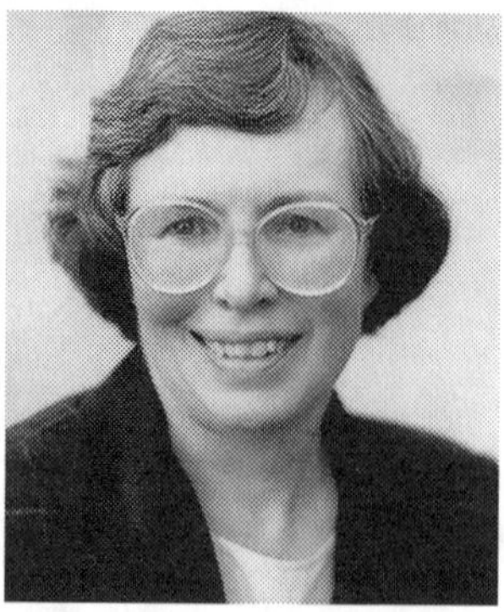

Anne A. Brewer, M.D. Dr. Brewer is Faculty and Assistant Director at the Stamford Hospital/Columbia University College of Physicians & Surgeons, Program in Family Practice in Stamford, CT. She is a graduate of Brown University, University of Vermont School of Medicine, and Episcopal Divinity School. She completed her residency in family practice at the University of Connecticut. She is a Diplomate of the American Board of Family Practice and holds the certificate of Added Qualifications in Geriatrics and Sports Medicine. She is married and has two children.

Primary Care Psychiatry and Behavioral Medicine

Brief Office Treatment and Management Pathways

Robert E. Feinstein, MD
Anne A. Brewer, MD
Editors

Springer Publishing Company

Copyright © 1999 by Springer Publishing Company, Inc.

All rights reserved

No part of this publication may be reproduced, stored in a retrieval system, or transmitted in any form or by any means, electronic, mechanical, photocopying, recording, or otherwise, without the prior permission of Springer Publishing Company, Inc.

Springer Publishing Company, Inc.
536 Broadway
New York, NY 10012–3955

Cover design by Janet Joachim

Acquisitions Editor: Bill Tucker

Production Editor: Jeanne Libby

99 00 01 02 03 / 5 4 3 2 1

Library of Congress Cataloging-in-Publication Data

Primary care psychiatry and behavioral medicine : brief office treatment and management pathways / Robert E. Feinstein, Anne A. Brewer, editors.
p. cm.
Includes bibliographical references and index.
ISBN 0-8261-1224-2
1. Psychiatry. 2. Primary care (Medicine) I. Feinstein, Robert E. II. Brewer, Anne A.
[DNLM: 1. Mental Disorders—therapy. 2. Primary Health Care. 3. Behavorial Medicine. 4. Critical Pathways. WM 400 P952 1999]
RC454.4.P726 1999
616.89—dc21
DNLM/DLC
for Library of Congress 98-42017
CIP

Printed in the United States of America

To my father, the late Harold R. Feinstein, M.D. He was a devoted family physician, who may not have fully appreciated his major contributions to my life and his patients.

To my wife, Marilyn Sommer Feinstein, for her editorial assistance, support, and encouragement. Her uplifting sense of humor and good cheer were welcome nourishment.

To my patients, medical students, residents, and colleagues, who have taught me that learning is not possible without an exchange of listening and caring.

— Robert E. Feinstein, M.D.

To all of my teachers, and especially my patients, whose willingness to allow me into their lives has taught me much of what I know.

To my family, Jim, Becky, and Matt Kowalski who provided inspiration, encouragement, and technical assistance in the writing and editing of this volume.

— Anne A. Brewer, M.D.

Contents

Part III Psychosocial Treatments in Primary Care

Foreword

Gifted clinicians throughout the ages have cared for patients by combining current knowledge of diseases and treatments with a genuine concern for the patient. The past 100 years has brought an explosion of understanding of the pathophysiology of disease. This has been accompanied by spectacular advances in diagnostic techniques, surgical modalities, and pharmacology. The logarithmic increase in information and knowledge put increasing pressure on medical school curricula as professors coped with conveying more information in the limited available time. Primary care, although not yet labeled as such, and psychiatry became increasingly marginalized as they took a back seat to the dramatic and more politically powerful medical and surgical specialties. Caring about patients seemed to become less important than curing patients in the medicine practiced and taught in the middle of the twentieth century.

Patients, physicians, and other health professionals became increasingly frustrated by the limits inherent in the disease-oriented biomedical model of medical practice. The pharmacologic, surgical, and public health victories over many of mankind's most feared killers had indeed lengthened life spans. Taking the place of these vanquished diseases were chronic illnesses that either killed more slowly or caused prolonged suffering. Heart disease, cancer, and mental illness are examples of these illnesses. A curative, biomedical approach to these diseases can be frustrating to patients and health professionals alike.

The specialties of Family Practice, specifically, and primary care and behavioral medicine, in general, developed as a reaction to the constraints of the traditional biomedical model. Popular writers like Norman Cousins and Bernie Siegel spoke eloquently to the public about the limitations of the disease-oriented approach. Medical writers like Michael Balint, George Engel, and Eric Kandel championed new approaches to the patient and the physician-patient relationship. Other models of health care such as holistic medicine, chiropractic, homeopathy, alternative medicine, and many others developed independently of mainstream medicine.

Mainstream medicine is now responding to the need for new knowledge and skills for optimal modern medical practice. Courses in preventive medicine, nutrition, and behavioral medicine are finding their way into the previously sacrosanct bastions of preclinical medical training. Many, if not most, medical schools now require primary care experiences during the clinical years. Partly driven by new forms of reimbursement, residency programs in family medicine, internal medicine, and pediatrics have new-found popularity.

Primary care psychiatry and behavioral medicine have recently developed within mainstream medicine. They are evidence-based, patient-centered, and multidisciplinary. They focus on psychiatric conditions, psychosocial symptoms, prevention-oriented behavioral change (e.g., smoking cessation, exercise, nutrition, etc.), and biopsychosocial interventions.

At The Stamford Hospital/Columbia University Family Practice Residency Program, our own efforts to integrate behavioral medicine into the lives of our family practice physicians have been assimilated into the structure of our residency. We have developed multidisciplinary outpatient, inpatient, and nursing home rounds. We have begun joint behavioral medicine and family practice precepting in the model office, a one-month behavioral medicine rotation, a Balint group, and formal lectures and workshops integrating behavioral medicine principles.

The resources needed to integrate family practice, primary care psychiatry, and behavioral medicine led to the development of the book *Primary Care Psychiatry and Behavioral Medicine: Brief Office Treatment and Management Pathways*. This book belongs in the library of many types of practitioners. It is a joint effort itself, between practitioners and teachers of family medicine and psychiatry. It will be very useful to training sites for medical students, medical residents, health psychology, and behavioral medicine students. It will be helpful to faculty in family practice, internal medicine, and other specialties (such as obstetrics/gynecology) that incorporate primary care into their training. It is a practical book with convenient tables, algorithms, and brief treatment approaches. It will be beneficial to social workers, psychologists, wellness professionals, nurses, and midlevel practitioners such as nurse practitioners and physician assistants.

The editors and authors of *Primary Care Psychiatry and Behavioral Medicine: Brief Office Treatment and Management Pathways* have done an excellent job of synthesizing recent information about the most common psychiatric and behavioral issues that arise in primary care. Application of the knowledge in this book is likely to result in more satisfied patients and physicians as clinicians handle the pervasive psychosocial problems of patients with greater skill and comfort.

Joseph V. Connelly, M.D.
Residency Director
The Stamford Hospital/
Columbia University
College of Physicians & Surgeons
Program, in Family Practice
Stamford, CT

Preface

The idea for this book emerged out of a unique collaboration among psychiatric faculty in behavioral science, family practice faculty members, and residents at the St. Joseph's Family Practice Residency Program in Stamford, CT (recently renamed The Stamford Hospital Columbia University College of Physicians & Surgeons, Program in Family Practice). Our approach to primary care psychiatry and behavioral medicine grew out of a need to improve and discover practical approaches to working with our patients on the psychosocial, lifestyle, and prevention-oriented care that is so easily neglected during an office visit.

At our practice site, the William Pitt Family Medicine Center, we see an ethnically diverse lower- to middle-income patient population. Our family practice physicians and residents offer pediatric, obstetrical, adult, and geriatric general medical care. Our local experience seems to match national statistics in that upwards of 30% of our patients have psychiatric symptoms or disorders that are either primary conditions or complications to the management of a medical condition. If we more broadly define the prevention and lifestyle change needs of our patient population, we estimate that 60% to 70% of our patients can benefit from prevention or behavioral medicine approaches.

We developed this book as part of our efforts to better meet the psychiatric, psychosocial, prevention, and lifestyle change needs of our patients and to meet the educational needs of our family practice residents, primary care medical students, and family practice faculty. This book was mostly written by faculty affiliated with our residency and with members of the Department of Psychiatry at Columbia University College of Physicians and Surgeons in New York City. We believe that the material we have developed is readily accessible to the wider scope of primary care professionals, which includes other primary care physicians, social workers, psychologists, nurse practitioners, nurses, physician assistants, behavioral medicine professionals, health educators, and wellness professionals.

The choice of the content for this book was based on the prevalence and incidence of conditions and issues that present in a primary care setting. Consequently, the text focuses on those disorders and conditions that are either the most common or the most problematic for clinicians.

The book begins with an introduction to many models of primary care. These models, or a combination of these models, were used by our authors as the basis of a framework for suggesting an office-based approach to a disorder or patient problem, or as part of a need for prevention, lifestyle change, medical adherence, or counseling. The introductory chapter also includes a newly conceptualized host versus environmental model of primary care that was developed principally by Dr. Rabinowitz, with assistance from Dr. Feinstein and other faculty.

Most chapters in the book were cowritten by a primary care physician and a mental health professional. All chapters were reviewed and edited several times by a family physician and psychiatrist. The tension in writing this text was fostering the collaboration between disciplines. We were asking the mental health professionals to distill and simplify complex clinical approaches and asking the primary care physicians to strive beyond the biomedical view to the widest practical view of office-based psychosocial and prevention-oriented care.

The book is divided into three sections:

1. **Psychiatric Disorders in Primary Care.** This section reviews the most common disorders or problems treated in primary care. It is loosely based on the DSM-IV Primary Care Version and, when required, DSM-IV. One of the many unique features of this section is our effort to suggest a longitudinal approach to patient care that moves beyond problem identification, differential diagnosis, and acute brief treatment. Our yearlong critical pathways and summary tables emphasize our office-based continuity approach to primary care psychiatric problems. The chapters on anxiety disorders, depression, and schizophrenia and other psychotic disorders provide a detailed review of basic psychopharmacology for the primary care physician. Chapter 8, Personality Disorders in Office Practice, suggests how to manage the most difficult patients for the purpose of improving the delivery of medical care. It should be read in conjunction with chapter 16, Consulting and Counseling in Primary Care. Read in sequence, the two chapters provide a basic approach to working with difficult patients.

2. **Behavioral Medicine in Primary Care.** This section focuses on prevention and some important issues for patients. Chapters 12 and 13 have

a special focus on cardiovascular and psychosocial risk factors and offer an office-based model for providing prevention-oriented primary care and lifestyle modification. The original work in these two chapters was, in part, developed from a federally funded grant written by Dr. Rabinowitz and Dr. Feinstein entitled "Biopsychosocial Life Support Curriculum for Family Practice Residents." This grant, from the Department of Health and Human Services, Bureau of Health Professions (# 5D15PE10297-030), was sponsored by the St. Joseph Medical Center and its Family Practice Residency Program. These two chapters represent 3 years of a collaborative effort from our entire faculty and resident group. Especially unique are our yearlong critical pathways for hypertension, hypercholesterolemia, smoking cessation, weight reduction, exercise, depression, and anxiety. They were developed out of a wonderful (yet sometimes tension filled) collaboration among family physicians and a cardiologist, psychiatrist, psychologist, nutritionist, and exercise specialist/grant coordinator. The remaining two chapters in this section cover issues of women's health and death and dying.

3. **Psychosocial Treatments in Primary Care.** The last section describes office-based counseling and psychosocial treatment approaches. Psychosocial treatment, though frequently offered, is rarely taught as a regular part of the primary care physician's training. Chapter 16, combined with chapter 8, covers the basics of managing difficult patients, suggests management interventions geared toward facilitating the delivery of medical care, describes the principal differences between consultation and counseling, and reviews different models for intervention and counseling. Chapter 17, Crisis Intervention in Office Practice, describes an underutilized form of primary care counseling. This form of treatment is accessible to primary care physicians for handling emergencies such as violence, suicide risk, and other health care or psychosocial crises. Chapter 18, Family Counseling, suggests a practical approach to involving families in office visits and health problem solving. Chapter 19, Behavioral Counseling and Medical Adherence, suggests a cognitive-behavioral approach to fostering lifestyle change, prevention, and improving patient adherence to medical care.

It was important to us that this book be practical, office-based, and comfortably accessible for use by students, residents, faculty, and the wider scope of primary care professionals. Please let us know your reaction to or comments about our work, as this kind of dialogue was the energy source for this book and will ultimately help us determine the book's usefulness.

Acknowledgments

We were delighted to work with the many chapter authors and other contributors. We are especially appreciative of the good-natured and productive dialogue that emerged during the editorial process. Our authors seemed to understand the inherent tension between the psychiatric and primary care approach to patient care. By the end of the process, the psychiatric professionals were starting to sound like primary care physicians and vice versa. This was not really surprising as, ultimately, patient care requires input from both perspectives.

We are especially grateful to Joseph V. Connelly, M.D., Residency Training Director at The Stamford Hospital Columbia University College of Physicians & Surgeons Program in Family Practice in Stamford, CT. He has always encouraged a behavioral science approach, sponsored our federally funded grant, and continues to encourage the entire faculty and residents to see patient care in the broadest possible terms.

We are indebted to the grant team who authored chapters 12 and 13 and the Family Practice Residents at our program who made sure that the approaches we were suggesting were usable and practical in the real world of primary care. Our grant team set the overall tone in our residency for a superb multidisciplinary collaboration. We want to extend a special thanks to Joyelle Gallicano, grant and curriculum coordinator, for all of her hard work and leadership in the implementation of the grant and our critical pathways. She kept us all organized, productive, and focused. We also want to thank Dr. Peter Rabinowitz, who was one of the early driving forces behind the grant and the principal developer of our Health Risk Appraisal. He was the major originator and contributor to the development of the office-based model described in chapter 13.

Rosemarie Perrin, our cyberspace editor from Atlanta, was exceptionally helpful. She reviewed the entire book for style, format, and consistency. Her kindness, encouragement, expertise, and efficiency made it a tremendous pleasure to edit this book. We will miss her daily e-mail.

We would also like to thank Springer Publishing Company for believing in our work and ultimately making this publication possible.

Robert E. Feinstein, M.D.
Anne A. Brewer, M.D.

Contributors

Abraham Bornstein, M.D., F.A.C.C.
Associate Clinical Professor of Medicine
New York Medical College
Valhalla, NY

Anne A. Brewer, M.D.
Assistant Director of Residency Training
Stamford Hospital
Columbia University College of Physicians & Surgeons
Program in Family Practice, Stamford, CT
Faculty
Columbia University College of Physicians & Surgeons
New York, NY

Dewees H. Brown, M.D.
Former Director of Residency Training
Middlesex Family Practice Residency Training Program
Middlesex, CT

Eve Caligor, M.D.
Associate Clinical Professor of Psychiatry
Columbia University College of Physicians & Surgeons
New York, NY

Laurel Carey, M.A.
Behavioral Scientist
Stamford Hospital
Columbia University College of Physicians & Surgeons
Program in Family Practice, Stamford, CT

Rita Charon, M.D.
Associate Professor of Clinical Medicine
Director of the Program for Humanity and Medicine & Medical Interviewing Course
Columbia University College of Physicians & Surgeons
New York, NY

Joseph V. Connelly, M.D.
Director of Residency Training in Family Practice
Stamford Hospital
Columbia Unversity College of Physicians & Surgeons
Program in Family Practice, Stamford, CT
Adjunct Assistant Professor of Medicine
Columbia University College of Physicians & Surgeons
New York, NY

Charlotte Creech, M.D.
Family Practice Resident (PGY III)
Stamford Hospital
Columbia University College of Physician & Surgeons
Program in Family Practice
Stamford, CT

Dr. Janis L.Cutler, M.D.
Assistant Director: Medical Student Education
Associate Clinical Professor of Psychiatry
Columbia University College of Physicians & Surgeons
New York, NY

Brian A. Fallon, M.D.
Associate Clinical Professor of Psychiatry
Columbia University College of Physicians & Surgeons
New York, NY

Robert E. Feinstein, M.D.
Director of Behavioral Sciences
Stamford Hospital
Columbia University College of Physicians & Surgeons
Program in Family Practice
Stamford, CT
Associate Clinical Professor of Psychiatry
Columbia University College of Physicians & Surgeons
New York, NY

Joyelle Gallicano, M.H.A.
Curriculum Development /Grant Coordinator
Stamford Hospital
Columbia University College of Physicians & Surgeons
Program in Family Practice
Stamford, CT
Health Education Coordinator
Scripps Memorial Hospital
La Jolla, CA

Marion Hart, M.D.
Adjunct Assistant Professor of Psychiatry
Cornell University Medical School
New York Hospital Cornell Medical Center, Westchester Division
White Plains, NY

Stanley Kaye, Ph.D.
Director of Psychological Services
Brooklyn Center for Psychotherapy
Professor Emeritus Graduate Program of Psychology: Brooklyn College
Brooklyn, NY

Pamela F. LeDeaux, M.D.
Clinical Assistant Professor,
Department of Family Medicine
SUNY at Stony Brook
Residency Site Director
St. Charles/Mather Health System
Port Jefferson, NY

Lewis A. Opler, M.D., Ph.D.
Medical Director New York City
Region, New York State Office
of Mental Health
Clinical Professor of Psychiatry
Columbia University College of
Physicians & Surgeons
New York, NY

Marian Ormont, M.D.
Assistant Professor of Psychiatry
NCP Hahneman
School of Medicine
Allegheny University of the Health
Sciences
Wayne, PA

Joseph S. Pachman, M.D., Ph.D., M.P.H.
Adjunct Faculty Department of
Psychiatry
Yale University School of
Medicine
New Haven, CT

Leslie Prusnofsky, M.D.
Clinical Assistant Professor of
Psychiatry
Cornell University Medical School
New York Hospital Cornell
Medical Center, Westchester
Division
White Plains, NY

Peter M. Rabinowitz, M.D., M.P.H.
Clinical Faculty
Stamford Hospital/ Columbia
University College of Physicians
& Surgeons
Program in Family Practice
Stamford, CT
Assistant Professor of Medicine
Yale University School of
Medicine
New Haven, CT

Gerald D. Roberts, M.D.
Former Clinical Director of
Liberation Programs, Inc.
Stamford, CT

Roberta Stiel, Psy.D.
Psychologist in Private Practice
Stamford, CT

Susan Vanderberg, M.D.
Program Director: Rush Illinois
Mesanic Family Practice
Residency Program
Associate Professor of Family
Medicine
Rush Medical College
Chicago, IL

CHAPTER 1

Psychosocial Aspects of Primary Care: Theoretical Models of Practice

Peter M. Rabinowitz

The practice of medicine is in the midst of major upheavals. As the forces of managed care and the marketplace reshape the traditional relationships of patients, providers, insurers, and communities, there has been a renewed interest in the role of primary care clinicians in the general health care system. Although this has produced a welcome emphasis on reorienting medical training toward increasing the size of the primary care workforce, it has also produced some conflicting visions of what primary care is and what it should consist of in the future. As Engel (1980) has noted: "How physicians approach patients and the problems they present is very much influenced by the conceptual models around which their knowledge and experience is organized" (p.585). Therefore, any discussion of the role of psychosocial interventions in primary care must begin with a clear definition of primary care and a theoretical basis for how psychosocial concepts fit into it. This chapter will review the development of major theories of primary care practice, with a focus on their psychosocial aspects.

THE INSTITUTE OF MEDICINE'S DEFINITION OF PRIMARY CARE

The Institute of Medicine Committee on the Future of Primary Care (IOM) has published a new definition of primary care, which extends a previous definition proposed in the IOM's 1978 study, "A Manpower Policy for Primary Health Care." The current version states that "primary care is the provision of integrated, accessible health care services by clinicians who are accountable for addressing a large majority of personal health care needs, developing a sustained partnership with patients, and practicing in the context of family and community" (Donaldson, Yordy, Lohr, & Vanselow, 1996, p.1).

The committee noted that despite all the changes that have taken place in primary care, its central feature remains the patient-clinician interaction. It therefore stated that "personal health care needs," which clinicians need to address, include "physical, mental, emotional, and social concerns that involve the functioning of an individual" (Donaldson et al. p.33).

Clearly, a great deal is being asked of today's primary care practitioners. In addition to maintaining competence across a wide spectrum of medical knowledge, they must know how to work effectively with individual, family, and community issues of a more psychosocial nature. How is this possible for the busy clinician who must see a different patient every 5 or 10 minutes? And how can students and trainees in primary care best develop skills in so many different areas?

Studies show that many primary care clinicians are falling short of the lofty goals of the IOM report in their daily work. Many fail to counsel adequately on prevention issues (U.S. Department of Health & Human Services, 1994). The rates of malpractice claims indicate that patient-doctor communication is often incomplete or insufficient. A large and growing interest among patients in alternative and complementary therapies is another indication that traditional medical practitioners are not meeting all of their patients' needs.

Part of the reason why today's primary care practitioners find it hard to master and implement psychosocial skills has been the continuing dominance in medical education and training of the "biomedical model" of care. The biomedical approach is the reductionistic and empiric grounding of medical practice in pathophysiology. This approach, championed by Flexner (1925) as a reaction to the turn-of-the-century quackery and therapeutic nihilism that abounded, has led to impressive research discoveries and therapeutics. Yet it has done so at the price of a relative devaluing of the humanistic and psychosocial aspects of medicine. Today, even in primary care training programs, the skills of psychosocial assessment, counseling, health promotion, disease prevention, and community intervention are often treated as curricular add-ons compared to the more medical core skills of diagnosis and treatment.

For primary care practitioners to consistently do a good job with the psychosocial demands of their work, the types of skills that this book discusses must assume an importance equivalent to such skills as physical diagnosis or choosing the right antibiotic. For this to take place, there should be some organizing principles that integrate and include all aspects of effective primary care practice.

EXISTING THEORETICAL MODELS RELEVANT TO PRIMARY CARE: THE BIOPSYCHOSOCIAL MODEL

George Engel, a psychiatrist, proposed in 1960 a biopsychosocial model for health care in reaction to the biomedical reductionism he saw in medical education and training. The biopsychosocial approach, based in systems theory, sets up a vertical hierarchy of levels of interactions that could be taking place in any clinical situation, ranging from the lowest (atomic level) through molecular, tissue, organ, and individual levels, and beyond this to two-person, family, community, and society levels. For example, the syndrome of cardiac chest pain can involve both molecular derangements in the heart and effects on a couple's sex life or, in the case of a world leader, the security of an entire nation. Engel pointed out that other levels in the vertical hierarchy may be operating at the same time and may be much more important than the biomedical level.

Case Example: Biopsychosocial Model

Michael I., a 40-year-old man, presents to the emergency room complaining of substernal chest pain. The patient is a busy financial officer for a large company and has recently suffered the loss of a close cousin from a heart attack. His primary care physician comes to the emergency room to examine him. Using a biopsychosocial approach, the physician attempts to assess the patient not only at the organ level of the heart and lungs (through auscultation) but also at the myocardial tissue level (through tests such as cardiac enzymes, troponin levels, and an electrocardiogram). Proceeding up the hierarchy of systems, the physi-

> cian also tries to understand the chest pain in terms of the patient's psychological coping, job stresses, and marital support. After the laboratory results indicate that no acute myocardial infarction is taking place, the patient is hospitalized for observation. Over several hospital visits, the physician is able to reassure both Michael I. and his wife that the pain was not caused by a heart attack and to discuss the fear and emotional pain that the loss of the patient's cousin brought about. The patient is able to leave the hospital and return to work.

Engel's coining of the term *biopsychosocial* was an important step in the attempt to define an integrated approach. The term continues to be the most popular one in use in the field of medicine to pay lip service to holistic considerations or describe curricula or medical worldviews that are something more than biomedical. In this way, it has served as a constant reminder that there is more to patient care than physical examination, laboratory tests, and medications.

Nonetheless, the model has several practical shortcomings. Splitting the clinical situation into numerous system levels of interaction can appear overly complex and make it difficult to gain a holistic appreciation of the patient. In addition, the hierarchical model does not always overcome the conceptual mind-body split that it set out to integrate. For example, the biopsychosocial model's hierarchy of levels neatly divides at the person level. Systems placed below the person level (all the way down to the atomic particle level) appear to be biological or biochemical, whereas systems higher on the hierarchy than a person (up to the society-nation level) appear to be psychosocial in nature. A further difficulty is that the proponents of the model have often been behavioral scientists rather than primary care clinicians; therefore, practical applications of the model have focused on the psychosocial aspects of a particular case. Thus the biopsychosocial model, as commonly presented, tends to underemphasize biological, chemical, and physical factors that could be at work on many of Engel's levels, such as environmental and occupational exposures to toxins taking place on the community level. For all these reasons, it is tempting to look further for a model that will consistently encourage the integration of biological and psychosocial factors in primary care.

THE FAMILY PRACTICE MODEL

Another approach, which has been more implicit than explicit, is the family practice model of care. Family practice, the youngest of the American medical specialty boards, grew out of the general practice tradition. The archetypal family doctor was proficient in a broad range of skills, from delivering a baby to comforting the dying. This comprehensive care often took place in the patient's home. The family doctor interacted with the community on a variety of levels, from house calls and hospital visits to community politics and involvement with the occupational work sites located in the community. The family doctor's role of caring for all family members from cradle to grave was a natural extension of the limited availability of specialists and the broad scope of practice expected of primary care clinicians. As a result, this physician could intuit the health concerns of one member of a family through knowledge of the rest of the family.

It has been the challenge of modern family practice to transfer the positive aspects of the general practice tradition to the modern medical context. This has involved ensuring that trainees in family practice develop competencies in both outpatient and inpatient care settings. Such broad competency is an ever-increasing task, given the recent explosion of medical knowledge and the increasingly specialized approaches to many of the functions once performed primarily by general practitioners. To provide a unifying focus to family practice care, the curriculum of family practice residency programs has introduced trainees to biopsychosocial, family system, and community medicine concepts.

Case Example: Family Practice Model

> Olivia M. brings her 2-year-old in for a fever. The family practice physician, while examining the infected ear, notes that this is the fourth infection this winter. He also remembers that Olivia's husband, who is also his patient, is a heavy smoker. As a physician for the whole family, he is a trusted medical adviser. After he has made the diagnosis of acute otitis media, he writes a prescription for antibiotics but also spends several minutes with Olivia explaining the relationship between second hand smoke and respiratory infections. She agrees that her husband will make an appointment for smoking cessation counseling.

Physicians entering family practice careers now face a work environment vastly different from that of their predecessors. Many family physicians are spending the majority of their clinical time in busy outpatient clinics quite removed from the communities they serve. A typical patient visit usually lasts less than 15 minutes. The physician rarely, if ever, makes a house call (Grumbach & Fry, 1993) or a visit to a patient's work site. The family physician, although trained to practice in the context of families, may not be seeing multiple members of the same family, because in the increasingly competitive medical marketplace there may be several other clinicians, such as pediatricians, internists, and gynecologists, taking care of them. In these situations, the traditional family practice model may not provide a sufficiently clear framework for the kind of integration of biological and psychosocial skills that the Institute of Medicine has proposed. Psychosocial issues may be overlooked because of the time pressure to diagnose and treat biomedical disease. Yet many family practice physicians are still able to incorporate, over a series of visits, psychosocial aspects into the patient's care.

THE FAMILY SYSTEMS MODEL

The discipline of family practice is one of the primary care fields that has drawn on family systems theory (Ramsey, 1989). Family systems theory attempts to explain health events through an understanding of the psychoneuroendocrine/immune interactions of a dynamic family system. On a practical level, this could involve use of genograms, family circles, family mapping, and other techniques of describing family systems at work in an individual patient.

Case Example: Family Systems Model

John T. is a teenager with a bad case of atopic dermatitis. His skin condition has proved resistant to the usual approach of emollients and topical steroids. Although he is a somewhat guarded historian, his family physician suspects that much of the problem lies in family stress. From talking with the patient and his parents in a series of family counseling sessions, it becomes evident that John is the child in the family most sensitive to his parents' high expectations. He also has the most trouble expressing his emotions. The family has recently been in turmoil because the father lost his job and is having frequent outbursts of anger. The physician senses the relationship between such interpersonal conflicts and the pattern of somatization and neurotic behavior in John. When John's father lost his job, he lost self-esteem and his role as family provider. This led John and other family members to challenge his authority, leading to the father's increasing outbursts and John's worsening skin condition. A family session helps reframe the situation. The physician helps members of the family reassure John's father about their continued need for his leadership. John is able to express his desire to work to help the family in need. With this intervention, the family begins to work together, the anger decreases at home, and John's atopic dermatitis improves.

A family systems approach has been advocated for other professionals who work with families, such as social workers, psychiatrists, and psychologists. Primary care clinicians, however, may not receive in-depth training in such interventions. In addition, studies of the impact of family systems interventions on medical outcomes have been disappointing. Partly because of the pressures of daily medical practice described above and the consequent limited interaction of the clinician with families as opposed to individual patients, this approach to primary care has been difficult for clinicians to implement. However, clinicians may refer patients to mental health professionals who are capable of providing family therapy.

THE COMMUNITY-ORIENTED PRIMARY CARE (COPC) MODEL

In part as a response to the growing isolation of health care providers and institutions from the communities they serve, community-oriented primary care (COPC) developed as a system of health care delivery that sees the community as the unit of care (Wright, R. A., 1993). This primary care model uses practice-based epidemiology to make a community diagnosis (assessment), which can be used to help tailor medical services to meet the needs of the community. This form of population-based medicine has several powerful advantages. It formalizes the feedback between providers and communities, helping ensure that resources are spent on the most appropriate needs. This in turn helps build trust between communities and medical institutions.

Case Example: Community-Oriented Primary Care

Patrick F. is seen by a physician assistant in a community health center. Patrick is a 10th grader complaining of a nonhealing oral sore. Upon examining the patient, the physician assistant notes a similarity to other cases that the clinic had seen recently. Upon further history-taking, the clinician learns that Patrick has been using smokeless tobacco, which has recently become fashionable at the local high school. After treating Patrick's ulcer, the physician assistant and her supervising physician search the clinic's computerized database and discover five similar cases in the past 3 months. They decide that it would be worthwhile to do a community needs assessment about the use of smokeless tobacco among youth. Through focus groups and a written survey, they and several of the clinic's outreach workers discover that smokeless tobacco is a concern of many of the parents in their community as well as school officials. They also determine some of the patterns of smokeless tobacco use in the community, and the health center uses this information to design an educational program in the high school about the dangers of smokeless tobacco.

Managed care, by increasingly pooling physician and patient data, is using similar approaches to get feedback from patients (consumers) and use it to reorient health care provider services (products). Managed care's focus on cost rather than health outcomes, however, is not what the originators of community-oriented primary care envisioned.

Although managed care has adopted certain aspects of COPC, physicians have been slow to accept this model for care (O'Connor, 1989). The physician's view is that it is impractical for clinicians to spend time doing community assessment. In addition, as an overall model for primary care, COPC falls short, partly because its emphasis on population-based care is too depersonalized to encourage the strong bonds between providers and individual patients that the Institute of Medicine report considers central to primary care.

PREVENTION-ORIENTED PRIMARY CARE (HOST/ENVIRONMENT MODEL)

In an attempt to meld some of the most important aspects of these various models to better fit new developments in primary care, this book will refer at times to a "prevention-oriented primary care model" that looks at a clinical encounter in terms of host and environment interactions (see chapters 12 and 13). This new model views disease as arising from the interaction of two main spheres: an individual's host factors (that individual's specific genetic, medical, and behavioral makeup that makes the host either more immune or more susceptible to disease) and the individual's functional environment (social, biologic, physical, and chemical). Health implies a state of balance between host immunity and environmental stressors, whereas illness and disease result from either impaired host immunity to disease, increased environmental stress, or both.

The driving force behind this model is the growing emphasis on preventive rather than strictly curative health care services. Practicing preventively requires a reorientation of priorities and skills, and the task of the primary care physician in this preventive, host/environment model is to assess at each patient visit the state of host defenses and environmental stressors and to determine what, if any, interventions are in order to help put the system back in balance.

Case Example: Prevention-Oriented Primary Care (Host/Environment Model)

Robert M., a 50-year-old machinist, comes to his primary care clinician complaining of fatigue and muscle aches. His medical history reveals that over the past year, he has had a complete neurological work-up for his fatigue and weakness and has been diagnosed with fibromyalgia. Screening for infectious, rheumatologic, and thyroid disease has been negative. He has taken non-steroidal medications without much effect. He is sleeping poorly and has little appetite. His lifestyle is fairly sedentary because he "just doesn't have any energy." He is concerned that exposures to cleaning solvents at work give him headaches and make him feel dizzy, and he believes that others in the workplace are also being exposed. Formerly a good worker, his relationship with his supervisor is now deteriorating. His wife has been supportive but is frustrated by his lack of improvement.

A case like this defies simple biomedical approaches. Fibromyalgia is one of a number of common syndromes that are poorly understood from a pathophysiological point of view and that are difficult to treat with medication alone. At the same time, although this patient appears to be clinically depressed, it is overly simplistic to say that his only problems are psychosocial. Primary care clinicians, unlike mental health professionals, must take responsibility for comprehensively assessing all aspects of a patient's health.

Using a prevention-oriented, host/environment model, the clinician can search for those aspects of the patient's condition that are causing the bulk of the illness and that can most effectively be modified.

Through a standard medical evaluation, with special emphasis on modifiable risk factors, the clinician arrives at a profile of the patient's host status. Robert M.'s age places him at risk of midlife adjustment difficulties as well as increased susceptibility to physical stressors at work. His sedentary lifestyle is making it hard to break the fibromyalgia cycle of pain and restricted activity. His depression stands in the way of any preventive lifestyle changes. At the same time, the fact that he has up until recently been healthy is a positive indicator of his potential to recover.

Years ago, a primary care physician would have assessed Robert M.'s environment through home visits (where the spouse and other significant family members might be encountered). The clinician might also have familiarity with the work site. Because this may be impractical under the current health care delivery system, the clinician can attempt to characterize the patient's environment through a series of screening questions about home and workplace.

The clinician learns that while the home situation appears generally supportive, the patient's fatigue and muscle pains have interfered with his sexual relationship with his wife. In addition, Robert M.'s work is increasingly a source of stress. He is concerned not only about himself and his exposure to solvents but also about the health of his coworkers. The clinician knows that solvent exposures can lead to transient changes in mental status and feels this is an important factor in the patient's care that may have been overlooked.

Having identified multiple risk factors that could be contributing to his condition, the clinician discusses with Robert M. which factors are most important, which problems are of highest priority to the patient, and which have the greatest chance of being successfully modified.

The clinician's medical priorities are the patient's depression, lack of exercise, and the solvent exposures at work. The patient's priorities, as they emerge during the discussion, are his sexual dysfunction, his poor work performance, and whether he or others at work are being harmed by the solvents.

The prevention-oriented primary care approach draws upon the priorities of both clinician and patient to choose several agreed-upon areas for intervention. Through this informed sharing of the decision-making process, the clinician and patient arrive at the plan of action described in the Figure 1.1.

Over a course of several months, the patient's depression and fatigue improve. Through exercise, he is able to raise his pain tolerance and perform more of his job duties. An industrial hygienist visits the work site and makes recommendations about the ventilation system in the areas where solvents are used. Robert M. is able to express his concerns to the plant management in a

Interventions to Improve Host Status

- Begin exercise program
- Begin counseling for depression
- Antidepressant medication (choosing agent that will also help pain threshold but that will not adversely affect sexual function)

Interventions to Reduce Environmental Stressors

- Refer patient to occupational/environmental medicine clinic for assessment of solvent exposures in workplace and identify other possible cases.
- Suggest job restriction from solvent exposures and physically demanding labor.
- Brief counseling of patient regarding coping skills with supervisor, to follow up with counselor.

Figure 1.1 Host/Environment Treatment Plan for Robert M.: Fibromyalgia.

> constructive way. Changes to the ventilation system are made, and a number of workers, including Robert M., notice a decrease in symptoms of headaches and dizziness at work. Through ongoing counseling sessions, the patient and his wife are able to improve their relationship.

This prevention-oriented approach hearkens back to what family doctors once did unconsciously by virtue of their intimate familiarity with the homes, families, and workplaces of patients. It requires the awareness and competency to assess and intervene with community health problems as well as psychosocial ones while remaining firmly based in the context of the individual patient-clinician interaction. Prevention, in this model, involves fostering both strong host defenses and healthy environments.

A key difference between this model and the biopsychosocial model is that it lumps aspects of the patient's condition into two categories, host and environment, whereas the biopsychosocial model splits these aspects into three levels and a far greater number of subsystem levels. Both lumping and splitting approaches to the infinite complexity of a patient and his or her environment run the risk of obscuring the most important problems at hand, by either excessive generalization or excessive detail. In a brief office visit, both clinician and patient can rarely deal with more than one level of interaction. Yet usually over the course of several visits, and certainly over several years of caring for a particular patient, the clinician develops an overall sense of the patient and his or her surroundings that most closely resembles the host/environment model. As computers increasingly find their way into the medical record, it will only become easier to assimilate and prioritize multiple risk factor information for both individual patients and an entire panel of patients for which the clinician is responsible. The prevention-oriented approach allows for shared interventions on the highest yield issues at hand.

OTHER CONSIDERATIONS

Although the use of a conceptual model can help the primary care clinician better assess and integrate psychosocial aspects into the daily care provided, the clinician will need to be well prepared with intervention strategies dealing with all the issues raised. Subsequent chapters in the book will address specific interventions.

An example is the patient with full-blown psychosis or serious personality disorder who needs specific psychiatric interventions that may be beyond the scope of the primary care clinician. Another is the patient with a significant addiction who may benefit from a mutual-aid self-help group approach, such as Alcoholics Anonymous. In such situations, it is important that the clinician identify the problem and appropriately access other members of the health care team or other community resources. At the same time, these patients are generally in need of excellent primary care services in addition to their specialized treatments, and the primary care clinician can play a vital role in the ongoing care of these patients.

The narrowly focused biomedical model of disease clearly fails to take into account the vital importance of psychosocial factors that are in fact central to primary care. However, creating an integrated model of primary care practice that incorporates psychosocial concepts with biomedical principles has been difficult. A major barrier is the limited time that primary care clinicians can spend with individual patients as well as the fact that, in this country, clinicians rarely make visits to their patients' homes or workplaces. To be useful for the primary care clinician, psychosocial assessments and interventions must be time-efficient and effective.

In this book, the reader will find a mix of approaches to the psychosocial aspects of primary care that reflect some of the schools of thought previously described in this chapter. The reader will notice that some of the chapters in this book follow a biopsychosocial approach; others take more of a community-oriented primary care approach or an implicit family practice tack. Several chapters refer to a prevention-oriented (host-environment) model of care. This diversity of approaches and techniques reflects the current eclecticism of primary care theory and practice in this country. Each of the various models presented in this book should be judged on how effectively it helps clinicians uncover the most important psychosocial forces at work in a particular patient and how well it sets the stage for effective interventions to resolve current health problems and prevent future illness.

REFERENCES

Engel, G. L. (1960). A unified concept of health and disease. *Perspectives in Biology and Medicine, 3*, 459–485.

Engel, G. L. (1980). The clinical application of the biopsychosocial model. *American Journal of Psychiatry, 137*, 535–544.

Donaldson, M. S., Yordy, K. D., Lohr, K. N., & Vanselow, N. A. (1996). *Primary care: America's health in a new era.* Washington, DC: National Academy Press.

Flexner, A. (1919). *Medical education in the United States and Canada, a Report of the Carneqie Foundation of the Advancement of Teaching, No. 4.* Boston: Updyke.

Grumbach, K., & Fry, J. (1993). Managing primary care in the United States and in the United Kingdom. *New England Journal of Medicine, 328*, 940–945.

O'Connor, P. J. (1989). Is community oriented primary care a viable concept in actual practice? An opposing view. *Journal of Family Practice, 28*, 206–208.

Ramsey, C. N. (1989). Toward a theory of family medicine. In C. N. Ramsey (Ed.), *Family systems in medicine.* New York: Guilford Press.

U.S. Department of Health and Human Services. (1994). *Healthy people 2000 review, 1993* (DHHS Pub No. (PHS) 94-1232-1). Washington, DC: U.S. Government Printing Office.

Wright, R. A. (1993). Community oriented primary care: The cornerstone of health-care reform. *Journal of the American Medical Association, 269*, 2544–2547.

PART 1

Psychiatric Disorders in Primary Care

CHAPTER 2

Anxiety Disorders

Robert E. Feinstein

Anxiety disorders are the most common psychiatric diagnosis in the United States today. According to the 1984 Epidemiological Catchment Area Survey conducted by the National Institute of Mental Health (Gorman & Papp, 1992), approximately 15.4% of the community samples in the study have a diagnosis of an anxiety disorder. Anxiety is the fifth most common clinical diagnosis in primary care, accounting for approximately 11% of all visits to physicians (Kanton & Geyman, 1995). In addition, anxiety disorders are often precipitated by, or are comorbid conditions with, medical illness.

Although they are exceedingly common, anxiety disorders often go unrecognized. Untreated, they can have serious consequences. For example, patients with panic disorders or panic symptoms have high rates of suicidal ideation and suicide attempts. Nevertheless, clinicians often miss anxiety disorders entirely in examination and evaluation of patients, especially some of the most common ones, such as social phobias, which have a 10% to 13% lifetime prevalence rate (Davidson, 1994); obsessive-compulsive disorder, with a 2.1%, 1-year prevalence rate (Jenike, 1992); and posttraumatic stress disorder, with a 7.8% lifetime prevalence rate in the general population of adults (Friedman, Charney, & Deutch, 1995). In addition, patients with anxiety disorders use approximately twice as much nonpsychiatric medical care as the general population of patients (Kanton & Geyman, 1995). Because more than half of all patients in the United States with a mental disorder receive their sole treatment from a primary care physician, it is vital that clinicians in primary care practices be informed and equipped to recognize and deal with psychiatric disorders, including anxiety and panic.

This chapter will review a biopsychosocial approach to anxiety disorders and will provide the following: an anxiety disorder algorithm and guidelines for differential diagnosis, a clinical review of anxiety disorders, screening instruments for anxiety disorders, a discussion of the physiological and psychological basis of anxiety disorders, recommendations for office-based treatment, a critical pathway for treating panic disorders, and patient education and resources.

ANXIETY DISORDER ALGORITHM AND DIFFERENTIAL DIAGNOSIS

Diagnosis

The first step in the work-up and treatment of anxiety disorders is to evaluate the patient for general medical conditions and substance-induced anxiety disorders. The anxiety disorder algorithm in the fourth edition of the American Psychiatric Association's *Diagnostic and Statistical Manual of Mental Diseases Primary Care Version* (1995, DSM-IV-PC) describes the general approach toward the work-up and differential diagnosis of anxiety disorders. Figure 2.1 summarizes the algorithm.

General Medical Conditions Producing Anxiety Symptoms

There are many medical causes for anxiety symptoms. The most common are hyperthyroidism, hypoglycemia or diabetes, cardiovascular disorders (arrhythmias, myocardial infarction, congestive heart failure, cardiomyopathy, cardiac transplantation, mitral valve prolapse), audiovestibular disorder, partial-complex seizures, Parkinson's disease, and pheochromocytoma.

The work-up for anxiety disorders should include a detailed medical and psychiatric history, physical examination, mental status examination, and relevant laboratory testing. The latter may include (1) common laboratory studies such as glucose, calcium, phosphate, and thyroid studies (more rarely used are arterial blood gases, catecholamines and cortisol levels, autoimmune screening, and ceruloplasmin if clinically indicated); (2) urine drug screens as appropriate; and (3) common diagnostic testing,

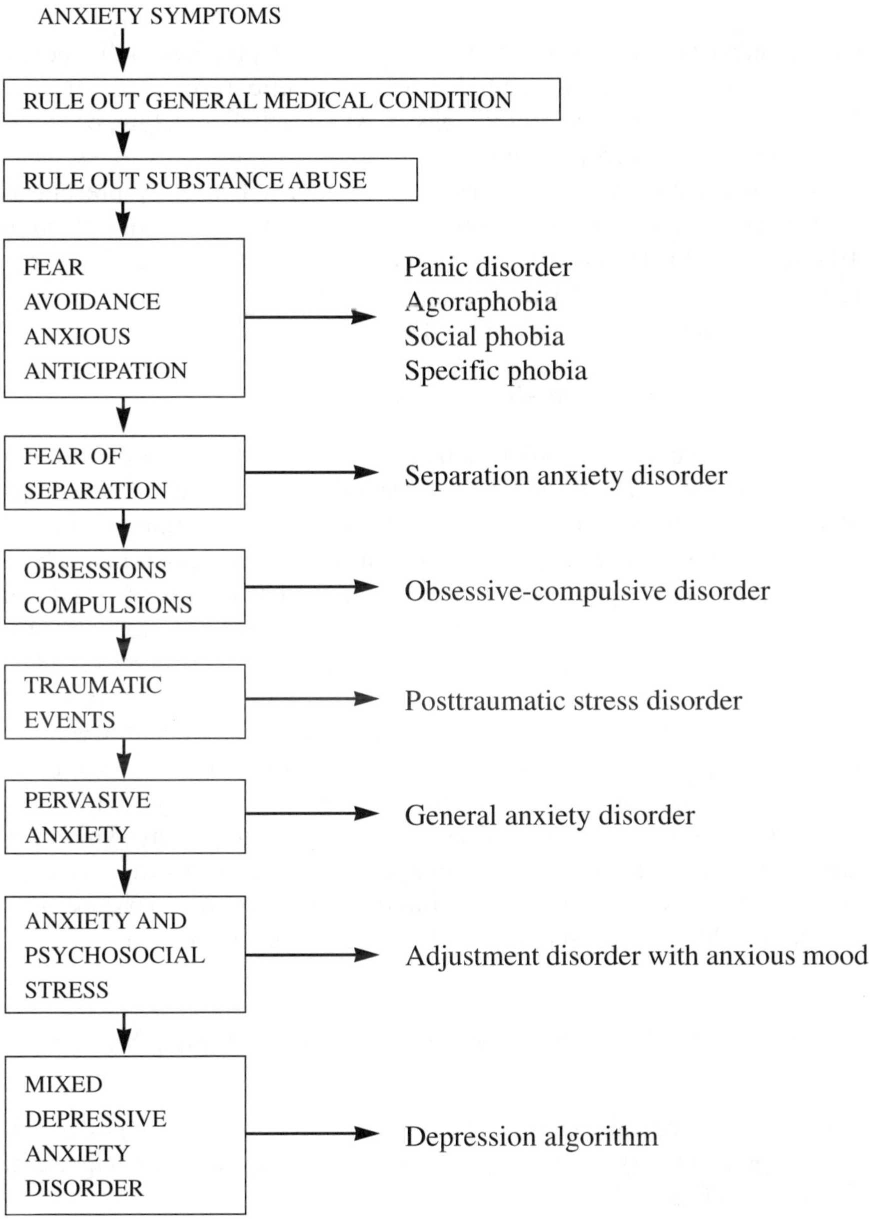

Adapted with permission from the Diagnostic and Statistical Manual of Mental Disorders, Fourth Edition, Primary Care Version. Copyright 1995 American Psychiatric Association.

Figure 2.1 Anxiety Algorithm.

such as electrocardiogram and, when indicated, sophisticated diagnostic testing, such as electroencephalogram, magnetic resonance imaging (MRI), computer assisted tomography (CAT), vestibular testing, echocardiography, and a sleep work-up.

In a primary care setting, anxiety disorders will usually present as somatic complaints or in association with another medical condition. From 10% to 83% of patients with general medical conditions suffer from anxiety disorders. Table 2.1 lists common medical conditions and the incidence of anxiety disorders associated with them.

Substance-Induced Anxiety Disorders

Drug-induced anxiety disorders can be caused by drug intoxication, drug withdrawal, medications, and environmental toxins. Table 2.2 lists drugs that are known to produce anxiety symptoms. The most common of these is caffeine. Two or more cups of coffee or its equivalent in caffeinated beverages can produce symptoms of generalized anxiety disorder (GAD) and panic. Nicotine withdrawal, especially during smoking cessation, can produce anxiety symptoms, especially in smokers who also consume caffeine. This is because nicotine enhances the metabolic breakdown rate of caffeine. Thus a person who used to smoke and drink caffeinated beverages and who stops smoking will experience a much greater effect from the same amount of caffeine as consumed prior to smoking cessation.

The most commonly abused drugs that can produce anxiety syndromes are cocaine and alcohol. It is extremely important to distinguish drug abuse–induced anxiety disorders from other anxiety disorders, as management is different from treatment for psychiatric anxiety disorders.

CLINICAL PRESENTATION OF ANXIETY DISORDERS

Once general medical conditions and substance abuse have been ruled out, evaluation of anxiety disorders proceeds along the *DSM-IV-PC* algorithm described in Figure 2.1.

Panic Attacks With/Without Agoraphobia Disorders

Signs and Symptoms

The essential feature of this disorder is one or more unexpected panic attacks followed by at least 1 month of worry. The panic attack appears

Table 2.1 Medical Conditions Associated with Anxiety Disorders

Medical Condition	Associated Anxiety Disorder	% Patients with Anxiety Disorder
Cardiac conditions		
Atypical chest pain seen in the emergency room	Panic disorder	16%
Chest pain and normal coronaries	Panic disorder	34%
Negative cardiac work-up	Panic disorder	55%
Cardiologist office	All anxiety disorders	57%
ICU patients	Panic disorder	33%
Postinfarction failure	Panic disorder	16%
Cardiomyopathy	Panic disorder	83%
Cardiovascular transplantation	Panic disorder	16%
Respiratory conditions		
COPD	Panic disorder	24%
Asthma (children)	All anxiety disorders	43.2%
	Separation disorder	32.4%
Gastrointestinal		
Primary biliary cirrhosis (PBC)	Panic & phobia	10%
Irritable bowel	All anxiety disorders	29%
Irritable bowel	Panic disorder	18%
Neurological		
Parkinson's disease	Panic/social phobia	21%/17%
Sydenham's chorea	Obsessive compulsive	13%
Tourette's syndrome	Obsessive compulsive	35%–50%
Tics	Obsessive compulsive	20%
Seizures	Panic/GAD	Unknown
Postconcussive/TIA	Panic/GAD	Unknown
Endocrine		
Thyroid disease	GAD/Panic	62%
Adrenal disease	GAD/Panic	Unknown
Others		
Pheochromocytoma	Panic attacks	Common
Porphyria	Panic attacks	Common
Sjogren syndrome	Phobia	10%
	Panic attacks	16%
Chronic pain	Panic attacks	Occasional
Sleep disorders	Posttraumatic stress	Unknown
Toxic gas	All anxiety disorders	Rare
Infections	All anxiety disorders	Rare

Table 2.2 Drugs Known to Produce Anxiety Symptons

Drug Intoxications	Drug Withdrawal	Medications	Psychiatric Medications	Exposure to Environmental Toxins
• Caffeine • Alcohol • Cocaine • Amphetamines • Cannabis • Hallucinogens • Inhalants • Phencyclidine	• Alcohol • Sedatives/hypnotics • Opiates • Cocaine	• Antihypertensive and cardiovascular medications • Calcium channel blockers and digitalis • Sympathomimetics and bronchodilators • Anesthetics • Analgesics • Anticholinergic and anti-Parkinson's agents • Insulin • Thyroid preparations • Oral contraceptive and/or hormone replacements • Antihistamines • Anticonvulsants	• Lithium • Antidepressants • Antipsychotics	• Gasoline • Paint • Organophosphate insecticides • Carbon monoxide • Carbon dioxide • Nerve gas

abruptly without a stimulus and is experienced as an intense fear, discomfort, or panic that develops quickly and peaks within 10 minutes. Symptoms of a panic attack can be cardiac, autonomic, gastrointestinal, neurological, or psychiatric in nature. The most common symptoms are noncardiac chest pain, shortness of breath, fear of impending doom, fear of going crazy, and feeling dizzy or faint. Less common symptoms of panic, which may go unrecognized, include fear of choking, nausea or vomiting, sweating or hot flashes, feelings of unreality or detachment from oneself, trembling, and paresthesias.

When patients present to a primary care physician, physical complaints often get all the attention. It is important to remember that panic can present with cognitive symptoms: the fear that something catastrophic will happen; affective symptoms including terror, heightened arousal, anticipatory anxiety, and feelings of depression; and behavioral symptoms, such as withdrawal, dependency, and avoidance of the phobic situation.

Some patients who have panic attacks may also develop agoraphobia. Agoraphobia is anxiety about being unable to exit or escape. Common agoraphobic symptoms include a fear of riding buses or planes; a fear of open spaces, such as supermarkets; a fear of elevators, subways, or bridges; or a more global and severe fear of leaving home. *DSM-IV-PC* describes three possible forms of panic disorder: panic attacks with agoraphobia, panic attacks without agoraphobia, and panic attacks within the context of other anxiety disorders.

One system for understanding the relationship and overlap of panic disorder, phobia, agoraphobia, and depression has been described as the seven stages of the natural history of endogenous anxiety (Sheehan, 1983). Many patients progress through an anxiety sequence by experiencing subpanic attacks (stage 1), which typically progress to full panic attacks (stage 2). With many panic and/or subpanic attacks patients develop a somatic preoccupation that becomes hypochondriasis (stage 3). Patients often progress and become avoidant of the location of the attack and develop a single phobia (stage 4), such as fear of riding a bus. If panic attacks continue, there is further avoidance of multiple sites of panic, and the patient progresses to more general avoidance of social situations, or social phobias (stage 5). As new phobic situations develop, the patient becomes polyphobic and agoraphobic and at the extreme may be homebound (stage 6). When undiagnosed or untreated, these panic and polyphobic states easily progress to depression (stage 7).

Course of the Illness

Panic attacks usually present between adolescence and the 30s, although some patients have new onset symptoms in childhood or after 45 years of age. Panic symptoms may come and go, and some patients may have total remission for years. Others follow a chronic course of unremitting symptoms. Agoraphobia typically develops within the first year of panic symptoms but can also be present without panic attacks. Long-term follow-up studies indicate that after the initial attack, 30% to 80% of patients will go through a 6-month panic-free period within 6 months to 7 years (Pollack & Smoller, 1995).

Epidemiology

Worldwide studies show lifetime prevalence rates for panic disorder between 1.5% and 3.5% and 1-year prevalence rates between 1% and 2%. According to the *DSM-IV* (1994), approximately 40% of patients with panic disorder also have agoraphobia.

Clinical Issues

Patients who suffer panic attacks usually are quite vocal about their symptoms. These symptoms should prompt a physician to ask about phobias, agoraphobia, hypochondriasis, depression, and suicidal history. Remember that chest pain, fainting, nausea, and vomiting are often symptoms of a panic disorder. Appropriate medical evaluations are important for these complaints, but it is equally important when working up these physical complaints to be aware that many physical symptoms can have a neurochemical, neurological, or psychiatric basis. Clinicians need to avoid telling patients after a medical work-up is negative, that nothing is wrong. Instead, it is better to comment that there may be an abnormal firing of the anxiety center in the central nervous system, which is controlled by genes, neurotransmitters, cognitions, life situations, and memories. It is vital to let patients know that their symptoms, along with a negative physical work-up, suggest panic attacks and that specific medical treatment is available and should be pursued.

It is also often helpful to tell patients that the abnormal panic and anxiety response, although terrifying, will not harm them physically. Clinicians can try to elicit a patient's "hot thoughts," the precipitating thoughts that usually accompany a panic attack. In general, patients with panic disorder interpret physical sensations, such as a rapid heart beat, in the most catastrophic way (e.g., as meaning they are having a heart attack). They may interpret a mild fainting sensation as a stroke. Making the patient aware that every bodily sensation need not be catastrophic can go a long way to reducing a patient's symptoms.

A common clinical mistake in treating patients with panic disorder is to undertreat or undermedicate patients, then become annoyed at their repeated calls for help. Panic patients typically need frequent, brief contact with their clinicians for the first week or two following the initial clinician contact.

PHOBIAS

Social Phobia Signs and Symptoms

Social phobia is the third most common psychiatric disorder, after depression and alcohol dependence (Davidson, 1994). A social phobia is a fear of one or more social or performance situations in which the person is fearful of public scrutiny. This pubic exposure produces an immediate anxiety response that can be fear, worry, or a full-blown panic attack. The typical anxiety is a fear of being criticized, laughed at, embarrassed, or humiliated in public for the whole world to see. Typical social phobias are a fear of public speaking; fear of meeting new people or strangers; fear of eating, choking, or writing in public; an inability to urinate in a public lavatory; and the inordinate fear of saying something foolish. Patients suffering from social phobias recognize them as unreasonable and either avoid public situations totally or endure them with high anxiety.

Social phobias usually interfere with daily functioning in school, at work, or in relationships with others. Fifty percent of patients with social phobias report at least moderate interference with their education (Davidson, 1994). As a group, persons suffering from social phobias are underemployed and have difficulty forming personal relationships and pursuing other social interests. In addition, substance abuse is common as a comorbid condition. Social phobia is also commonly seen as a comorbid condition with simple phobia and agoraphobia. The social phobic is often financially dependent on others because he or she is fearful of public work environments. In addition, social phobics have a much greater risk of suicidal ideation, suicide attempts, and substance abuse.

Course of Social Phobia

Patients who develop social phobias may have a childhood history of social inhibition or shyness. The social phobia typically develops in the mid-teens, either emerging insidiously or, conversely, emerging acutely after an incident, such as a publicly humiliating experience. This disorder is typically lifelong and may fluctuate with stress, specific phobic situations, and demands placed on the individual. It is sometimes clinically difficult to distinguish a social phobia from a feeling of embarrassment over a ritual or a public panic attack.

Specific Phobia Signs and Symptoms

A specific phobia is a persistent fear, anxiety, or panic attack that is precipitated or cued by a specific object or nonsocial situation. Individuals suffering with a specific phobia recognize that their fear is excessive or unreasonable and avoid those things or situations that provoke the anxiety. Typical specific phobias are fear of animals, most commonly dogs; fear of the environment, typically heights, water, or the weather; fear of blood, or injection injury; and fear of certain situations, such as planes, elevators, and tunnels. Traumatic events often precipitate a simple phobia. For example, a dog bite can precipitate a dog phobia.

Course of Specific Phobia

A specific phobia usually begins in childhood but can also emerge as new symptoms in the 20s. Phobias are exceedingly common in children but with so little impairment that no psychiatric diagnosis is warranted. In adults, phobias are also common and may not result in any impairment. To meet the criteria for a specific phobia, a phobia must cause significant daily distress and/or social and occupational dysfunction.

Epidemiology

Social phobia has a lifetime prevalence of 13.3%. It is the third most common psychiatric disorder in the United States. Specific phobia has a prevalence rate that varies with the threshold used to determine distress and social or occupational dysfunction. In community samples reported in the *DSM-IV* (1994), lifetime prevalence rates were 10% to 11.3%, and the 1-year prevalence rate was 9%.

Clinical Issues

The primary care clinician often misses or only incidentally discovers a phobia during a medical encounter or during diagnostic testing. Patients who have phobias to blood, injections, injuries, dental phobia, or even claustrophobia are often terrified by medical procedures or settings. Phobic patients may also confront the physician with unanticipated problems, such as severe distress during procedures such as colonoscopy or pelvic or rectal exams, or may develop claustrophobic panic during a CAT scan or MRI test. Patients undergoing these procedures may experience a marked distress and/or a panic attack and may be unable to complete the requested diagnostic testing or procedure.

On the opposite side of the spectrum, when there is no phobic stimulus present, a clinician may have no idea that a phobic disorder exists. Patients may actively avoid discussing phobias. This is not out of a desire to withhold information but rather the primary defense of avoidance, which attempts to make phobic symptoms disappear from view.

Clinicians should suspect phobias when they hear about difficulties at work, at school, in interpersonal relationships, or when the patient describes panic or anxiety in public situations. The clinician should specifically ask about fear of blood, injections, procedures, water, and claustrophobia and encourage the patient to acknowledge any fears of flying, elevators, bridges, tunnels, heights, animals, and storms. It is common for an adult to have a history of a phobia as a child, and a history of a parental death before the age of 17 is associated with increased risk for phobias.

Social phobia with panic can be differentiated from panic disorder. Panic episodes with panic disorder are unexpected and not cued by the environment, whereas panic attacks from phobias occur in social situations or are precipitated by the feared objects.

Social phobia and specific phobia may need to be differentiated from avoidant personality disorder. This differentiation can be difficult and often requires referral to a mental health professional.

Obsessive-Compulsive Disorder

Signs and Symptoms

Obsessions are recurrent thoughts, impulses, or images that cause marked distress or anxiety. Repetitive thoughts are intrusive, unwanted, and may even feel senseless, and they go beyond worry about real-life problems.

Common obsessions include thoughts of contamination or germs and repeated doubts (e.g., worrying about whether the lights or stove are off or if the door is locked). Some obsessions, such as counting, are designed to block distress. Others, such as repetitive thoughts of violence or recurrent blasphemous or sexual thoughts, can produce marked distress and anxieties.

Compulsions are ritualistic behaviors or mental acts that are performed in response to an obsession or are behaviors that need to be rigidly carried out in a certain sequence or fashion. Compulsions are designed to ward off dangerous impulses or anxiety or distress. Anxiety is most obvious when you ask a patient to disrupt a rigid routine. Most common compulsions include compulsive cleanliness, hand washing (up to 50 times a day), checking rituals (Did I lock the door?), and dressing and undressing rituals. Compulsions generally bind aggressive impulses that may produce distress. For example, compulsive number counting may prevent the patient from conscious awareness of his wish to hurt or harm someone.

Course of Obsessive-Compulsive Disorder

This disorder usually begins in adolescence or early adulthood, but it is not uncommon for it to begin in childhood. Males often have an earlier onset of the disorder, between ages 6 and 15, whereas females are more likely to show symptoms between ages 20 and 29. The onset of this disorder is typically slow. Most patients have a chronic fluctuating course, 15% deteriorate (*DSM IV*, 1994), and 5% undergo periods of complete remission (Jenike, 1992).

Epidemiology

The lifetime prevalence of OCD in the general population is 2.5%, and 1-year prevalence rates are 1.5% to 2.1%. The prevalence in the primary care setting may be as high as 10%, which approaches the prevalence of depression and other anxiety disorders. Patients with obsessive-compulsive disorder have a 5% to 7% incidence of Tourette's syndrome, and 20% to 30% report a current or past history of tics. In patients suffering with Tourette's syndrome, 35% to 50% also have obsessive-compulsive disorder (Jenike, 1992, 1996).

Clinical Issues

The recent success of effective psychopharmacological treatment of OCD has created a role for the primary care physician in treating these disorders.

However, the secretive nature of this illness means that the primary care physician has to have an index of suspicion and a knowledge of this disorder. Recognition of OCD in a primary care practice is often difficult, because few physicians are inclined to review a symptoms checklist. Screening for OCD should be considered in patients who are depressed, somatic without medical cause, compulsively buying, binge eating, or who report a recent obsessive love. If you suspect OCD, it is important to differentiate it from depression, body dysmorphic disorder, hypochondriasis, social phobia, and compulsive personality disorder (see also chapter 6, Somatoform Disorders). In some patients, OCD symptoms mask an underlying psychotic disorder.

Once OCD is recognized, the physician can look for precipitants and stressors that make the symptoms worse. As many as 65% of women with OCD relate the onset or exacerbation of their symptoms to pregnancy, childbirth, or parenting. The next step is to determine the patient's interest in treatment. The challenge to the clinician is to reframe the patient's medical complaints or to portray their obsessive-compulsive symptoms in a medical context that is both accurate and acceptable to the patient. Framing obsessions and compulsions as disorders of the basal ganglia or dysregulation of serotonin neurotransmitters or referring to the genetic overlap with Tourette's syndrome will allow some patients to see their OCD as a medical condition worthy of treatment. If the patient does not request treatment, many physicians will not offer it or even suggest a referral. For patients and physicians who are willing, treatment with selective serotonin reuptake inhibitors (SSRIs) can be extremely helpful and gratifying. For those patients who might be motivated for treatment or request further assistance, a referral to a psychiatrist is indicated.

Posttraumatic Stress Disorder (PTSD)

Signs and Symptoms

Any patient who is exposed to a highly traumatic event can develop an acute stress disorder that may or may not lead to posttraumatic stress disorder (PTSD). An acute stress disorder has symptoms similar to PTSD with a duration from 2 days to 4 weeks. If symptoms related to a trauma persist beyond 4 weeks, the disorder is classified as PTSD.

The symptoms of PTSD include persistent reexperiencing of the trauma through distressing recollections, dreams, a sense of reliving the event, flashbacks, or psychophysiologic reactions when exposed to cues that may represent the event. In addition, the patient avoids stimuli associated with the trauma, reports a numbing of general responsiveness, and may also experience an increase in arousal such as insomnia, startle response, or hypervigilance. These symptoms must last for at least 1 month and can cause significant distress and/or impairment in social or occupational functioning.

Traumatic events involve actual threatened death or injury, a threat to bodily integrity such as rape, or natural disasters such as floods. Traumas can be experienced directly or may be observed. Patients often describe survival guilt and avoidance of any situation or people that bring back memories of the traumatic event. Patients suffering with PTSD often develop interpersonal difficulties such as marital conflict, divorce, occupational and social dysfunction, and substance abuse. Many researchers believe that childhood PTSD, from child abuse or neglect, can lead to the development in adults of borderline personality disorders and dissociative identity disorders (formerly multiple personality disorder).

Course of Posttraumatic Stress Disorder

PTSD can occur at any age, even in childhood. Symptoms usually begin within 3 months of the trauma but can begin months and sometimes years later. Complete recovery occurs within 3 months in 50% of patients, but others can have symptoms for years. The severity, duration, proximity, and repetitions of multiple traumas increase the likelihood of developing the disorder. The magnitude of the trauma, the persistence of community devastation, the real-life sequela from the trauma, and the patient's coping capability affect the ultimate outcome of this disorder (see chapter 17, Crisis Intervention in Office Practice).

Epidemiology

The lifetime prevalence of PTSD is 1% to 14% in community samples and varies with the population and methodology of the studies. People at risk, such as military personnel and natural disaster victims, have higher prevalence rates.

Clinical Issues

One excellent approach to interviewing patients with PTSD is the crisis intervention approach, as detailed in chapter 17.

Generalized Anxiety Disorder (GAD)

Signs and Symptoms

Generalized anxiety disorder (GAD) is an illness of chronic worry. *DSM-IV-PC* diagnostic criteria for GAD specify excessive worry that is pervasive and difficult to control, that lasts for at least 6 months, and that occurs for more days than not. Associated symptoms include trembling, muscle tension, dry mouth, palpitations, and symptoms of hyperarousal such as a startle response or insomnia. These symptoms must cause clinically significant distress and impairment in social and/or occupational functioning.

A diagnosis of GAD should be considered only if the anxiety is not better accounted for by another disorder, because GAD symptoms are often present with panic disorder, obsessive-compulsive disorder, social phobia, hypochondriasis, posttraumatic stress disorder, and depression.

Course of the Illness

Many patients with GAD report lifelong histories of worrying with the onset occurring in childhood or adolescence. GAD may have more of a personality component than other anxiety disorders. The course is typically chronic and is worsened by acute stress.

Epidemiology

DSM-IV indicates that GAD has a lifetime prevalence rate of approximately 5% and a 1-year prevalence rate of 3%. In specialty services for anxiety disorders, approximately 12% to 15% of patients present with GAD.

Clinical Issues

One problem with the classification of anxiety disorders in both the *DSM-IV* and *DSM-IV-PC* is that it focuses on anxiety syndromes as illnesses or diseases. GAD appears to be more of a psychological illness than a disorder with genetic underpinnings. Rather than approaching GAD as an illness or disease, the clinician can work with the patient to try to understand the source of the patient's anxiety. GAD often can be linked to separations or fear of separation. Anxiety symptoms may arise from fear of loss of love, fear of bodily harm, pangs of conscience, or anxiety over not living up to an internal moral code. It is important to recognize that GAD is very responsive to psychotherapy provided by a mental health professional.

The cognitive approach to treating GAD is the assumption that anxiety results from a chain of events that begins with an external threat followed by an appraisal of that threat and then coping with the threat. According to this model, patients become anxious because of hot thoughts that represent a misappraisal of external dangers. The patient's worry is created by exaggerating dangers, underestimating his or her own ability to cope, and having an underlying belief that he or she is very vulnerable.

Hot thoughts are typically concerns over what horrible results will occur if this or that event takes place in the patient's life or work. Interviewing patients with this model, a clinician may try to uncover the most troubling "what ifs " and demonstrate to the patient his or her tendency to exaggerate the dangers or to underestimate his or her own capacities. More in-depth work with the cognitive model usually requires a referral to a mental health practitioner.

Mixed Anxiety-Depressive Disorder

Signs and Symptoms

In primary care settings, many patients may present with a mixture of both anxiety and depressive symptoms. Research is currently under way to determine if this might be a distinct category of patients or if anxiety and depression are so common that patients frequently present with comorbid disorders. *DSM-IV* has listed distinct research criteria for this combination disorder to help resolve this controversy. The criteria for mixed anxiety-depressive disorder include a dysphoric (uncomfortable) mood lasting at least 1 month that is accompanied by four of the following symptoms: difficulty concentrating, sleep disturbance, low energy, irritability, worry, weeping, hypervigilance, anticipating the worst, feelings of hopelessness, and low self-esteem. These mixed depressive and anxious symptoms cause significant distress and/or interfere with social or occupational functioning. This disorder cannot be diagnosed if the patient has suffered previously from depression, dysthymic disorder, panic, or generalized anxiety disorder.

Course of the Illness

Not much is known about the course of this disorder, and it is currently undergoing research validation studies. However, the clinical impression is that patients with this mixed disorder have greater psychological, physical, social, and occupational dysfunction than those suffering from major depression, panic, or generalized anxiety disorders alone.

Epidemiology

There is no detailed epidemiology for this mixed disorder because it is unclear whether the mixed disorder is a distinct entity from depression syndromes with anxiety, on the one hand, or anxiety syndromes with depression, on the other. If we examine patients with a diagnosis of depression, we find that 60% of patients will have moderate anxiety, 20% to 25% will have severe anxiety, and 15% will have a social phobia. If we examine patients with a diagnosis of anxiety disorder, we find that 10% have depression as well.

Clinical Issues

Patients with a mixed anxiety-depressive disorder are less responsive to conventional treatment and have a longer course and a poorer prognosis. They suffer with greater symptomatology and often require additional time from the primary care clinician and his or her staff. These patients have a higher risk of suicide (19.5%) than those suffering from either depression (7.9%) or anxiety (7%) alone. Suicide attempts after hospitalization are 3% to 12%.

Differential diagnosis in mixed anxiety-depressive disorder can be difficult, especially because the diagnostic criteria have not been validated. However, depressive disorders are distinguished by negative affect, feelings of hopelessness, anhedonia, and early morning awakening, whereas anxiety disorders have more autonomic symptoms associated with fear, agitation, anxiety, and difficulty falling asleep.

When treating this disorder, the clinician should focus on the depressive symptoms, because these symptoms convey the greatest risk of morbidity and mortality. Psychotherapy for this mixed disorder has not been studied. Clinical experience suggests that the treatments are often longer and more complicated than with patients suffering from either disorder alone.

SCREENING FOR ANXIETY DISORDER IN PRIMARY CARE

Probably the most common screening for anxiety disorders in primary care is done clinically. A clinical approach will often uncover panic disorders, agoraphobia, generalized anxiety disorders, posttraumatic stress disorder, and mixed anxiety-depressive disorder. One physician screening and research instrument for detecting anxiety is the Hamilton Anxiety Rating Scale, which screens for generalized anxiety, panic, and social phobic symptoms. Patient-driven self-reports include screens such as the Beck Anxiety Inventory Scale or Burns Anxiety Scale, both of which are helpful in screening for panic, social phobia, and generalized anxiety disorders. Additional research screening instruments include the Sheehan Panic Attack Scale, the Fear Questionnaire, the Yale Brown Obsessive-Compulsive Scales, and PTSD scales such as the Impact of Events Scale.

BIOLOGICAL AND PSYCHOLOGICAL BASIS OF ANXIETY DISORDERS

Biology of Anxiety Disorders

The biology and physiology of anxiety disorders is complex and incompletely understood. Preliminary genetic studies reveal a spectrum of genetic input that varies from one disorder to another and depends somewhat on how anxiety disorders are classified. For example, clinical anxiety has a monozygotic twin (MZT) concordance rate of 36% to 41%. Phobic neurosis has an 80% MZT concordance rate, and panic shows a 31% MZT concordance rate. These three measures of anxiety illustrate a significant genetic input for anxiety disorders. On the opposite side, preliminary studies show that genetic factors are minimal for GAD and PTSD.

Somewhere in the middle domain is obsessive-compulsive disorder. In some pedigrees (Jenike, 1996), Tourette's syndrome and OCD may represent different presentations of the same genetic abnormality, while in other samples, OCD appears to be genetically distinct.

The weight of biological research in the spectrum of anxiety disorders is focused primarily on the locus ceruleus, raphe, limbic (amygdala), and paralimbic cortex. It appears that generalized anxiety disorders, panic disorders, and phobias are most associated with the locus ceruleus and raphe nuclei dysregulation, whereas OCD is more often associated with limbic system dysfunction.

The leading biologic theory of panic disorder is called the suffocation false alarm. This theory suggests that in panic disorders there is a central respiratory control derangement that causes the nervous system to read an abnormal threshold of suffocation. Patients with panic disorder seem to suffer from a compensatory chronic state of respiratory hyperventilation.

They have a low baseline arterial PCO_2, a high PO_2, a decreased phosphorous level, and a respiratory alkalosis that allows them to maintain a normal pH. This state of chronic alkalosis makes patients susceptible to panic attacks. Common panic-inducing substances include sodium lactate and sodium bicarbonate. It seems likely that serotonin-activating drugs such as fluoxetine and imipramine exert their anti-panic effect through serotonin, which down-regulates the suffocation alarm system.

Psychology and Anxiety Disorders

The most common psychological theories that attempt to explain anxiety disorders include the cognitive-behavioral theory and the psychodynamic theory. These are reviewed in the treatment section of this chapter.

OFFICE-BASED TREATMENT OF ANXIETY DISORDERS

The treatment of anxiety disorders in an office setting has six basic components: (1) exercise; (2) relaxation response training; (3) pharmacology, with special attention to blocking panic attacks; (4) desensitization to the feared object or situation; (5) cognitive restructuring; (6) psychotherapy; and (7) family interventions and social support building.

Exercise

Exercise has been shown to be a beneficial adjunct to treatment for anxiety disorders. In deciding about how to prescribe exercise for a patient with different anxiety symptoms, it is probably useful to separate patients into a group with physical symptoms versus a group with cognitive symptoms.

Those patients suffering with palpitations, chest pain, neurological symptoms, or gastrointestinal symptoms may respond well to exercise. Those suffering with worry and obsessions may first need other psychiatric interventions. Exercise alone, without some cognitive explanation, can make some patients worse. For example, patients with panic-induced palpitations may be frightened by an increased heart rate from exercise. For these patients, it may be important to tell them before they begin mild exercise that a fast heartbeat from exercise does not mean heart attack. They also need to know that exercise will reduce the risk of all heart diseases. Many patients with cardiac panic may need to have their panic blocked with relaxation-response training or medication before they begin to exercise.

In suggesting an exercise program, it is important to tell patients that they might notice an initial increase in anxiety as they begin the workout; after exercise, they can expect to be less anxious. Exercise helps anxiety levels in the short term, for 4 hours postexercise. For most patients, anxiety levels typically return to their high post-exercise baseline levels within 24 hours. This means that daily exercise is probably required to see a prolonged anxiolytic effect. Exercise for anxiety symptoms should be prescribed with an individual's particular needs in mind. Those nervous at their jobs do better if they exercise in the morning, whereas those who worry at bedtime do better when exercising in the early evening.

Relaxation Response Training (RRT)

Relaxation response training (RRT) has been shown to be an effective complementary treatment for many medical conditions and may be particularly helpful in the treatment of panic attacks and anxiety disorders. RRT is basically one antidote to the "flight or fight" response. When practiced two or three times a day for 10 to 20 minutes, RRT can lower anxiety levels. It is a necessary part of anxiety disorder treatment when used in combination with desensitization therapy.

Relaxation response training can take many forms, including controlled diaphragmatic breathing, meditation training, and visual imagery. Tables 2.3 and 2.4 describe controlled diaphragmatic breathing and simple forms of relaxation response, respectively.

Psychopharmacology

The choices of appropriate psychopharmacology for the spectrum of anxiety disorders are described in Table 2.5.

Panic Attacks

If panic attacks are severe and frequent, the initial choice of medication should be geared toward blocking the acute panic attacks. This is usually done by use of the benzodiazepines. Clonazepam, often the first-line, intermediate-acting medication, can be initiated at .25 mg bid with anti-panic effects in the daily dose range of 1 to 2.5 mg and a daily maximum of 5 mg/day. Alprazolam is a shorter-acting medication, which can be started at 0.25 mg tid or qid with anti-panic effects at 3 to 5 mg/day and

Table 2.3 Controlled Breathing

1. When *not* anxious, count breaths/min.
   (normal is 8–12 breaths/min.)
2. When panicked/anxious, count breaths/3 min.
   (e.g., 90 breaths in 3 min. is 30 breaths/min.)
3. If 30 or > breaths, slow to 12 breaths/min.
   Inhale and think "expand" for 2 seconds.
   Exhale and think "let go" for 2 seconds.
   Pause for 1 second.
   Repeat for 5 minutes.
4. If < 30 breaths, slow to 8 breaths/min.
   Inhale and think "expand" for 3 seconds.
   Exhale and think "let go" for 3 seconds.
   Pause for 1 second.
   Repeat for 5 minutes.

Table 2.4 Relaxation Response

1. Choose a quiet time and environment.
2. Sit or lie comfortably.
3. Close your eyes. Pick a focus word phrase (e.g., *relax, one*, or *Omm*).
4. Relax your muscles.
5. Breathe slowly and naturally. Exhale, repeat your focus word.
6. Assume a passive attitude toward your thoughts. If worry sets in, release the worry and exhale. If troubled thoughts return say, "let it go" and go to your focus word.
7. Continue for 10 to 20 minutes, 2 or 3 times a day.
8. Practice the technique 1 to 2 times a day.

Source: Benson, H., & Stuart, E. M. (1993). *The wellness book*, pp. 45–46. New York: Fireside Simon & Shuster.

Table 2.5 Sequence of Medication Trials for Anxiety Disorders

Anxiety Disorder	Medication Sequence
Panic disorder	1. Try to use SSRI or TCA for primary treatment and/or maintenance. 2. Use clonazepam, alprazolam, lorazepam PRN if a supplement to the antidepressants is needed. 3. For acute severe panic symptoms, begin with clonazepam bid or alprazolam tid and add antidepressant later. 4. Taper off the benzodiazepines immediately.
Generalized anxiety disorder	1. If symptoms are chronic, begin with buspirone.* 2. For acute symptoms, first try benzodiazepines PRN. 3. If acute symptoms don't resolve, use trazodone, SSRI, or TCA. 4. If no response, use long-acting benzodiazepines (e.g., clonazepam or chlordiazepoxide).
Adjustment disorder and anxiety	1. Try benzodiazepine PRN. 2. If no relief, use buspirone* tid. 3. Trazodone, SSRI, or TCA
Separation anxiety disorder	1. TCAs, imipramine 2. SSRIs
Social or performance anxiety, specific phobia	1. Beta-blockers: Inderal, Atenolol, or Metoprolol** 2. MAOI best treatment responses*** 3. SSRIs 4. Imipramine (school phobia)
Obsessive-compulsive disorder	1. SSRIs best tolerated, effective. 2. Clomipramine best studied, effective 3. If treatment resistant, combine SSRIs. 4. Clonazepam (occasionally used as adjunctive)
Posttraumatic stress disorder	1. MAOIs or SSRIs*** 2. TCA 3. Anticonvulsants for irritability or aggression 4. Beta-blockers for startle 5. Trazodone/Ambien for sleep 6. Lithium

* Has its effects 1 to 6 weeks later.

** Trial dose with imagery used before the event.

*** Some prefer SSRIs as first line and MAOIs as second.

maximum daily doses of approximately 10 mg/day. These medications are often prescribed acutely but need to be prescribed cautiously to patients with an addiction history. It may take a few days to bring the panic attacks under control. During the first 2 weeks of panic medication treatment, patients need frequent and regular contact with their physician.

If panic attacks are not severe or acute, it is preferable to begin treatment with the SSRIs or antidepressants. Fluoxetine 5 mg or a low dose of other SSRIs are effective. Alternatively, the tricyclic antidepressants (TCAs) imipramine or nortriptyline can be utilized. Most antidepressants work well for panic with the exceptions of trazodone, bupropion, and probably nefazodone. Those patients who begin on SSRIs or TCAs may initially experience a mild worsening of symptoms followed by relief. They may repeat this pattern with subsequent dose increases. Beneficial effects occur within 1 to 3 weeks. The doses of these medications can be increased every 3 to 7 days as tolerated and should be brought to antidepressant levels for a response. The fluoxetine maintenance dose is typically 20 to 40 mg/day, whereas imipramine doses are 150 to 300 mg/day.

The SSRI or TCA regimen should be maintained for approximately 1 year. Relapse rates are 83% if discontinued within 6 months and 25% if discontinued at 18 months.

Phobic Symptoms

The psychopharmacology of phobic symptoms is different for agoraphobia, social phobia, and specific phobia/performance anxiety.

AGORAPHOBIA. Patients with agoraphobia with or without panic will benefit from SSRIs following the same approach as that described for panic attacks. Alprazolam 3 to 6 mg/day, clonazepam 1 to 3 mg/day, and imipramine 150 to 300 mg/day are alternatives. Monoamine oxidase inhibitors (MAOIs) are still probably the most effective agents for agoraphobia treatment, but their potential drug interactions and the need for a special diet have unnecessarily scared most primary care physicians away from their use.

SOCIAL PHOBIA. SSRIs are becoming the first-line psychopharmacology for social phobia despite the fact that MAOIs and clonazepam have a better established efficacy. Beta-blockers are not helpful for these patients. In open trials, fluoxetine has had a 70% response rate, which is comparable to phenelzine and clonazepam. The pharmacological treatment for phobic disorders often takes 6 to 10 weeks to achieve a complete effect.

When prescribing for patients with social phobia, it is important to remember that these patients frequently are self-medicating. One recent study showed that patients suffering from social phobias and those with performance anxiety use other medications with the following frequencies: hypnotic 22%, tranquilizer 23%, antidepressants 10%, alcohol 41%, and B-blocker 27%.

MAOIs such as phenelzine at 45 to 90 mg/day can reverse the most severe forms of social phobia, often within 6 weeks. MAOIs have a 70% chance of reversing the major avoidant symptoms associated with avoidant personality disorder within 3 to 12 months. Clonazepam in average daily doses of 2.4 mg is also very effective, with 70% of patients showing improvement in 6 weeks. Buspirone is also effective in the high daily dose ranges of 45 mg and up but may take 12 weeks or longer for a response.

SPECIFIC PHOBIA AND PERFORMANCE ANXIETY. Both of these disorders are responsive to beta-blockers, which decrease the "flight or fight" response. They are especially effective in controlling the physical anxiety response and less effective at controlling psychological fears and symptoms.

Beta-blockers should be tried first without any fear stimulus and, subsequently, in the real-life feared situation. Propranolol can be given in a single dose of 10 to 100 mg 2 hours before exposure to the phobic stimuli. Prior to the real-life situation, have the patient start with a 10-mg dose and visualize the feared object or situation. Adjust the dose according to the patient's response.

Metoprolol 25 to 50 mg or atenolol 30 to 100 mg can be used as alternatives. If exposure to a specific phobia is unpredictable, a patient may need long-term B-blocker treatment or MAOI medications.

Obsessive-Compulsive Disorder

The medication treatment of OCD has made it possible for primary care physicians to offer treatment to this difficult patient group. Approximately 70% of patients will show some response to drug treatment. The average patient will have a 40% decrease in symptoms, and 10% to 15% will have a full remission. Obsessions are generally more responsive to drug treatment than are compulsions, and comorbid depression does not predict response. The presence of tics or Tourette's syndrome makes patients less responsive to SSRIs alone. Poor responders are those patients with pure obsession and no compulsions, those who have a delusional belief that their compulsions are required, and patients suffering with severe depression.

Clomipramine is the best documented and most effective treatment for OCD. A typical starting dose is 50 mg/hs, and daily doses may be increased every 3 to 7 days with a target dose of 200 to 250 mg/day. Doses above 250 mg/day increase the risk of seizures. This medication, which is a serotonergic TCA, produces anticholinergic side effects, sweating, weight gain, and tremor, and can cause a serotonergic syndrome. Long-term drug treatment for years is often recommended for patients with OCD.

SSRIs are also efficacious in the treatment of OCD and have a better side effects profile. Fluoxetine and fluvoxamine have been best studied and therefore have become the most commonly used first-line medications for treatment of OCD. Sertraline and paroxetine are probably also efficacious. The doses used to treat OCD are usually higher than those used to treat depression, and the response time is often 12 weeks to 6 months. Fluoxetine may be given in daily doses from 20 to 100 mg/day; fluvoxamine, 200 to 300 mg/day; sertraline, 100 to 200 mg/day; and paroxetine, 40 mg/day. High doses may be required for a response, but this can also increase the drop-out rate and serotonergic side effects. About 40% to 60% of patients will respond to monotherapy. Patients requiring combination therapy should be referred to a psychiatrist.

MAOIs can be used if a patient suffers with OCD and panic, social phobia, or refractory depression. Clonazepam at 4 to 6 mg/day and buspirone at 30 mg/day may help some patients; however, these drugs are more often used in combination therapy.

Patients who have tics, Tourette's syndrome, or a tendency to schizo-obsessive features often do best on a combination of pimozide or another neuroleptic and an SSRI.

Posttraumatic Stress Disorder

The psychopharmacology of PTSD is not definitive. Patients with PTSD symptoms of increased arousal and flashbacks respond better to medications than those patients with avoidance and withdrawal symptoms. Successful drug treatment can take from 2 to 6 months and works well on intruding thoughts and numbness. MAOIs, SSRIs, and amitriptyline are effective. Doses of all these medications are in the antidepressant ranges. If these drugs do not work, patients can be referred to a psychiatrist for trials of anticonvulsants, benzodiazepines, beta-blockers, clonidine, lithium, and other drugs.

Generalized Anxiety Disorder

Sixty-six percent of patients suffering with GAD respond rapidly within 1 to 2 weeks to benzodiazepines. Most physicians will first try short-acting medications PRN such as lorazepam 1 to 4 mg PRN; alprazolam, 0.25 to 1 mg PRN; or oxazepam, 10 to 40 mg PRN. The PRN approach is efficacious in part because in the short term, patients with GAD have a high placebo rate of approximately 50% to 60%. If the short-acting PRN approach doesn't bring relief, then a switch to long-acting, potent benzodiazepines is suggested. Clonazepam at 0.5 to 2 mg/day or chlordiazepoxide at 25 to 75 mg/day are often used.

If symptoms of GAD are not acute or severe, buspirone can be a very effective alternative. There are no acute effects of buspirone except for the placebo effect. The initial effect of buspirone is in 1 to 2 weeks, and a full effect may take 4 to 6 weeks. This medication works better when the patient is free from benzodiazepines for 1 month. Typical starting doses are 5 mg tid for the first week, with increases of up to 5 mg every 2 to 4 days until a dose of 30 mg/day is reached within 2 weeks. Doses can go as high as 60 to 80 mg/day.

Several studies have also shown that imipramine, 10 to 300 mg, and trazodone in doses of 25 to 600 mg are also effective for GAD, independent of depression or panic.

Many patients with GAD may require long-term maintenance therapy, because 50% of these patients have symptoms for more than 5 years. There have been no long-term studies that address the duration of therapy. Psychotherapy may provide a better long-term treatment result if the patient is willing and able to undertake it.

DESENSITIZATION: EXPOSURE TO PHOBIC SITUATIONS OR OBJECTS

Once panic and acute anxiety symptoms are under control with medications, breathing control, or relaxation response training, it is important to help the patient to cease avoiding phobic situations and objects. Medications control panic but do not treat the avoidance behaviors themselves. The patient must be reintroduced to fearful situations or objects once the panic attacks or severe anxiety are markedly reduced, to overcome phobic or avoidant behavior. The two major methods of exposure are called graduated desensitization and flooding.

Graduated desensitization is exposing the patient to the phobic object or fearful situation, initially through imagery and eventually through real contact with the phobic situation. This graduated exposure to the fear is under the patient's control. Have a patient (who may or may not be on medication) imagine the fearful situation (e.g., public speaking) while practicing relaxation techniques. It is important that the patient practice, often several times a day, imagining the situation or phobic object while practicing relaxation. Repeated imagined gradual exposures will diminish the patient's fear.

After imagined exposure, the patient needs to use the relaxation techniques during a graduated exposure to the real-life situation. Some patients need a friend, family members, or a mental health professional to assist them in confronting the situation.

Flooding is an intensive total immersion in a phobic situation or continuous contact with the phobic object. For example, treatment of an eating-in-public phobia or germ phobia requires eating in public or continuous exposure to dirt for several days or weeks. Flooding is an exceedingly quick and rapidly effective treatment for phobias and obsessive-compulsive rituals. Patients learn relaxation techniques first, may be given medication, then are flooded with the phobic stimuli. This is an intensive experience that can be emotional and frightening. It is usually accomplished with the aid of a mental health professional over a period of several days to weeks.

COGNITIVE-BEHAVIORAL THERAPY

Cognitive behavioral therapy is a very effective treatment for all the anxiety disorders. Cognitive theory suggests that anxiety symptoms are caused by a patient's basic belief system, a stimuli, a cognitive or mental misappraisal of the stimuli, and a hot thought, all of which lead to emotions such as anxiety, fear, phobia, and obsessions/compulsions. An example of a cognitive behavioral diary for anxiety is illustrated in Figure 2.2 and discussed in detail in chapter 19, Behavioral Counseling and Medical Adherence. Hot thoughts that are associated with various anxiety disorders are summarized in Table 2.6.

Triggers of Distress	Anxiety or Fear	Physical Symptoms	Anxious Thought	Pros of Thought	Cons of Thought	Revised Thought	Anxiety Fear Physical symptoms
Who? What? When? Where? Why?	What is your anxiety or fear? Rate the severity 1=severe to 5= minimal	List your physical symptoms (e.g., heart racing, short of breath).	Write down one of your most anxious or fearful thoughts.	Write down the evidence that supports your fear or anxiety.	Write down the evidence that does *not* support the fear or anxiety	Write down a more realistic thought about your fear or anxiety.	Is your anxiety fear or symptoms improved? Rate the improvement 1=greatly to 5=no improvement

Figure 2.2 Cognitive Diary for Anxiety.

PSYCHODYNAMIC THERAPIES

Psychodynamic approaches to therapy have made major contributions to the understanding and treatment of symptoms of anxiety. In a dynamic framework, anxiety is considered a normal internalized response to perceived dangers. Anxieties can be aroused from fear of failure, fear of criticism, anxiety dreams, or anxiety from angry or sexual thoughts. Anxiety can be aroused from the outside by certain situations or phases of development. Psychodynamic theorists describe five basic domains of anxiety based on a fear of some kind of separation or loss: separation anxiety, stranger anxiety, castration anxiety, impulse anxiety, and superego or moral anxiety.

Separation anxiety is tension or fear resulting from separation from a loved one or a support system. When taking a history from anxious patients, it is important to obtain a detailed separation history, because recent separations may trigger unresolved fears of earlier separation.

Stranger anxiety appears at approximately 9 months of age. This anxiety appears to be a hard-wired capacity that only emerges when a child can differentiate caretakers from all others. An adult version of stranger anxiety is often reported in social phobics who are terrified of meeting new people.

Castration anxiety is a fear of loss of bodily parts, not simply fear of genital mutilation. Patients suffering with panic, blood, or wound phobias

Table 2.6 Charged Thoughts and Manifestations of Anxiety Disorders

Anxiety Disorder	Charged Thoughts	Manifestation
Panic disorder	**Catastrophic** Misreading of physical sensations	A racing heart = a heart attack
Social phobia	Expects psychological **humiliation** in public	Public speaking = being naked in public
Specific phobia	**Exaggerates harm** from external dangers	Sees a dog and thinks, "The dog will bite me"
Generalized anxiety disorder	**"What if"** thinking	Job criticism = "What if I were fired?"
Obsessive-compulsive disorder	Dangerous sexual, **aggressive, or fearful** thoughts	"If I stop washing = I will get germs, disease, and die
Postraumatic stress disorder	**Nightmares Flashbacks**	Rape or war memories

may reveal fears or fantasies about bodily damage. A patient who sustains a minor laceration may become hysterical because this superficial cut is unconsciously connected to a fear of bodily damage.

Impulse anxiety is the fear that our drives or urges will overcome us. Patients suffering with obsessive compulsive disorder, PTSD, compulsive gambling or shopping, sexual addictions, binge eating, or exercise addictions often feel overwhelmed by their internal desires.

Superego or moral anxiety is the tension felt when we feel we have broken our own moral code. A harsh judgmental attitude toward ourselves is a common manifestation of underlying guilt or shame. Treatment of excessive moral anxiety or harsh self-judgment is often a major focus with obsessive-compulsive and PTSD patients.

FAMILIES

When working with patients who suffer from an anxiety disorder, it is important to recognize that families suffer when a member has an anxiety disorder and that families can both help and hinder effective treatment.

Families Suffer

Living with someone who suffers with panic attacks, agoraphobia, OCD, PTSD, and other anxiety disorders can have profound interpersonal consequences for the patient's marital partner and children. Patients with anxiety symptoms may not be able to drive, appear in public, develop friends, or work and may avoid intimacy or be unable to experience life's pleasures. Children of anxious parents may develop a marked fear of the world, which can pave the way for the next generation of anxiety disorder and interpersonal, social, and occupational dysfunction.

Families Can Help

Families can be a tremendous aid in treating patients with anxiety disorders. Family members can offer additional information that can facilitate diagnosis, describe the major problematic areas, provide a buffer for the patient during times of fear and stress, act as health advocates, help the patient access community resources, and be invaluable therapy assistants, especially as cotherapists for behavioral/exposure treatment.

Families Can Hinder Treatment

Sometimes, families inadvertently or consciously support an illness or a phobia in a family member, because aspects of an individual's illness may help the family. When treatment of an anxiety disorder is not successful or is only partially helpful, it is necessary to examine the positive aspects of the illness for the family. Once these issues are addressed with the family, the patient may then be able to recover. For example, a phobic housebound woman was encouraged by her husband and working-age sons to stay home, cook, clean, and care for her family. Her efforts to overcome her agoraphobia were actively discouraged, because her leaving home meant additional work for the other family members.

CRITICAL PATHWAYS: PANIC DISORDER

A panic disorder critical pathway is illustrated in Table 2.7, which provides primary care guidelines for screening evaluation, psychopharmacology, and psychosocial treatment of panic over a 1-year time period.

Table 2.7 Critical Pathway: Panic Disorder

	Initial Visit	Week 2	Week 3	Week 4	Weeks 8–10	Months 6–9	Months 9–12
Assessment tools	Beck & Steer,[a] Burns,[b] or Hamilton[c] stress scale;[d] GAF[e] or GARF[f] scales	Anxiety algorithm,[g] GAF,[d] anxiety scale,[g] or cognitive behavior diary[h]		GAF,[e] anxiety scale[g] or cognitive behavior diary[h]	Beck & Steer,[a] Burns,[b] or Hamilton[c] stress scale[d]	GAF;[e] anxiety scale;[g] or cognitive behavior diary[h]	Beck & Steer,[a] Burns,[b] or Hamilton[c] stress scale; GAF,[e] GARF[f] anxiety scale;[g] or cognitive behavior diary[h]
Physical/lab/ diagnostic tests	1. Full PE 2. Chemistry panel 20, Drug screen, Electro cardiogram (EKG), Venereal Disease Research Laboratory Test (VDRL), Thyroid Function Test (TFT), Thyroid Stimulating Hormone (TSH).	Check lab results and treatment. Consider ECHO.		Check labs. Drug screen? Labs: VMAs, EEG? CAT/MRI?	If (-) responses, reevaluate diagnosis.		

continued

Table 2.7 *(continued)*

	Initial Visit	**Week 2**	**Week 3**	**Week 4**	**Weeks 8–10**	**Months 6–9**	**Months 9–12**
Diagnosis	1. Rule out medical disorder 2. Rule out drug-induced disorder 3. Primary anxiety disorder? 4. Suicidal?	Confirm diagnosis. Use anxiety algorithm.		Any response? If not, reassess treatment options.	Expect response If not, reassess.	Full recovery? Partial recovery?	Full recovery? Partial recovery?
Time	45 minutes	30 minutes	Patient calls	15 minutes	30 minutes	15 minutes	15 minutes
Objective	Diminish panic attacks.	Diminish panic attacks.	Diminish panic attacks.	Diminish panic attacks.	Panic attack blocked? Begin desensitization.	Desensitization.	Desensitization.
Educational materials	Anxiety info. Med. sheet	Patient/family education Anxiety scale[g] Cognitive behavior diary[h] Self-help		Phobia education materials Self-help	Education: drug maintenance Self-help	Education: relapse prevention Medication maintenance Self-help	Education: relapse prevention Medication maintenance Self-help

	Initial Visit	Week 2	Week 3	Week 4	Weeks 8–10	Months 6–9	Months 9–12
Treatment or Physician Clinician counseling/ intervention	1. **Educate** about work up/treatment options; discuss stress, and suggest social support. 2. **Counsel**: Reduce or discontinue caffeine, smoking, alcohol; relaxation response training (RRT); breath control (BC); discuss separation stress and supports. 3. **Medications** a. SSRI or new antidepressants	1. **Educate** about panic/phobia/ anticipatory anxiety. 2. **Counsel** RRT, BC, rate anxiety, cognitive behavior diary,[h] stress/worry, interpersonal problems, and social support. 3. **Medications** adjust q3–5day stress/supports	1. Extra phone availability. 2. **Counsel** Medication side effects, if any. 3. **Medication** adjustments PRN	1. **Educate** about phobic symptoms; discuss stress and need for support. 2. **Counsel** desensitization; discuss exposure to fearful situation; discuss exercise; review RRT, BC, problems. 3. **Medications** a. SSRI in therapeutic	1. Discuss stress, supports. 2. **Counsel** desensitization, relapse prevention, exercise, RRT, BC, anxiety scale,[g] cognitive behavior diary;[h] psychotherapy needed? 3. **Medications** a. Solely on antidepressants,	1. **Educate** about drug maintenance, relapse prevention. 2. **Counsel** desensitization; discuss stress, support, exercise, RRT, BC; anxiety scale;[g] cognitive behavior diary;[h] psychotherapy? 3. **Medications** a. If symptom-free for 6	1. **Educate** about drug maintenance, relapse prevention. 2. **Counsel** desensitization; discuss stress support, exercise, RRT, BC, Stress and Anxiety scales,[g] cognitive behavior diary;[h] psychotherapy? 3. **Medications** Consider: a. Drug taper

continued

Table 2.7 *(continued)*

	Initial Visit	**Week 2**	**Week 3**	**Week 4**	**Weeks 8–10**	**Months 6–9**	**Months 9–12**
Treatment *(continued)*	b. If severe panic, alprazolam tid or clonazepam bid. c. If mild or occasional panic, lorazepam PRN or oxazepam PRN. d. TCAs. e. MAOIs.			range? Adjust PRN b. Change or add a new antidepressant? c. Taper/ d/c benzo PRN if possible. d. If necessary, use clonazepam or alprazolam maintenance.	if possible b. Combination benzo and antidepressant maintenance required? c. Dose adjustments PRN.	months, consider taper b. No benzo if possible c. Maintain antidepressants or combination as necessary New medications, if appropriate.	b. Discontinue all drugs. c. Drug maintenance as necessary. New medications, if appropriate.
Consultations	If suicidal, consider psychiatric consultation.	Medical specialist, if required.	Consider family visit and/or psychiatric consultation.	Consider psychiatric consult and/ or referral to psychotherapy.	If (-) response, **DEFINITE TREATMENT REFERRAL**	Referral? Psychotherapy? Psychopharmacology?	Referral? Psychotherapy? Psychopharmacology?
Physician or clinician counseling/ intervention	1. Breath control (BC). 2. Relaxation response training (RRT).	GAF[e] review: 1. BC 2. RRT 3. Stressors 4. Social support	As necessary.	GAF[e] review/ Mood rating Cognitive behavior diary[h] Meds	GAF[e] review Review cognitive *mood rating* Cognitve diary[h]	GAF[e] review Review cognitive behavior diary/ medications.	GAF[e] review Review cognitive behavior diary/ medications.

	Initial Visit	Week 2	Week 3	Week 4	Weeks 8–10	Months 6–9	Months 9–12
Counseling/ intervention *(continued)*	3. Social support. 4. Stresses. 5. Decrease caffeine, smoking.	5. Mood rating. 6. Cognitive behavior diary.[h] Extra phone availability.	Extra phone availability.	Review: 1. BC. 2. RRT. 3. Stresses. 4. Separation issues. 5. Exercise.	Social support. Medications. Antiphobia Rx. Review Rx. (-) Response: reassess. diagnosis and treatment.	Continue to treat phobic symptoms.	Continue to treat phobic symptoms.

Developed by: Robert E. Feinstein

[a]Beck, A. T., & Steer, R. A. (1990). *Beck anxiety inventory*. San Antonio, TX: Psychological Corp. Harcourt Brace.

[b]Burns, D. (1989). *The feeling good handbook*. New York: Penguin Books.

[c]Hamilton, M. A. (1959). The assessment of anxiety states by rating. *British Journal of Psychiatry, 32*, 50.

[d]Holmes, T. H. & Rahe, R. H. (1967). Stress scale: Social readjustment scale. *Journal of Psychosomatic Research, 2*, 213.

[e]GAF (Global Assessment of Functioning) scale. American Psychiatric Association. (1994). *Diagnostic and statistical manual of mental disorders* (4th ed., p. 200). Washington, DC: Author.

[f]GARF (Global Assessment of Relational Function) family assessment scale. *DSM-IV*, pp. 758–759.

[g]Anxiety algorithm; see Figure 2.1.

[h]Cognitive behavior diary; see Figure 2.2.

Prescreening

The symptoms of panic attacks often emerge during the course of a regular office visit for other medical complaints. At the first awareness of panic symptoms, the primary care physician can take a clinical history and can also provide the patient with self-report screening instruments that can help the physician get a great deal of information in a minimum amount of time. It is helpful if the patient fills out one of several screening questionnaires and returns one to the physician before the next office visit. The Beck and Steer (1990) or Burns (1989) anxiety scale and a Global Assessment of Functioning (GAF) scale allow the clinician to rate the severity of the anxiety symptoms in the patient and the patient's global functioning. These scales also provide measurable benchmarks to assess how the patient is responding to treatment and to follow the patient's symptoms from one office visit to another. If the patient cannot complete the self-report scale, the clinician could complete the Hamilton rating scale and use this at each office visit. The Holmes and Rahe (1967) scale will alert the clinician to stressful events in the patient's life and help predict future health risks to the patient. Scores under 150 mean that the patient has little stress. A score of 150 to 300 means that the patient has a 50% chance of developing a major physical or mental illness within the next 2 years. A score over 300 means that the patient has an 80% chance of developing a major physical or mental illness within the next 2 years.

Initial Evaluation Intake (45 Minutes)

The physician's initial work-up includes a history, physical exam, relevant laboratory work, and completion of the GAF and the Global Assessment of Relational Functioning (GARF) scale. Once the clinician becomes familiar with these scales, they take minutes to complete. The GAF scale yields a single number that describes the patient's level of symptoms and social and occupational functioning. The GARF scale also yields a single number that provides a quick assessment of the functioning of the patient's support network. These two numbers provide an additional way to follow the patient's functional progress over the next year.

During this initial intake, the physician's clinical work is to gather medical information and perform or order relevant medical tests that will help rule out medical and drug-induced anxiety states. When relevant, the clinician can counsel about reducing consumption of caffeine, alcohol, and nicotine. The clinician can then intervene with anxiety management techniques such as breathing control (see Table 2.3), RRT (see Table 2.4), and begin appropriate psychopharmacology (see Table 2.5).

Second Week (30 Minutes)

The patient should return in 1 week in order to bring panic symptoms under control as rapidly as possible. The focus of this session is to complete the medical anxiety work-up, reassess the patient's GAF scale, adjust medications, introduce a cognitive diary (see Figure 2.2), and give the patient appropriate educational material and information on community resources for support. If appropriate, the clinician should permit the patient to telephone the office over the next few weeks, as necessary.

Fourth Week (15 minutes)

At this visit, the clinician assesses the patient's GAF scale and reviews the patient's cognitive diary. The clinician should then suggest exercise, as appropriate, review anxiety management skills (breathing control and RRT), and adjust medications. Most patients' symptoms, at this point, should be coming under control and patients should be close to the therapeutic range of their medications.

Weeks 8 to 10 (30 Minutes)

This is a crucial office visit, as a major treatment response and a marked diminution of panic in most patients should be expected. Prior to this visit, the patient, while in the waiting area, should repeat a Beck and Steer or Burns scale or a new Holmes and Rahe scale. The clinician can complete new GAF and/or GARF scales to measure the patient's functional progress. If the patient has responded, the clinician may want to instruct the patient on the basics of antiphobia treatment. The physician should also review the section on graduated desensitization and continue appropriate treatment. If there is a partial response or no response, a psychiatric referral should be considered.

Long-term Follow-up

This should be determined by assessment of the patient's needs with clinician input.

REFERENCES

American Psychiatric Association. (1994). *Diagnostic and statistical manual of mental disorders* (4th ed.). Washington, DC: Author.

American Psychiatric Association. (1995). *Diagnostic and statistical manual of mental disorders: Primary care version* (4th ed.). Washington, DC: Author.

Beck, A. T. & Steer, R. A. (1990). *Beck anxiety inventory*. San Antonio, TX: The Psychological Corporation. Harcourt Brace.

Burns, D. (1989). *The feeling good handbook*. New York: Penguin Books.

Davidson, J. R. T. (1994). Social phobia: Outlook for the 90's. *Journal of Clinical Psychiatry, 55*, 503–510.

Friedman, M. J., Charney, D. S., & Deutch, A. Y. (Eds.). (1995). *Neurobiological and clinical consequences of stress, from normal adaptation to post-traumatic stress disorder*. Philadelphia: Lippincott-Raven.

Gorman, J. M., & Papp, L. A. (1992). Anxiety disorders (Foreword). In A. Tasman & M. Riba (Eds.), *Review of psychiatry* (Vol. 11, pp. 243–246). Washington, DC: American Psychiatric Press.

Holmes, T. H. & Rahe, R. H. (1967). Social readjustment rating scale. *Journal of Psychosomatic Research*.

Jenike, M. A. (1992). New developments in the treatment of obsessive-compulsive disorder. In A. Tasman & M. Riba (Eds.), *Review of psychiatry* (Vol. 11, pp. 323–346). Washington, DC: American Psychiatric Press.

——— (1996). Recent developments in neurobiology of obsessive-compulsive disorder (academic highlights). *Journal of Clinical Psychiatry, 57*, 492–503.

Kanton W., & Geyman, J. P. (1995). Diagnosis and treatment of anxiety disorder. In R. Rakel (Ed.), *Textbook of family practice* (5th ed., pp. 1469–1485). Philadelphia: W. B. Saunders.

Pollack, M. H., & Smoller, J. W. (1995). The longitudinal course and outcome of panic disorders. *Psychiatric Clinics of North America, 18*, 785–801.

Sheehan, D. V. (1983). *Anxiety disease*. New York: Scribner.

CHAPTER 3

Depression

Janis L. Cutler and Rita Charon

The syndrome of depression is one of the most common of all medical illnesses. Untreated, it has a high rate of morbidity and mortality; however, when recognized, it is highly treatable. Unfortunately, persons suffering from depression do not necessarily complain of feeling depressed. Instead, they frequently present to the physician with a lack of interest in life and with somatic or other vague complaints. The alert primary care clinician can readily recognize and diagnosis depression and offer treatment.

CLINICAL PRESENTATION

The primary care clinician may encounter undiagnosed unipolar depression as (1) new-onset depressive spectrum disorders, (2) depression associated with somatic complaints, or (3) depression associated with chronic illness. Depressive symptoms also may present as part of a bipolar disorder, and the primary care clinician should be able to recognize bipolar manifestations. This chapter will review diagnostic presentations of unipolar and bipolar illness and cover therapeutic considerations for treatment of unipolar depression. Patients with bipolar disease generally will be referred to psychiatrists for management.

Figure 3.1 provides a brief overview of the depressed mood algorithm, which can be used in primary care to guide differential diagnosis.

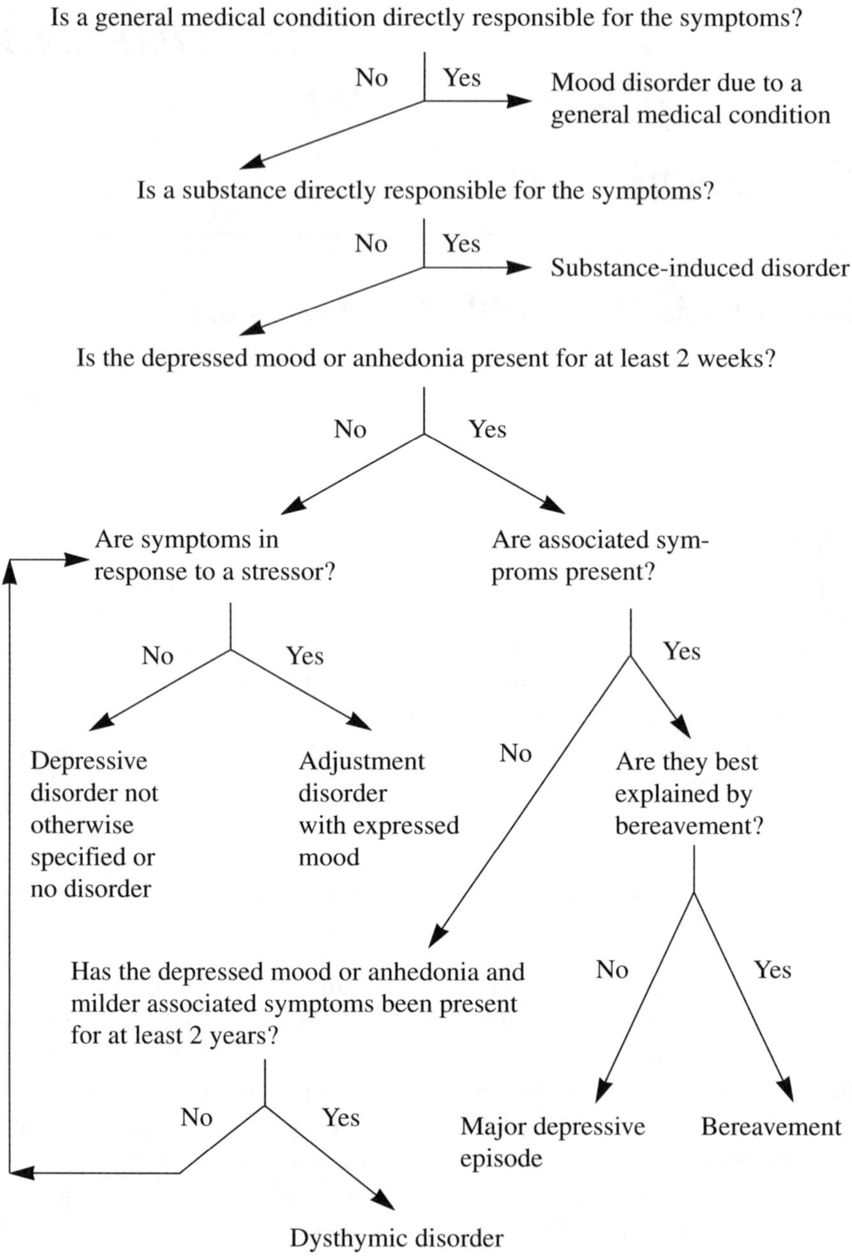

Figure 3.1 Depressed Mood Algorithm.

Unipolar Depression

New-Onset Depressive Spectrum Disorders

Mood disorder due to a general medical condition refers to alterations in mood that are pathophysiologically related to an underlying medical condition. Such diseases as hypothyroidism, hyperthyroidism, adrenal disease, Parkinson's disease, cerebrovascular disease, some metabolic diseases, autoimmune conditions, some infections such as Lyme disease, and certain cancers (notably pancreatic cancer and cerebral neoplasms) seem to bring about depressive changes independent from the psychological impact of the stress of illness on the patient. Other medical conditions such as chronic fatigue syndrome and fibromyalgia seem so intimately related to depressive disorders that the boundary between the physical disease and the psychiatric disease has yet to be defined.

Substance-induced depression is seen in relation to exogenous substances that, although ingested for recreation, mood alteration, or treatment of medical disease, result in depressive symptoms. Chronic use, intoxication, or withdrawal may precipitate a depressed mood, loss of interest in activities, or a functional daily impairment. The most common mood-altering agents causing depression are alcohol, sedatives, hypnotics, amphetamines, opiates, cannabis, cocaine, and psychotropic medications, including anxiolytics and antipsychotic agents. Prescription drugs that can cause a depressed mood include anticholinergics, some antihypertensives (notably reserpine and alpha-methyldopa), steroids, oral contraceptives, and some antineoplastic agents.

Major depressive disorder is a syndrome of depressed mood or anhedonia (loss of pleasure) and associated symptoms that are present every day for at least 2 weeks. Some patients may describe their mood as down, blue, or sad. Others may be more preoccupied with depressive ruminations and worries and identify their mood as nervous. The subjective experience of depressed mood may be unbearably painful. Some patients may have no noticeable abnormality of mood but instead have a loss of interest or pleasure in their usual activities. This anhedonia will frequently extend to activities and to relationships, even intimate ones. Thus parents may not enjoy their children, and husbands and wives may feel that it is a burden, rather than a pleasure, to be with their spouse.

In addition to depressed mood and anhedonia, the associated symptoms of major depressive disorder include an appetite disturbance (either anorexia or increased appetite, which may or may not be accompanied by a 5% change in weight) and a sleep disturbance. Some patients may sleep more than usual, whereas others will have difficulty falling and staying asleep and will sleep for fewer hours than usual. Whether suffering from hypersomnia or insomnia, patients often feel tired during the day. Patients also may note poor concentration, complain that they are a bit forgetful, or may notice that their mind drifts when watching television or reading. Other associated symptoms of major depression include psychomotor agitation or retardation, feelings of worthlessness, and suicidal ideation or recurrent thoughts about death. At least five of these findings must be present nearly every day for 2 weeks in order for the diagnosis of a major depressive episode to be made. Table 3.1 provides a list of criteria with a mnemonic.

A major depressive episode can be accompanied by associated features—*psychotic*, *melancholic*, or *atypical*—which also should be specified as part of the diagnosis.

Psychotic features, most commonly mood-congruent hallucinations and delusions such as somatic delusions or delusions of guilt, are typically present only in severe cases of depression. Patients with a psychotic depression are at high risk for suicide, even in the absence of suicidal ideation.

Patients with melancholic features report nearly complete anhedonia or disinterest for those activities that they usually find pleasurable. In addi-

Table 3.1 Diagnostic Criteria-Major: Depressive Episode

Mnemonic: Dr. Sig: E Caps

Dr: Depressed mood: most of the day for 2 weeks

S: Sleep: Insomnia or hypersomnia
I: Interest: Loss of interest/pleasure (anhedonia)
G: Guilty: Feelings of guilt, worthlessness, hopelessness

E: Energy: Loss of energy or fatigue

C: Concentration: Impaired concentration
A: Appetite: Decrease/increase in appetite/weight
P: Psychomotor: Agitation or retardation
S: Suicidal ideation

Source: Wise MG, & Taylor SE. Anxiety and Mood Disorders in Medically Ill Patients. *Journal of Clinical Psychiatry, 51*(Suppl. 1):27–32, 1990. Copyright 1990, Physicians Postgraduate Press. Reprinted with permission.

tion, patients with melancholia also have at least three of the following symptoms: a pervasive and irremediable depressed mood, diurnal variation (depression worse in the morning), early morning awakening, marked psychomotor retardation or agitation, significant anorexia or weight loss, and excessive or inappropriate guilt. Melancholic features predict a particularly robust response to psychopharmacological interventions. Psychotic and melancholic features frequently coexist in the same patient.

Atypical features tend to occur in patients with milder symptoms, although they seem to predict a lower level of response to tricyclic antidepressants. Patients with atypical depression experience mood reactivity as well as at least two of the following symptoms: overeating or weight gain, oversleeping, leaden paralysis (feels like an enormous effort just to move one foot after the other and walk a short distance), and rejection hypersensitivity (not just during episodes of depression).

A major depressive episode has a seasonal pattern if most of the patient's major depressive episodes occur with a change in season, particularly with the onset of fall or winter, when there is less natural light. The diagnosis should not be made if there is a clear psychosocial stressor that is related to the change in seasons. Although patients with this subtype of depression respond to standard pharmacological and psychotherapeutic interventions, they can also benefit from light treatment.

Postpartum onset depression occurs within 1 month postpartum. While the symptoms themselves do not differ from those of major depressive episodes that occur at other times, recognition and rapid intervention are indicated to protect both the mother and child. See chapter 15, Women's Health Through the Reproductive Cycle, for a full discussion.

Pseudodementia is a severe form of depression that looks like dementia. Patients suffer with erratic cognitive impairments, marked distress, and an inability to concentrate or focus on daily tasks. Pseudodementia is a variant of depression that can be readily confused with a dementia. See chapter 5, Psychiatric Symptoms Due to Medical Illness, for further discussion.

Dysthymic disorder is a chronic form of depression in which the signs and symptoms are milder than those of other depressive disorders but can cause significant distress and dysfunction. A history of at least 2 years of complaints occurring on more than half of the days is necessary to make this diagnosis. Patients often suffer from this disorder for years without realizing that they are depressed. Primary care physicians commonly see this disorder in association with many chronic medical illnesses. Making this diagnosis and treating the patient for this disorder can be especially helpful to patients suffering from chronic medical diseases. Like major depression, dysthymic disorder is associated with physiological changes, including appetite and sleep disturbances, low energy, and poor concentration. Patients also experience indecisiveness, low self-esteem, and hopelessness. These patients may appear to be chronic pessimists and complainers to friends and family.

Bereavement is typically accompanied by symptoms such as sighing, sadness, insomnia, decreased appetitie, and weight loss as a reaction to the loss of a loved one. Symptoms of normal bereavement generally resolve within 2 months and usually do not require medical or psychiatric treatment. If bereavement persists for longer than 2 months, then the diagnosis of major depressive disorder must be considered. Pathological symptoms of a major depressive disorder that may follow or interrupt normal bereavement include: excessive guilt, thoughts of death beyond the natural desire to be with the loved one, a pervasive and new sense of worthlessness, profound psychomotor retardation, persistent inability to fulfill ordinary duties, and hallucinations other than hearing the voice or transiently seeing the image of the deceased.

Adjustment disorder with depressed mood may be diagnosed when patients present with depressive symptoms within 3 months of an identifiable psychosocial stressor. For example, loss of a job, divorce, or academic failure may precipitate depressed symptoms that do not meet the criteria for major depression or dysthymic disorder. The treatment of choice for these patients is usually psychotherapy rather than pharmacological treatment.

Somatic Complaints and Depression

It is not uncommon for depressed patients to present with physical symptoms instead of with the catalogue of mood alterations and vegetative signs that would point to depressive disorders. Chronic headaches, gastrointestinal complaints, back pain, fatigue, sleep disorders, dyspnea, palpitations, and itch are some of the physical symptoms that may be clues to depression. Hypochondriasis and somatoform disorders, covered in detail in chapter 6, may include inattention to mental suffering, social proscription from declaring emotional pain, personal distaste of declaring disorders of feelings, lack of the language needed to describe emotional suffering, or such characterological factors as stoicism and rigidity that disallow one's claim of emotional distress. Posttraumatic stress situations, especially those involving sexual or physical abuse, can lead to specific depressive syndromes that present as complaints in the reproductive organ system, extreme social withdrawal, eating disorders, or body-image distortions.

Even in the absence of somatoform disorders, patients may hide behind their physical symptoms. In some instances, cultural factors color the sensation of depressive symptoms to mimic physical ones. In others, religious beliefs prohibit reporting all but physical manifestations of depression. Nonetheless, the primary care physician, committed to ideals of continuity and holism, will learn of his or her patient's burden of suffering, including emotional pain that is expressible only as physical pain. To adequately diagnose and treat such suffering, the primary care clinician must inform his or her understanding of individual patients with knowledge of gender-related, cultural, and religious dimensions of the experience of depression.

Chronic Illness and Depression

Any chronic medical disease implicating loss of bodily function or integrity may be accompanied in certain patients with mood changes. As with other stressors, medical diseases may precipitate episodes or relapses of depressive disorders. The primary care physician is often faced with patients suffering with chronic medical conditions who are discouraged and/or depressed in the face of their physical limitations or nearness to death. Clinicians in these settings should refrain from conceptualizing depression as an inevitable and untreatable aspect of the patient's illness. The clinician has to be careful not to misattribute symptoms, such as fatigue, solely to the medical condition and should strive to diagnose accurately mood disorders that coexist with medical illness. Treatment of the comorbid depression should be as aggressive as treatment of the underlying medical conditions. Although all medical conditions may be accompanied by depression, the following, because of their prevalence in the general population and their toll of physical suffering, are particularly likely to occur in concert with depression:

Stroke incurs not only physical and cognitive losses but also specific emotional tolls. Stroke patients with damage in the left dorsal lateral frontal cortex or left basal ganglia may experience depression because the brain injury is located where it can interfere with either language capacity or integrative functions governing emotions. Prospective studies examining depression following stroke demonstrate that the mean duration of depression after stroke is under 1 year.

Dementia may be closely associated with or mistaken for depression. The most prudent clinical course is generally to treat potential depression regardless of the possibility of associated dementia. See chapter 5, Psychiatric Symptoms Due to Medical Illness, for a more extended discussion of treatment of depression in the patient with dementia.

Diabetes, both insulin-dependent and non-insulin-dependent, is associated with higher rates of depression than are seen in the general population. Furthermore, the coexistence of diabetes and depression or dysthymia can significantly influence the clinical outcomes of patients, because patient autonomy and judgment, critical for effective treatment of diabetes, may be hampered by depression and dysthymia. Hence, the primary care physician needs to be especially alert to the symptoms of depression in diabetics.

Coronary artery disease, both with and without a history of myocardial infarction, seems to carry an additional risk of depression, and depression can increase mortality in some of these patients. See chapter 12, Cardiovascular and Psychosocial Risk Factors Reduction: Office-based Interventions, for an extended discussion of depression and heart disease.

Cancer, in North America and elsewhere, carries cultural burdens as well as medical ones. The diagnosis of cancer is often experienced as a sentence of prolonged and untreatable suffering, including disfiguring surgery and/or debilitating medical treatments. That the cure for cancer often remains elusive despite all scientific efforts makes each victim feel great anger and discouragement as well as great worry. Emerging findings about the genetic bases of some common malignancies may give some patients the additional burden of worry and guilt that their children may be similarly affected. The rates of depression documented among patients with cancer do not differ from those seen in patients with other severe chronic illnesses; however, they are considerably higher than in the general population. Several risk factors, including isolation, lack of support, and uncontrolled pain, may add to an individual cancer patient's likelihood of developing concurrent depression. At least in the acute phase, treatments for malignancies may require daily or weekly attendance for radiation or chemotherapy over periods of months. This arduous treatment can unduly interfere in the patient's work and home life, taking away the solace of continued functioning or interrupting times of blessed forgetfulness. Suicide risk among cancer patients is elevated in the face of prior history of depression, family history of suicide, poor social supports, physically disfiguring treatment, pain, advanced age, and advanced disease. The primary care physician is obliged to monitor patients with cancer closely for these risks and to treat concurrent depression aggressively. Sadly, recent movements toward patient autonomy in choosing the time of death may, in some cases, place additional burdens on patients with cancer to hasten their deaths or may raise doubts in their minds about the role of the physician in their terminal care.

Manic and Hypomanic Symptoms and Bipolar Disorder

Major depressive episodes can occur in association with manic or hypomanic symptoms. Patients with a history of mania or hypomania are at significantly increased risk of becoming manic when treated with antidepressants. Therefore, all physicians who diagnose and treat depression should be familiar with manic and hypomanic symptoms, including how to recognize their presentation and how to elicit a history of bipolar disorder.

Patients who are manic are commonly described as being euphoric, "high," or "on top of the world." The feeling state can actually be somewhat dysphoric, however, with irritability being the more apparent presenting affect. Manic patients feel and appear as though they are working on overdrive in some way. Their speech is fast, their thoughts are racing, they have lots of energy although they are sleeping less than what is normal for them, and their sexual appetite is increased. A clinician who finds himself or herself enjoying immensely an interaction with a patient or feeling entertained in some way should consider the possibility that the patient is manic. Of course, some patients are just naturally funny or seem somewhat "hyper." To discern this as well as other psychiatric conditions, it is extremely important to compare the patient's current presentation with his or her baseline.

The judgment of manic patients is frequently impaired. This clouded judgment, in combination with their increased appetite for excitement, pleasure, and stimulation, can result in impulsive decisions, such as spending sprees, unsafe sex, or poor business decisions, any of which may have major consequences. Manic patients who are irritable can become violent or, more commonly, provoke others to violence, thus again putting themselves at risk.

Hypomania is simply a milder form of mania. It presents with increased energy, decreased need for sleep, mild euphoria, fast speech, and rapid thought processes. By definition, patients are not hypomanic if psychotic symptoms are present or if psychiatric hospitalization is required. Otherwise, the distinction is a matter of degree: During a hypomanic episode marked impairment in social or occupational functioning should not occur.

Following is a summary of the major categories of manic disorders to provide primary care physicians with a foundation for diagnosis and referral.

MOOD DISORDER DUE TO A GENERAL MEDICAL CONDITION. This disorder includes manic or hypomanic sequelae of such medical conditions as hyperthyroidism, cerebrovascular disease, vitamin B12 deficiency, and certain cancers (e.g., cerebral neoplasm and pancreatic cancer). New manic symptoms should trigger diagnostic evaluations for underlying medical conditions.

SUBSTANCE-INDUCED MOOD DISORDER. Substance-induced mood disorder with manic features may be caused by legal and illicit drug use. Medically indicated substances with manic side effects include psychotropic medications, steroids, isoniazid, levodopa, and sympathomimetics such as those found in decongestant medications. The most common illicit drugs that may cause manic episodes are cocaine, phencyclidine, cannabis, and amphetamines.

BIPOLAR I DISORDER. This condition is defined as a mood disorder that includes a major depressive episode accompanied by a distinct period of mania that lasts for at least 1 week. Sometimes the depressive and manic periods coincide, with both depression and mania present every day during at least a 1-week period. This concurrence is diagnosed as a *mixed episode*. For example, a patient may have racing thoughts and high energy but also feel sad and tearful and have no appetite. Some patients with bipolar I disorder demonstrate psychotic features, with delusions, hallucinations, and thought disorder. Mood-congruent psychotic symptoms are most common and are characterized by grandiosity. Typical delusions involve the belief that one is a god, the president, or royalty. Voices might tell the patient that he or she will save the world or has special powers.

BIPOLAR II DISORDER. Bipolar II disorder is defined as recurrent major depressive episodes interspersed with hypomanic episodes.

CYCLOTHYMIC DISORDER. Cyclothymic disorder refers to a milder form of bipolar illness in which states of depressed mood fluctuate with states of elevated mood. However, the severity of the depression does not meet diagnostic criteria for major depression, and the elevation in mood is of shorter duration or lesser intensity than full manic states. Patients with cyclothymic disorder may develop bipolar disorder at a later stage of life.

EPIDEMIOLOGY

Depression is an extremely common disorder. A nationwide community sample recently diagnosed 4.9% of subjects with a current episode of major depression and an estimated lifetime prevalence at 17.1%. Other large sample studies have suggested that 20% to 25% of women and 7% to 12% of men will suffer an episode of major depression at some point in their lives. In primary care settings, the point prevalence of major depression among outpatients has been found to be between 4.8% and 8.6%. Among medical inpatients, the point prevalence is reported at 14.6%. The lifetime prevalence of dysthymic disorder is estimated at 4.1% of women and 2.2% of men. Depression commonly begins in early adulthood, with peak onset in the 20s and 30s. More than half of the people who experience one episode of major depression are at risk for recurrence.

Bipolar disorder is not as common as major depressive disorder, occurring in between 0.4% of men and 1.6% of women over their lifetimes. In contrast to depressive disorders, there is no gender difference with respect to prevalence.

ETIOLOGY

Genetics certainly seem to play a role in the development of mood disorders, particularly bipolar disorder. First-degree relatives have an estimated 12% lifetime prevalence of bipolar disorder, which is about 10 times that found in the general population. Recurrent major depressive disorder is associated with an increased risk among first-degree relatives as well, occurring 1.5 to 3 times more commonly than among the general population.

A number of observations suggest that neurotransmitter abnormalities play a key role in mood disorders. In particular, depression seems to be associated with an abnormal noradrenergic system. Serotonin, acetylcholine, gamma aminobutyric acid, and such second messengers as G protein and messenger RNA seem to be involved as well. Neuroendocrine abnormalities in depressed patients, particularly hypercortisolism, suggest the involvement of the hypothalamic pituitary-adrenal system. A number of abnormalities in the sleep architecture of depressed patients implicate an abnormally phase-advanced circadian rhythm in the pathophysiology of depression. The decreased REM latency seems to represent a state of chronic arousal.

Psychosocially, depression can be understood as a response to stress in vulnerable individuals. More specifically, the psychology of people who are at particular risk of developing depression suggests the influence of depressed or emotionally absent parents, childhood losses, and adult loss of a significant other who was ambivalently regarded. Thus depression can be seen quite commonly after the death of a parent or spouse with whom the patient was angry. Events that damage self-esteem, such as rejection after a job interview, being passed over for a promotion, or the presence of negative, distorted, or irrational thoughts about oneself, are common psychological precipitants as well. The impact of stressful events seems to be most significant in contributing to the first or second episodes of depression and less so to subsequent episodes. Stressors probably contribute to the onset of manic episodes as well, particularly in the earlier years of the condition.

CLINICAL INTERVIEW

Depressed patients, by definition, feel hopeless, helpless, or suffer from anhedonia. While outwardly harsh or judgmental toward themselves, depressed patients may feel inwardly critical of everyone, including their physician. Thus depressed patients can evoke feelings of anger and frustration in the clinician as well as feelings of sadness. Although it is unprofessional to share these feelings with the patient, it is necessary for the clinician to recognize and accept his or her own negative feelings. Recognition of the clinician's negative countertransference is important because it frees the clinician from inadvertently conveying anger to the patient. By processing his or her anger and frustration, the clinician protects the quality and kind of care that the patient receives.

The initial responses to a patient who presents with a depressed mood should be quiet listening and empathic understanding. The clinician's task is more difficult when the patient's chief complaint is not depression. Vague complaints without a clear physical basis or symptoms that do not respond to typical medical interventions should prompt the clinician to screen for depression. Similarly, persistent worries or anxiety about medical illness suggest the possibility of a major depression. The clinician should anticipate that anhedonia, not depressed mood, is the more common presentation of depression in the primary care setting. The clinician also must be careful not to ascribe symptoms of major depression to situational factors. Instead, mention of recent difficulties at work or home should raise the index of suspicion, because psychosocial stressors frequently contribute to the onset of depressive episodes.

Although the diagnosis of depression still carries a stigma, it is important for clinicians to address the issue openly. In the situation of a patient who is suffering significant psychosocial stress, an opening remark might be: "That sounds pretty rough. How are you handling all of this?" or, "Does this ever get you down?" A tone of voice that is caring, understanding, and nonjudgmental is at least as important as the content of the question. A patient is helped when the clinician is conveying appropriate concern and providing the opportunity for the patient to admit to symptoms of depression. When no acute stressor is present but the patient seems overly concerned about a medical condition, unduly pessimistic about the prognosis, or chronically worried, that patient should be approached in a somewhat different way. The clinician can encourage the patient to be open and diminish his or her concerns about being judged by introducing the topic with an educational statement, such as "People suffering from diabetes sometimes get overly discouraged," then continuing with the question, "Has that been happening to you lately?" Sometimes, instead of asking, it is necessary to make a statement, such as "It sounds like you've been getting pretty down recently." This remark gives the patient permission to be down and avoids any sense of judgment or disapproval from the clinician.

After establishing that the patient has a depressed mood, the clinician should move into a more active interview mode to review the differential diagnoses of the spectrum of depressive disorders, as outlined in the depressed mood algorithm (refer back to Figure 3.1). The clinician should then pursue further details to elicit the characteristics of the neurovegetative changes as carefully as possible, keeping in mind the symptoms of the melancholic subtype as well as those of major depression itself. Structured depression screening instruments, such as the Prime-MD Clinician Evaluation Guide (Spitzer et al., 1993), or depression screening instruments, such as the Beck Inventory (Beck, 1978), can sometimes be useful for the primary care clinician in organizing this history-taking process or in estimating the severity of the depression. The patient's functioning, both past and current, should be assessed to determine the extent to which the depression interferes with current functioning. The patient's past psychiatric history and family history of depression should be explored as well. If other episodes of depression have occurred, the course of those episodes, including the patient's response to treatment, will be important to help the clinician formulate a treatment plan.

It is important to elicit the presence of hypomanic or manic episodes in the patient's history, as this history has significant treatment implications. Episodes of flagrant mania can usually be elicited without much difficulty; however, milder hypomanic episodes can be more difficult to identify, because the behavioral abnormalities are more subtle or unrecognized. It may be more difficult to discover a history of mania when interviewing a patient who is in the midst of a depression and who may be unable to recall having felt well. If a psychiatric history was not obtained before the patient became depressed, then family members can be helpful in diagnosing a bipolar disorder.

A complete mental status examination must be performed on patients who appear to be depressed. This examination is necessary to confirm the diagnosis, because several criteria of a major depressive episode involve mental status findings: excessive guilt, suicidal ideation, and psychomotor agitation or retardation. In addition, several aspects of the patient's mental status will determine whether a psychiatric consultation or hospitalization are indicated and how aggressively treatment should be pursued: the presence or absence of psychosis, the presence and severity of suicidal ideation, the degree of cognitive impairment, and the patient's capacity for insight and judgment. The mental status examination includes assessment of depressive symptomatology and the degree of cognitive impairment using object recall, serial 7s, calculations, and general knowledge. Attention to the patient's level of concern with any deficits and degree of effort with the tasks will be helpful in differentiating pseudodementia from a dementia or from other disorders induced by a general medical condition.

Psychotic material is best obtained indirectly, exploring the content of the patient's concerns and worries. Once an area of possible delusional content is identified, the ability of the patient to "test reality" should be assessed. Somatic and guilt-ridden concerns in particular should be carefully explored for the possibility of delusions. The clinician should directly inquire about hallucinations and suicidal ideation. If hallucinations are present, one must ask if voices are commanding the patient to do anything or take any action. If the patient has command hallucinations to hurt or kill himself or herself or others or has suicidal risk, then a very intensive treatment approach is warranted. When in doubt, the primary care clinician should always obtain a psychiatric consultation, as discussed in the next section. A detailed review of the evaluation and management of these symptoms is presented in chapter 7, Violence and Suicide.

TREATMENT

Patients with a major depressive episode respond to initial attempts at treatment at a rate of about 75%. Treatment response is over 90% when modalities are combined. Standard treatment includes antidepressant medications and psychotherapy. Hospitalization is indicated for patients who are a significant suicide risk or are unable to care for themselves. Psychiatric consultation should be obtained in these situations if the patient is psychotic, because psychosis increases the risk of suicide even in those depressed patients who deny suicidal ideation. Electroconvulsive therapy (ECT) is an additional effective treatment choice for hospitalized patients, particularly when the depression is complicated by psychosis. All manic patients should be managed in consultation with a psychiatrist. Triggers for psychiatric referral include the following:

- Presence of psychotic symptoms
- Severe decrease in the level of functioning
- Recurrent depression
- Chronic depression
- Refractory depression
- Suicide risk
- Bipolar disorder
- Severe depression
- Diagnostic questions
- Cardiac disease that requires TCA treatment
- Need for psychotherapy
- Need for electroconvulsive therapy (ECT)

The mainstay of treatment of mood disorders recommended by the primary care physician will be pharmacological (see Table 3.2). Treatment with serotonin selective reuptake inhibitors (SSRIs) is less complicated than treatment with tricyclic antidepressants (TCAs) and monamine oxidase inhibitors (MAOIs). It is unclear whether SSRIs are as effective as TCAs in the treatment of patients with severe episodes of major depression that require hospitalization; however, in outpatients with mild to moderate symptoms, SSRIs and TCAs are equally effective.

The choice of antidepressant is made on the basis of medical conditions comorbid with depression (see Table 3.3) or the basis of the side-effect profile that the physician wants to exploit or minimize (see Table 3.4). The SSRIs (fluoxetine, sertraline, paroxetine) are all associated with gastrointestinal symptoms (nausea, diarrhea, vomiting), headaches, rashes, and sexual dysfunction (delayed ejaculation and orgasm). Overall, however, patients find them fairly easy to tolerate. The most troublesome side effect, a feeling of activation that can cause significant insomnia as well as daytime jitteriness, can be managed with morning administration or with adjunctive benzodiazepines or low-dose trazodone. This agitating effect may occur less with paroxetine which is more frequently sedating. If seda-

Table 3.2 Antidepressants

Medication	Starting Dosage	Maximum Dosage
SSRIs		
Fluoxetine	10–20 mg qd	80 mg qd
Sertraline	25–50 mg qd	200 mg qd
Paroxetine	10–20 mg qd	50 mg qd
Tricyclics		
Imipramine	25–50 mg qhs	300 qhs
Desipramine	25–50 mg qhs	300 mg qhs
Nortriptyline	25 mg qhs	150 mg qhs
Other Antidepressants		
Bupropion	75 mg bid	300–450 mg qd in divided doses
Trazodone	50–100 mg hs	400–600 mg qhs
Nefazodone	50 mg bid	400–600 mg qhs
Venlafaxine	75 mg qd	375 mg qd in divided doses

tion is a problem, the patient can be given the less sedating medication sertraline. Alternatively, sedation can be managed with bedtime dosing. Most side effects are dose-dependent or tend to resolve or diminish with time. The half-life of all of the SSRIs is sufficiently long to permit once-a-day administration. Fluoxetine has an extremely long half-life and increases the blood levels of many other medications. This can be a problem for patients wanting to discontinue the medication because of side effects or for those patients who are on other medications that interact with fluoxetine.

New antidepressants provide additional options for matching the most tolerable side-effect profile for a particular patient. Bupropion tends to be activating and has virtually no anticholinergic, cardiovascular, or sexual side effects. It does have an increased incidence of seizures associated with its use, particularly at higher doses (above 300 mg) or when the dosage is increased rapidly. No more than 150 mg should be prescribed in one dose. Nefazodone and trazodone are in the same molecular family and are similarly quite sedating, but nefazodone does not seem to cause priapism, a significant risk for men treated with trazodone. Venlafaxine has relatively few anticholinergic side effects but is associated with hypertension, particularly at higher doses.

The TCAs currently in use include nortriptyline (NT), desipramine (DMI), amitriptyline (AMI), and imipramine (IMI). TCAs are less effective for those patients with the atypical subtype of major depression. These medications are associated with anticholinergic side effects (dry mouth, constipation, blurred vision, and urinary hesitancy), cardiovascular effects (delayed cardiac conduction and orthostatic hypotension), sedation, weight gain, sexual dysfunction (delayed orgasm and ejaculation), and lowered seizure threshold. Thus the physician may want to avoid TCAs in elderly patients or patients with heart disease, who may be more susceptible to serious problems such as delayed cardiac conduction system effects or anticholinergic effects including urinary retention or delirium. Although all TCAs cause side effects, their profiles differ somewhat. DMI is the least anticholinergic and sedating, whereas NT causes less orthostatic hypotension.

Therapeutic serum levels are well established for IMI, DMI, and NT. NT is distinct in having a "therapeutic window"; above a certain point it loses its effectiveness. In practice, this window makes NT somewhat more difficult to use, as blood levels measurements are required for optimal management. On the other hand, DMI and IMI can be increased by one dosage increment every 3 to 4 days or weekly, titrating response against side effects and aiming for the maximum dose tolerated.

Table 3.3 Treatment of Depression With Comorbid Conditions

Disorder	Preferred	Avoid
Allergies (MH)	Doxepin*, trimipramine*	
Cardiac conduction problem (WH)*	Bupropion, fluoxetine, fluvoxamine, paroxetine, sertraline	TCAs[2]
Cataplexy (MH)	Desipramine*, fluoxetine, imipramine, protriptyline*, tranylcypromine*	
Congestive heart failure (WH)	SSRIs, bupropion	Nefazodone[3], trazodone, TCAs, venlafaxine?
Constipation (chronic) (MH)	Fluoxetine, fluvoxamine, sertraline, trazodone, venlafaxine	Amitriptyline, doxepin, protriptyline, trimipramine
Diarrhea (chronic) (MH)	Amitriptyline, doxepin, protriptyline trimipramine	Bupropion, SSRIs, venlafaxine
Diabetes Type II	Fluoxetine	Amitriptyline, doxepin
Epilepsy (WH)	Desipramine, doxepin, phenelzine, SSRIs	Amoxapine, bupropion, maprotiline, trimipramine
Partial impotence, organic (WH)	Bupropion (MH), trazodone	Fluoxetine, fluvoxamine, paroxetine, sertraline, phenelzine
Dementia, delirium, cognitive disorder (MH)	Bupropion, fluoxetine, fluvoxamine, nefazodone, paroxetine, sertraline, trazodone, venlafaxine	Amitriptyline, clomipramine, doxepin, imipramine, protriptyline, trimipramine
Irritable bowel syndrome (MH)	Amitriptyline, desipramine, doxepin, nortriptyline, phenelzine, trazodone	
Migraine headache (MH)	Amitriptyline,* doxepin*, fluoxetine imipramine,* paroxetine, phenelzine,* sertraline, tranylcypromine, trimipramine	
Narrow-angle glaucoma (WH)	Bupropion, fluoxetine, fluvoxamine, nefazodone, sertraline, trazodone, venlafaxine	Amitriptyline imipramine, clomipramine, doxepin, paroxetine, trimipramine

Table 3.3 *(continued)*

Disorder	Preferred	Avoid
Neurogenic bladder (WH)	Bupropion, fluoxetine, sertraline, venlafaxine	
Parkinson's disease (MH)	Amitriptyline, bupropion, doxepin, imipramine, protriptyline, trimipramine	Amoxapine, SSRIs?
Peptic ulcers (MH)	Doxepin*, trimipramine*	
Sleep apnea (MH)	Protriptyline*, tranylcypromine*	
Tardive dyskinesia (WH)	Desipramine, imipramine, nefazodone, trazodone, trimipramine, venlafaxine	Amoxapine

1 MH = might help; WH = won't hurt
2 Although TCAs have quinidine-like, Type 1-A anti-arrhythmic effects, new studies suggest that in MI patients Type 1-A has increased mortality.
3 Beware of rare bradycardias.
* Efficacy established.
From *Psychotropic Drugs Fast Facts*, Second Edition by Jerrold S. Maxmen, M.D. and Nicholas G. Ward, M.D.. Copyright (c) 1995 by Nicholas J. Ward and the Estate of Jerrold S. Maxmen. Copyright (c) 1991 by Jerrold S. Maxmen. Reprinted by permission of W. W. Norton & Company, Inc.

The MAOIs are highly effective antidepressants that have declined in usage with the introduction of more easily tolerated drugs. Tyramine exposure from the diet and interactions with sympathomimetics and meperidine put patients who are on MAOIs at risk for the development of hypertensive crisis. Commonly associated side effects include weight gain, orthostatic hypotension, and sexual dysfunction.

All antidepressants have a lag time of 3 to 6 weeks before a response can be expected. Occasionally, patients can begin to notice improvement in the first week or two of treatment, although rapid improvement is ordinarily an unsustained placebo response. If a patient does not respond or has only a partial response after 6 weeks, the dose should be pushed to the maximum recommended dose, as tolerated. Adjunctive medications can be helpful, but their use should probably be limited to psychiatric consultants. Common strategies include the addition of lithium carbonate (usually 300 mg bid to tid will result in a serum level of 0.6 to 1.0), which is equally effective as an adjunctive therapy in unipolar and bipolar

Table 3.4 Managing Antidepressant Side Effects

Side effect	Management
Headache	Check for substance use or withdrawal (including caffeine): reduce dose.* Use analgesics (PRN).
Nausea	Take with meal and a large glass of water. Reduce dose.*
Insomnia	Take in the A.M. Reduce dose.* Add sleep aid.
Orthostatic	Rise slowly from reclining or seated position.
Hypertension	Sit down if light-headedness occurs. Maintain ample fluid intake. Reduce dose.*
Constipation	Increase fluid intake. Increase exercise. Increase fiber intake. Use stool softeners and bulk-forming agents.
Dry mouth	Use sugar-free candy, gum. Maintain fluid intake.
Appetite stimulation Weight gain	Exclude concurrent eating disorder or depressive relapse. Prescribe exercise and nutritional counseling. Reduce dose.* Switch medication.
Sedation	Take medication at night. Reduce dose.*
Treatment emergent anxiety	Reduce dose.* Switch medication.
Sexual dysfunction	Reduce dose.* Switch medication. Suggest a "drug holiday." Supplement with buspirone or bupropion.

*Reducing dose may decrease efficacy.

Source: McElroy SI, Keck PE, Friedman LM. Minimizing and Managing Antidepressant Side Effects. *The Journal of Clinical Psychiatry, 569*(Suppl 2):49–55, 1995. Copyright 1995, Physicians Postgraduate Press. Reprinted by permission.

depressed patients, with results within 10 to 14 days in most cases. Combining a TCA with an SSRI is another useful approach. Relatively low doses of the TCA should be used, because the SSRI increases the levels of the TCA. If a patient fails to respond to an adequately long trial at maximal dosages of one antidepressant, a switch to another class of antidepressant is most prudent.

Bipolar patients cannot be treated with an antidepressant without a mood stabilizer to protect them from switching to mania. Mood stabilizers are effective treatments for manic episodes as well. The treatment of the manic patient can be quite complex and requires the expertise of a psychiatrist. If a depressed patient appears to be becoming hypomanic during the course of antidepressant treatment, psychiatric consultation should again be considered.

Among the mood stabilizers, lithium carbonate has been used most extensively to treat bipolar disorder. For many bipolar patients, it is well tolerated and extremely effective. Primary care physicians should be aware of its low therapeutic index and the potential for renal and CNS toxicity above the therapeutic range of about 1.1 mEq/l. Dehydration can cause dangerously high lithium levels in previously stable patients, as can interactions with nonsteroidal anti-inflammatory medications and diuretics. Carbamazepine and valproic acid have excellent track records as secondary choices for patients who cannot tolerate lithium or for whom it is ineffective. These may even be prudent first-line medications in patients with mixed episodes and rapid cycling.

Six months of maintenance antidepressant treatment at the dosage required for the initial response is indicated for a single episode of depression, although dysthymia or recurrent episodes may require lengthier courses. To avoid physical withdrawal symptoms, discontinuation should occur gradually over about 2 weeks, depending on the initial dosage.

Medication management of the mood disorders will not be successful without careful attention to the therapeutic alliance with the patient as well as the relevant psychosocial factors. Adherence to treatment, an issue for all patients, requires particular attention in depressed patients. It is helpful to view your treatment plan through a depressed patient's eyes: The patient is in terrible pain and feels hopeless and helpless to change that distress. The physician recommends a medication with immediate side effects, warning the patient that it probably won't work for several weeks. Thus the patient may be left with the false impression that his or her situation is worse than before the consultation.

Several interventions can enhance adherence. First, the patient should participate in the choice of medications. Two medications might be presented to the patient, allowing the patient to select the more appealing side-effect profile. Second, exploiting desired side effects, such as the sedation of nefazodone for a patient with insomnia, is highly desirable. Although adding a benzodiazepine or low-dose trazodone to an SSRI can serve the same purpose, the patient may take only the sleeping pill and not the antidepressant. Third, the physician should approach the patient with quietly self-assured optimism, providing information and reason for hope. For example: "I know that the world looks bleak to you right now and that you can't believe that you'll ever feel better. Your depression makes everything seem more hopeless than it really is. I am confident that we can get you feeling much better, back to yourself. It will take some time, but it is likely that your depression will respond to medication." Guarantees for any one medication should be avoided, but the physician should convey optimism that a successful outcome will be found. Finally, the patient's complaints about side effects should be heard and addressed as much as possible. (See Table 3.4 for managing common medication side effects). When it is not possible to reduce or eliminate bothersome side effects, it is essential that the physician acknowledge the patient's difficulty in tolerating the symptoms. Physicians can sometimes dismiss a patient's concerns, particularly if the side effects are annoying but not dangerous. The patient's perception that the physician is unconcerned can be extremely destructive for the therapeutic alliance.

The frequency of visits during the induction phase of treatment for depression will vary, depending on the solidity of the patient's previous relationship with the primary care clinician, the severity of the patient's feelings of hopelessness, and ambivalence about treatment, and the quality of the patient's support network. Ideally, the patient should be seen weekly or every 2 weeks, even if briefly, until a clear positive response has been attained. The focus of these visits should be threefold: (1) assessing mood (a patient's use of a self-rating mood scale [see Figure 3.2] can be helpful to monitor the patient's response to treatment), (2) monitoring the patient for side effects, and (3) reassuring the patient and encouraging him or her to continue to comply with the treatment regimen.

Although pharmacological treatment is the most effective primary care approach to depressive disorders, the physician has many additional contributions to make. A detailed critical pathway for primary care treatment of depression is listed in Table 3.5. If the depression occurs in a patient with intercurrent medical illnesses, simultaneous forms of therapy must be offered for both the physical illness and the mood disorder. Care of the physical illness may act synergistically with the pharmacological treatment of the depression, both in supporting adherence to a drug regimen and in giving the patient assurances of improvement.

Primary care physicians often underestimate the importance of their supportive psychotherapy with depressed patients. The physician occupies a vital role of importance for all patients, as a dependable and insightful presence in the patient's life, and this transference of the medical relationship can be used to the patient's advantage. The primary care clinician can legitimize a patient's sense of discouragement, can acknowledge the

Figure 3.2 Depression Rating Scale.

0	1	2	3	4	5	6	7	8	9	10

Severely Depressed	Moderately depressed	Not depressed

Rate the best and worst mood on each day and record below.

Example:

Date:	Best Mood:	Time	Worst mood:	Time
10/23/98	6	4:00 P.M.	3	7:00 A.M.

burdens of an illness, and can allow the patient to articulate his or her own anger, fears, or worries. The physician is in an ideal position to assist patients in making sense and creating meaning from their medical and depressive illnesses. See chapter 16, Consulting and Counseling in Primary Care, for a detailed discussion.

Whether or not depressed patients have a comorbid medical illness, their primary care clinician can probe for the psychosocial accompaniments of depression (e.g., isolation, fear of abandonment, shame, unworthiness, or fear of burdening others). By inquiring about these emotional states and suggesting solutions, the clinician conveys, powerfully and concretely, that the patient deserves personal caring. Support groups may help patients through the initial stages of treatment of their depression. Family members or friends may be mobilized as allies of treatment.

Primary care physicians may choose to involve mental health professionals in their treatment of depressed patients. Clinicians should promptly refer patients to a psychiatrist for treatment of bipolar disease or of depression that is not amenable to primary care treatment. Because of the persistence of the stigma of mental illness, some patients resist a psychiatric referral. Skillful use of the therapeutic alliance can often overcome this resistance. If a patient refuses referral, the primary care clinician may benefit by discussing the case with a psychiatric colleague. If a depressed patient absolutely refuses to accept psychiatric referral and appears to be in danger, the primary care physician must be prepared to use the full force of his or her legal and professional authority to compel the patient to seek

Table 3.5 Critical Pathway: Depression

	Initial Visit	Week 2	Week 3	Week 4	Week 8–10	Month 6–9	Month 9–12
Assessment Tools	Beck,[a] Hamilton,[b] stress scale,[c] GAF,[d] GARF[e]	Depression algorithm,[l]		GAF,[d] mood scale,[j] cognitive behavior diary[k]	Beck,[a] Hamilton,[b] GAF,[d] mood scale,[j] cognitive behavior diary[k]	GAF,[d] mood scale,[j] cognitive behavior diary[k]	Beck,[a] Hamilton,[b] GAF,[d] GARF,[e] cognitive behavior diary[k]
Physical/lab/ diagnostic tests	Full physical exam, complete blood count, chemistry panel 20, drug screen, electrocardiogram, thyroid function test/thyroid stimulating hormone. Venereal disease research laboratory test.	Consider CAT, MRI, EEG, as needed.		Drug screen?	Reevaluate diagnosis; drug screen? other labs?		

	Initial Visit	Week 2	Week 3	Week 4	Week 8–10	Month 6–9	Month 9–12
Diagnosis	1. Rule out medical cause. 2. 2° drugs. 3. Comorbid medical/ psychiatric. 4. 1° depression.	Confirm psychiatric diagnosis; use depression algorithm[i]		Medical response? If not, reassess comorbid condition, diagnosis, and treatment.	*Expect response*; if not, reassess depression algorithm,[i] comorbid disorder, diagnosis/ treatment.	Full recovery? partial recovery?	Full recovery? partial recovery?
Time	45 minutes	30 minutes	Patient calls	15 minutes	30 minutes	15 minutes	15 minutes
Physician Emergency Risk Assessment	Emergencies; suicidal risk,[f] plan?	GAF[d] Emergencies? Extra phone availability	As necessary; extra phone availability.	GAF[d]	GAF;[d] check for suicide risk with a +Rx response.	GAF;[d] emergencies?	GAF;[d] emergencies?
Educational materials	Depression info, medication sheets, suicide risk.	Patient: mood scale[j] cognitive behavior diary,[k] Family education.		Education PRN, self-help.	Education: drug maintenance;[l] self-help.	Education: relapse prevention, self-help.	Education: relapse prevention, self-help.
Objective	Reduce somatic symptoms.	Reduce somatic symptoms.	Reduce somatic symptoms.	Expect mood anhedonia to improve.	Expect recovery from symptoms.	Discuss medications; taper, maintenance.	Depression remits; off all medications/or maintenance.
Treatment	1. Educate about depression, work-up, treatment options[g]	1. Educate about depression.	Extra phone availability.	1. Educate about recovery.	1. Educate about expected response.	1. Educate about relapse prevention maintenance Rx.	1. Educate about relapse prevention maintenance Rx.

(continued)

Table 3.5 *(continued)*

	Initial Visit	Week 2	Week 3	Week 4	Week 8–10	Month 6–9	Month 9–12
Treatment *(continued)*	2. Counsel: losses, stress social support. 3. Behavioral[h] 4. Medications a. Begin SSRI/ or new-generation antidepressants b. Sleep medications PRN c. No benzodiazepine alone	2. Counsel: losses, stress, problems, social support. 3. Behavioral[h] 4. Medications: adjust q 3–5 days.	2. Counsel medications or side effects. 3. Behavioral[h] 4. Medications a. Therapeutic dose range? b. Adjust meds. c. Discontinue benzodiazepines as soon as possible.	2. Counsel as needed. 3. Behavioral[h] 4. Medications a. Off benzodiazepines/PRN? b. Antidepressants alone, if possible. c. Combination drug treatment? d. Augmentation?	2. Counsel: + response, discuss maintenance - response, review treatment options.[g] 3. Behavioral[h] 4. Medications a. Maintenance? b. New medications? c. Off benzodiazepines/PRN? d. Combination drug treatment? e. Augmentations?	2. Counsel: + response, discuss maintenance - response, review treatment options.[g] 3. Behavioral[h] 4. Medications a. Drug taper? b. D/C drugs? c. New medications or augmentation? d. Drug maintenance?[l]	2. Counsel: + response, discuss maintenance - response, review treatment options.[g] 3. Behavioral[h] 4. Medications a. Drug taper? b. D/C drugs? c. New medications or augmentation? d. Drug maintenance?[l]
Consultations	Psychiatric consult if emergency requiring help or admission.	Medical specialist or psychiatric consult?	Family session? psychiatric consult?	Psychiatric consult? Referral to psychotherapy?	No response? Psychiatric referral. Reevaluate all options[g]; Electroconvulsive therapy?	Reevaluate treatment response. Options.[g] Psychiatric referral?	Reevaluate treatment response. Psychiatric referral?

Developed by Robert E. Feinstein.

[a] Beck scale (Patient self-report depression inventory. Beck, A.T. (1978). *Beck Inventory*. San Antonio, TX: The Psychological Corp./Harcourt Brace.

[b] Hamilton, M. A. (1960). Hamilton rating scale for depression: Physician assessment scale of the patient. *Journal of Neurology and Neurosurgical Psychiatry 23*, 62.

[c] Holmes, T. H., & Rahe, R. H. (1967). Social readjustment rating scale. *Journal of Psychosomatic Research,* 2,213–218.

[d] GAF (Global Assessment of Functioning). American Psychiatric Association. (1994). *Diagnostic and statistical manual of mental disorders* (4th ed., p. 200). Washington, DC: Author.

[e] GARF (Global Assessment of Relational Function) family assessment scale. *DSM-IV*, pp. 758–759.

[f] Suicidal risk. See chapter 7, Violence and Suicide.

[g] Treatment options: psychotherapy, family therapy, medications, combined treatments, ECT.

[h] Behavioral interventions: sleep hygiene, exercise, rate moods, cognitive behavioral diary, RTT, if anxious.

[I] Depression algorithm; see Figure 3.1.

[j] Mood scale. Patient rating of mood; see Figure 3.2.

[k] Cognitive behavioral diary

[l] Medication maintenance: If 1st episode, continue 6–12 months; 2nd episode, 1–2 years; 3rd episode, lifetime maintenance?

treatment. Options available to a primary care physician are discussed in chapter 7, Violence and Suicide.

Other mental health professionals play a major role in the medical care of depressed patients, especially those patients with chronic medical illnesses. Social work counseling, in conjunction with pharmacological treatment for depression, may offer the patient the support and skill unavailable from a busy physician. Teaming with a social worker or psychologist trained in family therapy may allow a physician to involve family members positively in the care of the depressed patient. Incorporation of a visiting nurse in the medical team may lengthen the attentive arm of the physician, allowing the patient to feel cared for between office visits.

Primary care clinicians can feel a great sense of satisfaction from their care of depressed patients. Responses to pharmacological treatment are gratifying. In addition, the profound results of the clinician's personal attentiveness and loyalty can, over time, develop lifelong relationships with patients, enabling their acceptance of medical treatment and improving their chances of recovery from depression.

REFERENCES

American Psychiatric Association. (1994). *Diagnostic and statistical manual of mental disorders* (4th ed.). Washington, DC: Author.

American Psychiatric Association. (1994). *Diagnostic and statistical manual of mental disorders: Primary care version* (4th ed.). Washington, DC: Author.

Beck, A. T. (1978). *Beck inventory*. San Antonio, TX: The Psychological Corp./Harcourt Brace.

Spitzer, R. L., Williams, J. B. W., Kroenke, K., Linzer M., Verloin deGruy, F., Hahn, S. R., & Brody, D. (1993). *Prime-MD: Primary care evaluation of mental disorders*. New York: New York State Psychiatric Institute.

CHAPTER 4

Substance Abuse

Gerald D. Roberts

There is a commonly held belief that substance abusers are difficult and unrewarding to help in primary care settings. Fortunately, this view is changing as primary care physicians and clinicians realize their unique position to identify, manage, help, and treat patients who abuse substances. Clinicians frequently see patients early in the development of substance abuse, and by acquiring the necessary knowledge and skills, can intervene to prevent further progression of the abuse. Also, clinicians can use their relationship with their patients to involve them in the process of evaluating and treating substance abuse.

THE MAGNITUDE OF THE PROBLEM

Alcohol is the most studied substance of abuse, because its abuse has consistently occurred at high rates in most societies for long periods of time. In primary care settings, the lifetime prevalence of "alcohol abuse" is between 16% and 35%, with the prevalence of current problems ranging from 5% to 20%.

The prevalence of alcohol abuse and dependence is directly related to the criteria used to make these diagnoses. Using the diagnostic criteria of the American Psychiatric Association, in the 5-year spread between 1980 and 1985, 8% of the U.S. population was alcohol dependent and 5% abused alcohol. In the 1-year spread from 1990 to 1991, 14% of noninstitutionalized adults between the ages of 15 and 54 were alcohol dependent (*DSM-IV* 1994). In primary care settings, 15 to 20% of patients seen in the office or hospital are alcohol dependent (Mayo-Smith, 1997).

The lifetime prevalence of substance abuse other than alcohol is between 7% and 9%, with the prevalence of current substance abuse approximately 3%. The magnitude of all forms of substance abuse is actually higher because abuse estimates are based on a diagnostic system that excludes large numbers of mild and moderate problem users who probably make up the largest number of substance abusers in primary care practices.

According to the Biopsychosocial Model of Substance Abuse (Engel, 1980), the problem of substance abuse stems from the dynamic interplay between the person and his or her unique mix of biological, psychological, and sociocultural factors (see Figure 4.1). Although the individual is influenced by biological, psychodynamic, and sociocultural forces, he or she is ultimately responsible for how he or she chooses to use or abuse substances.

THE ASSESSMENT AND TREATMENT OF SUBSTANCE ABUSE

The process of diagnosis, assessment, and intervention with a substance-abusing patient (summarized in Figure 4.2) has five steps: screening, involvement of the patient in the process, assessment, negotiation, and intervention.

Screening for Substance Abuse

Diagnosis of substance abuse begins with physician recognition that a patient may be abusing a substance. The clinician may obtain this information through screening, or from the patient or the patient's family or friends.

Screening Initiated by the Physician

The physician's right and responsibility to initiate a discussion of substance use is inherent in the physician-patient "contract." This contract involves an implicit agreement by both parties to work together in promoting the patient's good health. The primary care clinician needs to suspect substance abuse in order to make the proper diagnosis.

The first indications of a substance abuse problem often arise during the initial office visit. The clinician has to be attentive to the psychosocial

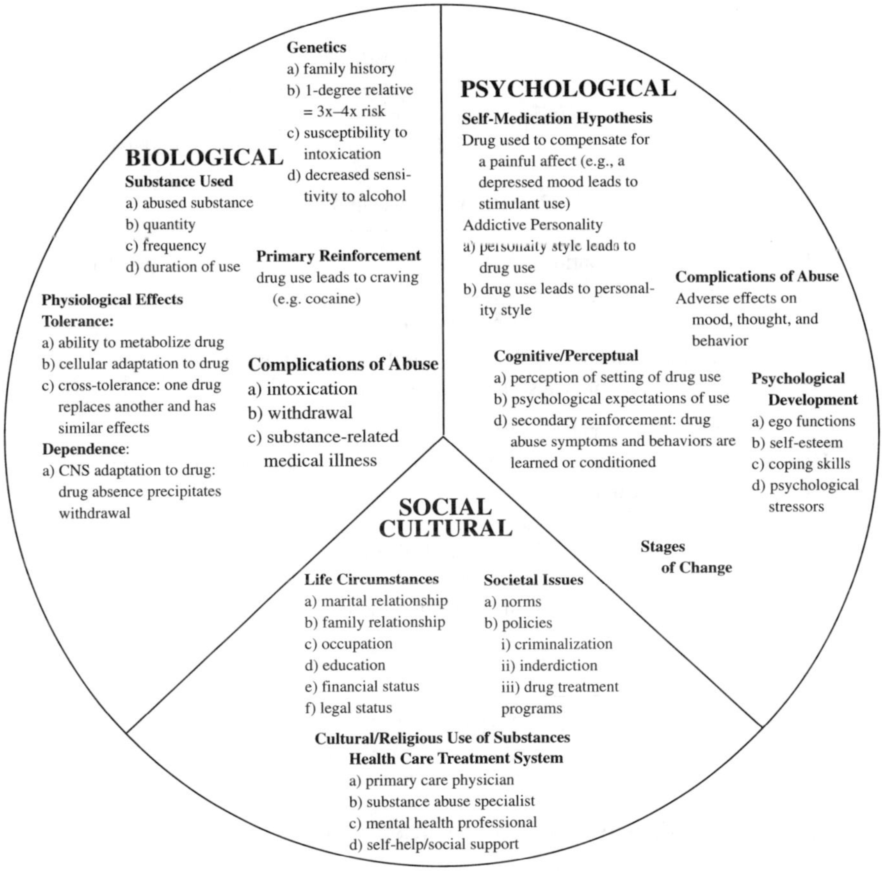

Figure 4.1 Biopsychosocial Model of Substance Abuse.

domain in order to learn about substance abuse problems. Inquiry about substance abuse and possible complications can be direct, by asking the patient outright if he abuses alcohol or uses illegal drugs, or may be indirect, by asking about problematic life events and any connection between these events and substance use. The earliest clinical indicators of substance abuse are behavioral and involve changes in mood, social or occupational functioning, and relationships. It is not unusual for patients to deny substance abuse when directly asked. Patient denial should not lead the clinician to collude in the assumption that a substance abuse problem does *not* exist. Rather, the clinician must ask questions from the perspective of oth-

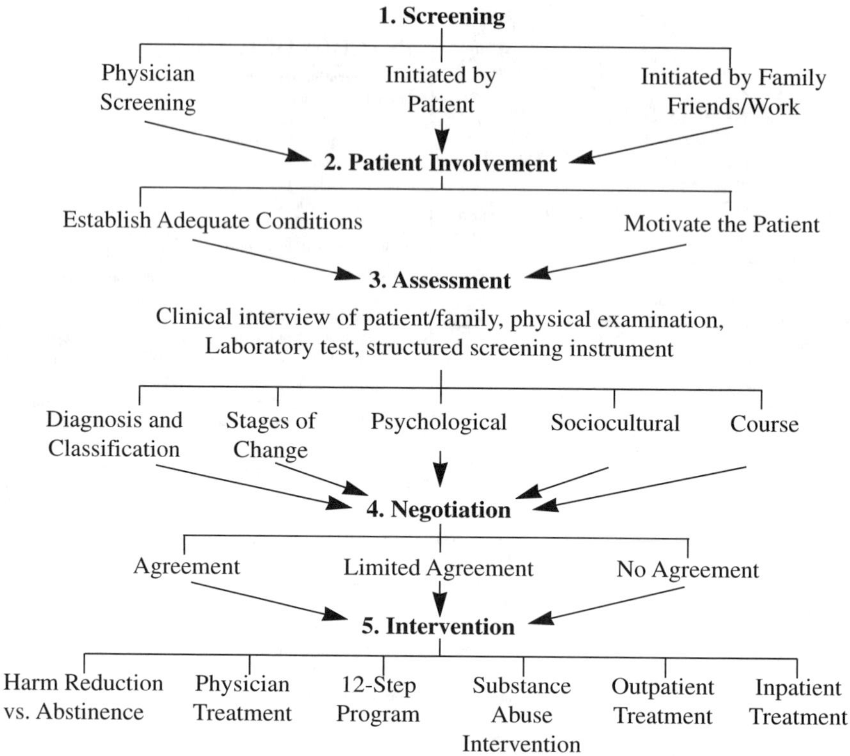

Figure 4.2 Substance Abuse Assessment and Treatment.

ers looking at the patient, for example, "Has anyone in your family, work life, or legal system ever thought you had a substance use problem?"

The physician can also utilize the CAGEAID (Brown, 1992) and AUDIT (Alcohol Use Disorder Identification Test) substance abuse screening tests. CAGEAID was originally developed to screen for alcohol abuse and later adapted to include other substances (see Table 4.1 for CAGEAID questions and scoring). AUDIT (Saunder, Aasland, & Babor, 1993) was developed by the World Health Organization and revised to include other substances. AUDIT is more comprehensive, but the time to administer this test may be prohibitive in some primary care settings. Both tests were validated using criteria for substance abuse, which tend to exclude mild abusers.

Once the substance abuse screening has been initiated, it is helpful to inform the patient of the clinician's concern and request the patient's

Table 4.1 CAGEAID Testing

Directions: Answer yes or no to the following questions.

- Have you felt you ought to **C**ut down on your drinking or other substance use?
- Have people **A**nnoyed you by criticizing your drinking or other substance use?
- Have you felt bad or **G**uilty about your drinking or other substance use?
- Have you ever needed an **E**ye opener in the morning to steady your nerves or other substances to get the day started?

Scoring: One "yes" response has a sensitivity of about 90 and specificity between 52 and 93. "Other substance use" has been substituted for "drug use" in the standard questionnaire.

Source: Brown, R. L. (1992). Identification and office management of alcohol and drug disorders. In M. F. Fleming & K. L. Barry (Eds.), Addictive disorders, p. 29. St. Louis: Mosby Year Book.

agreement to proceed. Respect for the patient's autonomy is a primary consideration when helping the patient deal with the fear of giving up control. If the patient does not consent to proceed further, the clinician can indicate he or she will raise the issue at a future time.

Substance Use Questions Initiated by Patient

Patients may indicate some concern or may have questions about their own substance use. The clinician should not assume that raising the subject means that the patient is fully open to the idea of quitting substance abuse. For example, the patient who is worried about having lost control over substance use may want reassurance rather than help in cessation. It is important to help the patient clarify his or her goals. This type of communication fosters a therapeutic alliance and protects against clinician-patient misunderstanding. Patients may seek help in the following areas: (1) discontinuation or reduction of substance use; (2) relief from the consequences of substance use; (3) ventilation of feelings of guilt or shame; (4) mollifying family or employer; (5) some source of external control or limit-setting; and/or (6) clarification, information, or referral for help. Another way to explore why the patient has raised the issue of substance use is to ask why the patient is interested now or what has led the patient to seek help at this point in time. Understanding the patient's motivation for help provides the clinician with the basis for involving the patient in his or her own treatment.

Substance Use Questions Initiated by Families, Friends, or Coworkers

Often, the family, friends, or people from work recognize the substance abuse problem before the patient and contact the clinician out of their concern. This can be a difficult situation, because the clinician needs to respect the patient's confidentiality and may not be able to discuss the patient with the concerned party. However, the clinician can listen to the information, ask the contact to directly express the concerns to the patient, and request that the contact accompany the patient to the next office visit. In addition, the clinician can broach the topic of substance abuse with the patient by mentioning that he or she was contacted by someone who was concerned about the patient's substance abuse. The clinician can also invite the patient to bring in other concerned parties for an open discussion.

Involvement of Patient in the Process

It is important to involve the patient in a collaborative effort to determine whether substances are being used in a harmful way. In order to communicate concern for the patient's health and seriousness of purpose and to establish the conditions necessary to engage the patient, the physician needs to provide privacy, confidentiality, and adequate time (15 to 30 minutes). The patient should be assured that the information exchanged in the consultation is private and that it will not be shared with others unless the patient's behavior presents a risk of serious harm to the patient or others. The consultation process is reviewed in chapter 16, Consulting and Counseling in Primary Care.

Miller and Rollnick (1991) offer a six-pronged approach to physician-patient communication called FRAMES, which stands for **F**eedback, **R**esponsibility, **A**dvice, **M**enu, **E**mpathy, and **S**elf-efficacy. Although each of these aspects is initiated by the clinician, the process is an interactive one, involving the patient.

Feedback

The clinician gathers information and impressions and presents them to the patient as organized feedback. For example, "I'd like to tell you what I've found in talking with you and doing the laboratory tests. Your family history suggests you may have a predisposition to excessive alcohol use. It seems to me, that sometimes you medicate your nervousness and compulsive work habits. You're able to stop using but quickly resume at a later time. Your lab tests indicate some impaired liver functioning, which is probably due to the alcohol use. How do you see your situation?"

The feedback portion of the interview helps the clinician and patient clarify their views and gives them both an opportunity to discuss areas of agreement and disagreement. This type of feedback can help patients see their behavior as meaningful and communicates a sense of the potential serious health consequences of substance abuse.

Responsibility

The physician presents patient-physician responsibilities for dealing with substance use problems. Some patients feel so helpless that they want the clinician to take over all their care and tell them what to do. At the other extreme are patients who are ambivalent or don't want to change their behavior. These patients will resist the clinician's attempt to take control. To foster a therapeutic alliance and respect the patient's rights, the clinician needs to encourage the patient to assume responsibility. It is optimal to specify what the clinician can offer and what the patient can do for self-care. For example, the clinician might say, "I understand your reluctance to face your substance use. You don't have to pursue this further, as that decision is yours. Whatever you decide, I think you might want to know some more about how alcohol affects you. I can help you with that, if you like. If we find a reason for concern, you have choices. You can continue to drink but be more aware of the effects of drinking on your feelings and behavior, or you can try to reduce your use and see if that helps, or you can stop all use now."

Advice

The physician needs to distinguish those patients who will respond best to clear, nonjudgmental advice. Sometimes, a nondirective approach can leave a patient confused and foundering. When giving advice, clearly identify the problem and risks, explain why change is important, and offer specific ways to effect this change. For example, "I've carefully evaluated your situation, and I'm concerned about your use of alcohol. You've been drinking out of loneliness and to deal with the loss of your wife. I understand this, but drinking is causing your headaches and memory loss and is interfering with your ability to cope. I feel strongly that you should stop drinking now. I can help you do this, and I believe you can." Even if advice in the near term has no immediate effect, it may become a motivating factor in the future.

Menu

The clinician can offer a "menu" of options for the patient's behavior, choice of a goal, or action. Offering the patient options enhances the patient's sense of control and allows the patient to make choices based on his particular situation.

Empathy

Empathy refers to the clinician's ability to experience emotionally what his patient is experiencing, making it possible for the patient to feel the clinician's warmth, respect, and support. Empathy suggests to the clinician hypotheses about the patient's substance abuse, which can be tested and discussed with the patient. For example, "You seem to feel the need to continue smoking marijuana because it gives you a break from work tension and enables you to go back to work the next day. So you're afraid to give up marijuana, because you believe it's necessary to your functioning. Is that really so?"

Self-Efficacy

Self-efficacy refers to the patient's belief that he or she can change. It is not enough for the patient to recognize a problem and want to do something about it; the patient needs to believe he or she can take effective action. The clinician's conviction that he can help and the patient's belief in his or her ability to change, play an important part in facilitating change.

Assessment of Substance Use

The clinical interview of the patient and family (if indicated and possible) is the most important means of assessing the patient. Assessment begins as soon as the issue of substance use is raised. Substance abuse plays an important part in so many medical and psychiatric conditions that it must be considered whenever a clinician is evaluating a patient. The physician must be knowledgeable about physical symptoms, psychiatric presentations, and sociocultural factors, which vary from substance to substance (see Shader, 1994, for a review). The initial assessment phase should focus on an evaluation of the acute complications of substance abuse, such as intoxication and withdrawal syndromes. These conditions often require immediate treatment, which take precedence over the more comprehensive substance use assessment.

Substance Intoxication

Substance intoxication is caused by the recent administration of a substance, which can, by its direct physiological effects, produce maladaptive medical, behavioral, or psychological changes. The signs and symptoms of intoxication are specific for each class of substance. Alcohol, cocaine, and opioid intoxication are commonly seen in primary care settings.

Alcohol intoxication produces mood lability, belligerence, impaired judgment, and impaired social or occupational functioning. The signs include slurred speech, incoordination, unsteady gait, nystagmus, delirium, and coma. The clinical picture varies with the dose, the duration or chronicity of use, the person's tolerance for the substance, expectations about the substance's effects, and other factors.

Amphetamine or cocaine intoxication produces euphoria or affective blunting, hypervigilance, anxiety, tension or anger, impaired judgment, or impaired social or occupational functioning. The signs include tachycardia or bradycardia, pupillary dilation, elevated blood pressure, perspiration or chills, nausea or vomiting, cardiac arrhythmias, delirium, seizures, and rarely coma.

The clinical picture of opioid intoxication includes initial euphoria followed by apathy, dysphoria, psychomotor agitation or retardation, sleep, impaired judgment, or impaired social or occupational functioning. The signs include pupillary constriction (or pupillary dilation due to anoxia from severe overdose), drowsiness or coma, slurred speech, and impairment in attention or memory.

Refer to Hyman and Tesar (1994) and Shader (1994) for a comprehensive review of substance abuse intoxications.

Substance Withdrawal

Physical dependence and withdrawal syndromes from substance abuse can develop with the use of alcohol, amphetamines, cocaine, nicotine, sedatives-hypnotics, and anxiolytics. A withdrawal syndrome is specific for each drug of abuse and can cause significant distress or impairment in social or occupational functioning (see Hyman & Tesar, 1994, and Shader, 1994, for a review).

The physician needs to be aware of several high-risk complications from withdrawal, including:

- Alcohol withdrawal from either abrupt cessation or from a dramatic decrease in intake of alcohol. Approximately 50% of patients in alcohol withdrawal have symptoms of tremors, and some patients may go on to develop delirium tremens (DTs). DTs have a mortality rate of less than 3% but may cause death from hyperthermia, status seizures, fluid electrolyte imbalances, or psychiatric symptoms that inadvertently lead to suicide or homicide. Failure to suspect impending DTs can result in preventable complications and unnecessary hospitalization. DTs can occur during a hospital stay, surgery, or even childbirth.
- A grand mal seizure may occur in as many as 20% to 30% of individuals undergoing withdrawal from alcohol, sedative-hypnotics, or anxiolytics. A single withdrawal seizure is not uncommon. More disturbing and potentially life threatening are status seizures, which sometimes cannot be interrupted by pharmacological intervention and result in death.
- After the heavy and prolonged use of opioids, opioid withdrawal syndrome can be precipitated by the administration of opioid antagonists such as naltrexone. Patients awakened by opioid antagonists can become belligerent, increasing the risk to the clinician.
- A typical pattern of cocaine abuse is many days of high-dose use ("runs" or "binges") followed by discontinuation. Abrupt discontinuation of cocaine use can result in acute withdrawal symptoms (a "crash") during which the patient is at significant risk for experiencing depression and/or suicidal behavior.

Physical Examination and Laboratory Testing

The medical work-up for substance abuse requires a comprehensive physical and psychiatric evaluation, as described in detail in chapter 5, Psychiatric Symptoms Due to Medical Illness. Physical examination and laboratory testing should be done to support the diagnosis of substance abuse, assess substance use complications, or evaluate for coexisting conditions. Laboratory tests, useful as markers for alcohol abuse, can also be clinically used to help abusers see concrete evidence of the complications of alcohol. They include liver function tests, gamma glutamyltransferase (GGT), aspartate aminotransferase (AST), mean corpuscular volume (MCV), and blood alcohol levels (BAL) (a level of 100 mg/dl in a routine office visit or a level of >300mg/dl at any time should alert the physician to alcohol use or abuse). A urine screen is useful only for recent significant alcohol or drug consumption. Laboratory tests for other substances can be helpful.

Physicians need to note in the chart when a patient agrees to toxicology testing. Serum or urine toxicology can be used as an additional means to establish abuse or monitor known substance abuse. Positive urine screens will not indicate the duration or frequency of use, nor will they help to rule out a withdrawal syndrome. To effectively use urine toxicology testing, it is important to know how long after use a substance can be detected. Cocaine's short half-life means that laboratory testing will not detect the substance unless the test is done shortly after use. However, cocaine's main metabolite extends the time it can be detected to 2 to 4 days. Detection after last use varies significantly among substances of abuse: 5 to 12 hours for cocaine proper; 1 to 5 days for amphetamines, short-acting barbiturates, benzodiazepines, and opiates; 2 to 8 days for acute cannabinoid use; and 14 to 42 days for chronic cannabinoid use.

The purpose of the assessment is to prepare the clinician and patient for the next step, which is to work toward an agreement about the nature of the problem and interventions.

Classification of Substance Use

A substance use classification scheme proposed for primary care settings describes the patient's patterns of use along a continuum of severity: normative, problematic, or dependent use. The clinician can categorize the patient's pattern of use, specifying the extent of use and complications (see Table 4.2).

Patterns of Use

Normative use includes use of small amounts of a substances, occasionally ingested for pleasure or to manage minor tensions or psychological discomfort. Normative use means that the patient can use it or not, without any significant consequence. Normative use is determined by sociocultural factors, which vary from culture to culture (Western Europe vs.

Table 4.2 Classification of Substance Abuse

	Normative Use	Problematic Use	Dependent Use
Definitions	• Occasional use. • Used to enhance life. • Established by sociocultural norms.	• Regular use: mild, moderate, or severe abuse. Use clinical judgment to assess severity. • Patient investment in continued use.	• Regular use: mild, moderate, or severe abuse. Use clinical judgment to assess severity. • Patient investment in continued use.
Boundary marker	• No complications.	• Complications or adverse effects. • No dependence.	• Physical dependence. • Complications or adverse effects.
Extent of use	• Based on norms. Guidelines: 0–30 glasses of wine or equivalent per month. • No more than 3 glasses at a time. • No safe amounts of tobacco, PCP, or hallucinogens.	• Based on norms. Guidelines: no more than 3 glasses/day. 1. Mild: 30–40 glasses of wine/equivalent/month. 2. Moderate: 40–60 glasses of wine/equivalent/month Severe: 60 or more glasses of wine/equivalent/month. • No criteria for illicit or IV drug use.	• Same as problematic user. • Patient uses more concentrated forms (e.g., crack, IV heroin, hashish). • Dependence possible with most substances.
Complication or adverse effects	• Generally none, but normative use can lead to car accidents. No use during pregnancy.	• Biopsychosocial complications. Mild, moderate, severe based on the impact on the patient's life and reversibility.	• Biopsychosocial complications with greater life-threatening risks.

Muslim countries), within the same culture (barbiturates prescribed for sleep vs. the same dosage used for a "high" in a social situation), and from period to period (19th-century use of opioids vs. 20th-century attitudes toward heroin).

Problematic use is on a continuum of severity of use from mild, moderate, to severe, with either a continuous or binge use pattern. Drug use becomes problematic if there are significant medical, psychological, or social consequences directly resulting from drug use. Clinical judgment should be used when assessing the severity of complications. For example, abuse of alcohol with a once-a-month episode of intoxication, mild gastritis, and some mood swings would be considered mild complications. A patient with weekly episodes of severe intoxication, peptic ulcers, and panic attacks would be experiencing severe complications.

Dependent use is distinguished from severe problematic use by the presence of physical dependence. Diagnosis, management, and treatment of withdrawal syndromes are a major aspect of the acute medical treatment approach.

Specify the Extent of Use

Once the clinician has identified the presumed pattern of use (normative, problematic, or dependent use), it is important to specify the following: (1) all substances used; (2) frequency of abuse (3) variations in the timing of abuse (e.g., is the use continuous, or does it have a binge pattern; is the substance used at night or on weekends; or is the use precipitated by separations?); (4) specific amount of each substance consumed on a typical day (ounces of alcohol, lines of cocaine, joints of marijuana, prescribed medications, over-the-counter preparations, etc.); (5) the route of administration (oral, snorting, skin popping, inhaling, or intravenous); (6) evidence of intoxication, tolerance, or physical dependence/withdrawal; and (7) risky behaviors associated with use, such as driving a vehicle, using machinery, or having unprotected sex.

Complications

The clinician can also make a biopsychosocial list of complications for each patient. This problem list can be used with the patient to demonstrate the many complications of the patient's substance abuse and can facilitate accurate and comprehensive medical record keeping:

- Biological complications can be formulated from a list of signs and symptoms based on the review of sytems. These include general effects of substance abuse, such as malnutrition, weight loss, fatigue, and insomnia, and specific complaints related to substance abuse, such as esophageal varices, gastritis, peptic ulcers, alcoholic hepatitis, cirrhosis, secondary hypertension, cardiomyopathy, peripheral neuropathy, Wernicke-Korsakoff syndrome, delirium, dementia, spontaneous abortion, birth defects, bone marrow suppression, drug interactions, vehicular accidents, and trauma. In addition, medical complications from the route of administration should also be described, including items such as puncture marks, sclerosed veins ("tracks"), thrombophlebitis, acute endocarditis, HIV infection, and nasal mucosal damage and septal defects due to intranasal use ("snorting") of cocaine or heroin.
- Psychological complications from substance abuse include alterations of mood, thinking, sense of self, and behavior. The patient may not recognize that his or her maladaptive behaviors interfere with learning healthier ways of coping. For example, a patient who comes home from work feeling tense and irritable may habitually drink two or three glasses of wine to relax. While this behavior works "too well" in terms of reducing tension, it prevents the patient from developing better solutions to work stress, which could improve his or her daily work life. It is important to consider substance abuse as a causal factor in the presence of any of the following psychological complaints: irritability, agitation, generalized anxiety, panic attacks, hostility, violence, depression, mood swings, dysphoria, psychosomatic symptoms, psychotic disorders, sexual dysfunction, sleep disorders, impaired judgment, reality testing, and regulation of drives, affects, and impulses. Behavioral problems associated with drug use include driving a vehicle or operating machinery under the influence, having unprotected sex, sharing needles, episodes of violence/criminal activity, and suicidal tendencies.
- Sociocultural complications of substance use include dysfunctional relationships with spouse, family, friends, employment, school, or financial and legal problems associated with substance abuse. When assessing sociocultural effects the clinician can be sensitive to the fact that substance use is woven into the very texture of many cultures. In Europe, the norm is to drink wine with most meals, and chewing cocoa leaves (cocaine) is part of some South American native cultures. In Japan, men drink sake as part of recreation within

the work culture, although women remain abstinent. In many religions, substances have been utilized as a symbol in religious rituals (wine has been a Judeo-Christian staple) and continue to be an inherent part of religious life.

Since the psychological and social symptoms or complications of substance abuse can mimic those of many mental disorders, a broad psychiatric differential diagnosis is required to determine which symptoms are due to substance abuse versus a mental disorder. The term "dual diagnosis" is used when a substance abuse problem and a psychiatric condition coexist. Psychiatric symptoms in the presence of substance abuse are assumed to be substance related until an extended substance-free period can prove otherwise. If psychiatric symptoms existed prior to drug use or persist long after the effects of drug use are expected to be gone, then the symptoms are likely to have been caused by a psychiatric condition.

Stages of Change

In preparation for an intervention, it is important to understand the patient's readiness for change. The six stages of change are precontemplation, contemplation, preparation, action, maintenance, and relapse. To evaluate the stage of change, see Table 4.3 for stage-specific questions that are helpful in a clinical situation. These stages are reviewed in detail in chapter 19, Behavioral Counseling and Medical Adherence. Table 19.1 in Chapter 19 specifically outlines clinician interventions that can help a patient progress from one stage of change to the next.

The Psychology of Substance Abuse

Khantzian (1985) developed the self-medication hypothesis, which states that substances are used as a way to cope with one's internal and external environment by regulating painful affects and related behaviors. Although individuals frequently use more than one substance, many seem to have a predilection for one substance, the "drug of choice." Patients may self-select those substances (by experience and experimentation) that relieve their particular state of distress and help to improve their functioning. For example, the anxious patient chooses alcohol for its inhibition-releasing or sedating effect; the depressed patient chooses cocaine for it energizing/antidepressant effect; the patient who seeks to control his or her impulses or pain may choose heroin for its hypnotic or analgesic effect.

Table 4.3 Stage of Change Questions for the Substance Abuser

The following questions can be used to place the patient in a particular stage:

Precontemplation
- Do you see your use of the substance as a problem?
- Do you see the complications as a problem?
- Do you see any connection between your use and the complications?
- Do you plan on doing anything about your use?
- Are you planning on *not* doing anything because you don't see a problem, you see a problem but have decided there's no risk, you don't like being told what to do, or you have given up on being able to change?

Contemplation
- Are you considering making a change?
- Do you have mixed feelings about giving up the use and what you see as the benefit of use?
- Do you have mixed feelings about being able to change?

Preparation
- Are you motivated to take action in the near future?
- Do you feel prepared to take action?
- Do you have a plan of action?
- Have you thought of what might get in your way?

Action stage
- What goals have you set for yourself?
- What actions are you taking to change your substance-using behavior?
- What indicators do you see that your actions are being effective?

Maintenance stage
- Are you maintaining the goals you reached?
- Are there any indicators of not being able to hold on to the change you've made in yourself, your life situation, or your use of the substances?

Relapse Stage
- Have you lapsed into drug use?

The premise of the self-medication hypothesis is that people do not use substances to get "high" but to feel normal. Khantzian (1985) suggests that the person turns increasingly to substance use as a basic and global way of adaptation. Substance abuse also prevents other healthier coping mechanisms such that the substance abuse takes on a life of its own and the patient becomes "locked in" to substance-abusing behavior. Patients do describe a feeling that they gain benefits from substance use. Perceived benefits include the management of anxiety, depression, anger, insomnia, and feelings of inadequacy. Substance abusers may state that substance use improves their ability to cope with intimacy, sexuality, socialization, and relationships; provides an escape from reality; and makes them feel confident, powerful, or "high." Discussing the patient's perception of these benefits makes it easier for the clinician to empathize with the reasons the patient has such difficulty giving up substance use. The self-medication theory also suggests that a patient with psychiatric problems has painful affects that lead to substance abuse and, thus, a dual diagnosis.

The challenge to the self-medication hypothesis is posed by those who believe that the reverse process occurs in most cases of substance abuse, that is, that substance abuse leads to psychopathology or the appearance of the "addictive personality" (Vaillant, 1995). This view is supported by studies that show that psychiatric problems are alleviated when abstinence is achieved. It is likely that both processes exist for different patients.

Psychiatric Symptoms/Strengths and Weaknesses/Sociocultural Factors

When evaluating substance abuse, the clinician needs to be aware of psychiatric symptoms and/or diagnoses that may complicate the substance abuse treatment. As part of the assessment, the clinician can routinely inquire about depressive/manic moods; anxiety symptoms or disorders; delirium, dementia, or other organic brain syndromes; sociopathy; and psychotic symptoms. The severity of these symptoms or disorders will greatly complicate management and treatment of substance abuse. If psychiatric symptoms are mild and substance related, they will likely improve with treatment of substance use problems. If psychiatric symptoms indicate a dual diagnosis, then the treatment is more difficult, and the patient may need to be referred to a mental health/substance abuse clinician and/or program.

It is also often helpful to have a sense of the patient's strengths and weaknesses. Patients with a better prognosis include:

- Patients who have been able to stop abusing substances in the past. (New attempts at cessation of abuse can be modeled on older, successful attempts. Past failures should signal a need for different approaches for the new attempt);
- Patients who have been generally able to deal with stress and adapt to life's problems;
- Patients with stable marriages;
- Patients with interpersonal support;
- Patients with higher socioeconomic status;
- Patients with a stable work history;
- Patients with less psychopathology.

Poor prognostic indicators include social phobia and/or a distaste for spirituality (which may preclude the use of Alcoholics Anonymous or other group support); patients who are unwilling to take medications; patients with severe psychopathology, including poor self-care, self-destructive tendencies, and/or sucidality; potentially violent patients; and patients who use pathological defenses. Other factors that can affect substance abuse treatment include cultural, racial, and ethnic perspectives on substance use.

Special Populations and Substance Abuse

Specific factors pertain to certain populations: adolescents, the elderly, men, and women. While a comprehensive discussion of substance abuse and these specific populations is beyond the scope of this chapter, the following can be considered.

Adolescence is a time of rapid change and experimentation with substances, and it is difficult to predict which adolescents will go on to abuse substances. All adolescents should be assessed for the presence of substance abuse, but clinicians should be particularly alert to those adolescents who are using substances to cope with themselves and their life and whose use is outside the norms of their peer group. Substance abuse in the older population is frequently missed, particularly the abuse of prescriptions and over-the-counter medications. Older people have increased sensitivity to substances unless tolerance has developed. Heavy alcohol use among males is common in the corporate business culture, where those who don't participate are often seen as not following the company norms. Issues specific to women relate to social stigma of drug use, deficiencies in gender-specific research, metabolism (e.g., gastric alcohol dehydrogenase is lower in women than men), and pregnancy.

Course

The course of the substance abuse over time is more variable than linear. Patients shift in severity of substance abuse and their motivation for change and may have periods where they are abstinent. Understanding how patients got to where they are helps the clinician plan substance abuse interventions that can have a major impact on the future. Although each patient's course is unique, it is possible to characterize the most typical courses:

- *People who reach some level of substance abuse and then discontinue that use without any intervention.* For example, a patient threatened by the loss of a significant relationship may fit this pattern.
- *Patients who reach a point of mild or moderate problematic use and remain in this position for years.* This course occurs when the complications of use do not reach an unacceptable threshold for the patient or for the people who support him or her. This also occurs when the physician either ignores or does not pursue indicators of substance abuse.
- *Patients who fit the stereotype of a progression that seems inevitably downward* (as dramatized in *The Lost Weekend, Days of Wine and Roses*, and *Long Day's Journey Into Night*). The patient seems to reach a point of no return, at which the substance abuse takes on a life of its own. At this point, only the person's family, physician, or the legal system has the power to alter the progression of the patient's course.
- *Patients who move along a spiraling course toward health or toward complications and disability.* Those who have achieved a reasonably secure recovery usually look back on starts and stops and the events that moved them backward and that can move them forward. Most patients fall into this category. Alcoholics Anonymous does not refer to someone as having recovered but as being "in recovery." This differentiation reflects the potential for spiraling in either direction.

Negotiation

Negotiation between physician and patient actually begins at the initial meeting and can be guided by the FRAMES approach described above or can follow the "Informed Shared Decision Making" model described in chapter 13, A Model for Office-Based Cardiovascular Risk Reduction and Behavioral Change. Negotiation progresses from initial acknowledgment of the patient's substance abuse to the assessment of the patient's stage of change. In order to negotiate a complete treatment plan, the patient must have reached the preparation stage, at which there is an acknowledgment of the need for treatment and a determination to proceed. Those patients who remain in either precontemplation or contemplation stages of change may be helped by specific interventions, which are outlined in Table 19.1, chapter 19, Behavioral Counseling and Medical Adherence. Patients in preparation or action stages can proceed to negotiate their treatment options with their clinician. After providing a choice of treatment options, the clinician can negotiate a specific treatment plan and a shared agreement about the need for support or community resources. Once the patient has reached the stage of preparation, a shared treatment plan can be negotiated, as in the following example.

CASE STUDY: NEGOTIATING A TREATMENT PLAN.

> Brad is a severe problematic alcohol abuser, evidenced by his daily consumption of four bottles of beer and episodic binge drinking. He also suffers with complications of intoxication, presumptive liver disease, impaired relationships, and depression. He is afraid to discontinue use entirely because it helps with his depression. He has many personal strengths and support from his mother and employer. Throughout the assessment he is clear that he has reached the stage of preparation and is determined to discontinue his alcohol use. The clinician begins negotiating a treatment plan by offering the patient the options of harm reduction (reducing alcohol consumption) or abstinence. Together, they discuss the pros and cons, and Brad decides he prefers to try to stop drinking. They discuss the treatment options within abstinence, which include (1) stopping on his own; (2) stopping with support of Alcoholics Anonymous (AA); (3) stopping with the support of medications (naltrexone); (4) stopping with the support of outpatient substance abuse treatment in an individual, group, or partial outpatient hospitalization program; or (5) inpatient substance abuse treatment. Brad decides he would like to try cessation and naltrexone. The physician agrees, adding that the support of AA with a sponsor might prevent a future need for hospitalization. The patient agrees to this treatment plan.

This phase of negotiation often blends easily into the intervention phases.

Intervention/Treatment

The physician's role in treating substance abuse operates on three levels of prevention: primary, secondary, and tertiary. The aim of primary prevention is to encourage normative use and prevent progression to the problematic level. Secondary prevention is focused on treating the biopsychosocial effects of substance abuse and preventing complications related to problematic use. Tertiary prevention is targeted for dependent users, whereby the purpose of intervention is to treat withdrawal and other reversible complications and to prevent future difficulties.

Three Tiers of Physician Involvement

The physician needs to place himself or herself at one of the three levels of clinician involvement and utilize a substance abuse intervention within his or her own comfort zone.

At the first tier, the clinician identifies the level of substance abuse, negotiates with the patient for additional evaluation and treatment (if indicated), arranges for additional help, and monitors the progress of the recommendations.

At the second tier, the clinician accepts some responsibility for treatment after negotiating a treatment plan with the patient. The physician may manage acute withdrawal, deal with some of the complications of abuse, involve the family in the plan (if indicated), refer to self-help groups, and support patient efforts toward abstinence.

At the third tier, the clinician accepts clinical responsibility for the treatment of the patient for as long as is needed (clinician involvement at this level is usually taken by a specialist, such as a psychiatrist, but is within the capability of the primary care physician with adequate interest and knowledge).

All substance abuse treatments are improved when the physician remains involved. Treatment options for patients with ongoing support from the clinician include: (1) harm reduction versus abstinence; (2) physician treatment with or without medications; (3) 12-step programs; (4) substance abuse interventions; (5) referral to an outpatient substance abuse/mental health service for individual, group, or partial intensive outpatient treatment; and (6) referral for inpatient treatment.

Harm Reduction/Moderation

Harm reduction or moderation as a goal of treatment refers to reducing the amount of the substance used in order to eliminate or reduce complications. The rationale for harm reduction/moderation is that some patients either will not accept abstinence as a goal or have failed to become abstinent after repeated attempts. Harm reduction, while not the ultimate answer to substance abuse, allows some patients to have health benefits from moderation and can reduce health costs. A recent randomized and controlled study (Fleming, Barry, Manwell, & London, 1997) examined 64 physicians at 17 practice sites, along with 482 men and 292 women identified as problem drinkers. Primary care physicians gave half of these patients two 10- to 15-minute alcohol counseling/harm reduction sessions over 1 year, using a scripted workbook. The 12-month follow-up revealed that this harm reduction approach significantly reduced the amount of alcohol consumed, the amount of binge drinking, the frequency of excessive drinking, and decreased the length of hospitalization for men in the harm reduction group. At a clinical level, harm reduction may be the only reasonable immediate intervention possible for the group of substance abusers in the precontemplation or contemplation stages toward abstinence.

Harm reduction applies to other ways of reducing harm caused by substance use, such as substituting methadone for heroin or supplying clean needles to IV substance abusers. This form of harm reduction is controversial and is, consequently, a political, social, and medical issue.

Although it is an effective model for some problem drinkers, harm reduction/moderation may not work well for many patients. In the adolescent and young adult population, moderation still leads to short-term risks of intoxication-related injuries and automobile accidents. For other patients, harm reduction is merely a license to continue drinking. Sometimes, a clinician's commitment to abstinence can bring better results than harm reduction can. The difficulty at this time is that there are not yet good criteria for deciding who will benefit more from harm reduction versus efforts toward abstinence. Harm reduction as a treatment modality is described in chapter 16, Consulting and Counseling in Primary Care.

Abstinence

The decision to choose abstinence as a goal versus harm reduction needs to be negotiated with each patient. The clinician can pursue abstinence when this seems to be in the patient's best interest. Total abstinence in a normative drinker may eliminate a health benefit, as a small amount of daily alcohol (less than 2 oz per day) probably reduces the risk of coronary artery disease. On the other hand, abstinence from other substances of abuse may be desirable, because the risk of substance abuse greatly outweighs any potential benefits from use. A single ingestion of alcohol or drugs may impair alertness and be a factor in a fatal motor vehicle accident, or a small amount of alcohol/drugs may be responsible for hypertension or adversely affect fetal development. Long term, normative users of substances do not have absolute protection from progression to problematic use at times of severe stress. Since most adverse consequences of substance abuse are roughly related to dose and duration of use, abstinence is often the most helpful recommendation for problematic and dependent users.

In clinical practice, the goals of abstinence need to be negotiated between patient and physician. Most of the time, clinicians need to respect the patient's choice. The more the patient takes responsibility for abstinence, demonstrates self-efficacy, or arrives at a stage of change where he or she can ask for help, the better the treatment prognosis. Occasionally, however, a clinician might need to choose to end the professional relationship with the belief that continuing to watch severe substance abuse merely gives the patient license to continue self-destructive behavior. If this drastic measure is required, the clinician needs to explain to the patient the reason for terminating, send a formal termination letter, and make a new referral. In a few circumstances, the physician may decide to act unilaterally, without the consent of the patient (e.g., with minors or emergency situations in which substance abuse creates immediate life-threatening problems). Substance abuse emergencies in which involuntary commitment is undertaken include a medical condition that is life threatening to the patient (delirium) and situations in which substance abuse contributes to suicide risk or violence potential (see chapter 7, Violence and Suicide).

Physician Treatment With and Without Medications

Physicians treat mild or moderate substance abuse problems and can treat mild intoxication and withdrawal syndromes. After acute medical management of these states, the physician may also encourage and support the patient's efforts toward abstinence. Some patients (e.g., cigarette smokers or patients who mildly abuse other substances) may wish to quit on their own. The physician can educate the patient about cessation/minor withdrawal symptoms and schedule a follow-up office visit within 1 week of cessation. Patients who meet criteria for outpatient treatment with a clinician include those who demonstrate preparation stage activities (express a desire or determination to stop and make plans); mild substance abusers; those who have been successful in the past in reducing or discontinuing substance abuse without help; those with coexisting psychological and sociocultural problems whom the primary care clinician determines can be managed without treatment by a mental health specialist; patients who begin to investigate or participate in 12-step programs; patients who have support from family, friends, or employers; and patients whose living environment is not characterized by pressure to use substances.

12-Step Programs

The physician may support abstinence with the use of a 12-step self-help group, such as AA or NA (Narcotics Anonymous). AA and other 12-step groups, such as Cocaine Anonymous, work in a similar way. These self-help groups comprise people who refer to themselves as "alcoholics" and who are in remission or trying to become abstinent. AA defines alcoholism in the first of the 12 steps: "We admitted we were powerless over alcohol, that our lives had become unmanageable." The only requirement for AA membership is a desire to stop drinking.

AA members distinguish between abstinence and sobriety. Abstinence means not using alcohol and is seen as a bridge to sobriety. Sobriety, on the other hand, refers to major changes in the recovering person's approach to physical and mental health, social relations, family life, work, love, and spirituality. Through its 12-step program, AA provides a means to reach sobriety. The organization is based on psychological processes, including catharsis, imitative behavior, instillation of hope, interpersonal learning, and altruism. The best way for a physician to understand AA is to go to a few open meetings. Having attended several meetings will also give the clinician credibility when he or she recommends AA to a patient. It is helpful to have copies of AA meeting schedules available and knowledge of how to contact an AA sponsor. In addition, clinicians who are interested and capable might provide brief individual or family substance abuse treatment, utilizing treatment approaches described in chapters 16, 17, 18, and 19. If the clinician feels the patient needs additional support, he or she can refer to an outpatient or inpatient substance abuse and/or mental health specialist or substance abuse/mental health treatment services.

Substance Abuse "Intervention"

When a patient refuses to acknowledge the severity of a substance abuse, a clinician or the patient's family can organize an intervention. An intervention prevents serious long-term harm to a patient or deals with an acute/emergency situation. When organizing the intervention, the clinician or patient's family involves all of the most important people in the patient's life. The group plans a time to confront the patient with care and concern about the medical necessity for treatment. The group of concerned friends, family, and professionals offers the patient the option of getting treatment or losing his or her relationship with them. This powerful tool can be considered with substance abusers whose continued use poses a danger to themselves or others or whose ability to protect themselves is markedly impaired. The techniques of conducting a substance abuse intervention are based on crisis intervention principles described in chapter 17, Crisis Intervention in Office Practice, and family therapy principles described in chapter 18, Family Counseling.

Outpatient Substance Abuse/Mental Health Treatment

If the patient needs treatment by a substance abuse or mental health specialist, or if the clinician wants to refer a patient, a private referral can be made to a psychiatrist, clinical psychologist, social worker, or substance abuse counselor who is qualified to treat substance abusers without supervision. Patients who need a more structured program can be referred to a hospital or a freestanding substance abuse clinic that offers outpatient treatment programs, individual counseling, 12-step groups, and a network of sponsors to assist the patient in his or her abstinence efforts. Often, these outpatient treatment services are available in the evening, so that many patients are able to continue working while in treatment.

"Partial"/Intensive Outpatient Substance Abuse Treatment Programs

"Partial" programs are designed for people who have not been able to succeed in a less structured outpatient program. Often, patients undergoing outpatient detoxification may do so in an intensive program. Other patients who may benefit from intensive programs include patients with questionable motivation to remain substance free, patients who have previously relapsed after leaving an inpatient facility, patients who are returning to high-risk communities or families, and patients with "dual diagnoses" (substance abuse combined with significant psychiatric problems).

Inpatient Substance Abuse Treatment

Some patients may require inpatient treatment. The physician may hospitalize his or her own patient in a general hospital for acute treatment of intoxication, withdrawal, overdoses, or because of acute medical complications from substance use, such as gastritis, ulcers, liver failure, or HIV disease. Once the acute medical problems are resolved, the patient may be referred to outpatient treatment, an intensive partial program, or an inpatient substance abuse/psychiatric unit. Inpatient treatment should be considered for the following patients: those who have had substance overdoses, patients experiencing complicated or difficult withdrawal, patients who have failed treatment in less intensive settings, patients with marked coexisting psychiatric conditions, and patients whose substance use poses danger to themselves and/or others.

Pharmacological Treatment of Substance Abuse

Medication plays an important part in the management of acute intoxication, withdrawal syndromes, and the maintenance of abstinence. Although medication may be one of the most critical aspects of acute medical treatment, it should always be used in conjunction with a comprehensive psychosocial approach aimed at harm reduction or abstinence.

Acute Intoxication

The experience of acute intoxication and withdrawal is determined not only by physiological processes but by psychosocial processes, such as the setting in which the substance was ingested, the expectations of the person, the patient's psychosocial strengths and weaknesses, and the kind of social support provided.

The pharmacological approach to the treatment of acute intoxication is based on administering an antagonist to block access of the substance to its receptor site on the neuronal membrane. At the present time, only opiate and benzodiazepine intoxication is routinely treated with an antagonist. The intoxicating, analgesic, and reinforcing effects of opiate substances are mediated by their binding to specific opiate receptors on nerve cell membranes. The opiate antagonist naloxone binds to the same receptors blocking the opiate's effects. Naloxone is administered intravenously and promptly and completely reverses acute opiate intoxication. Naltrexone is a longer acting compound, which acts in a similar way. Flumazenil (Mazicon) is a specific benzodiazepine receptor antagonist that can reverse a benzodiazepine overdose when given intravenously (it does not work on sedative-hypnotic medications).

Acute intoxications are also managed by seclusion and restraint. If necessary, intramuscular injections of haloperidol (Haldol) or lorazepam (Ativan) may be used to calm a patient when circumstances suggest an acute danger of harm to a patient or others. Chapter 5, Psychiatric Symptoms Due to Medical Illness, and chapter 7, Violence and Suicide, provide specifics on acute pharmacological management of intoxicated states.

Withdrawal Syndromes

There are many effective medications that ameliorate withdrawal syndromes. Prevention of substance abuse withdrawal is based on administration of a drug, either the abused substance itself or a drug from the same pharmacological class, that is cross-tolerant (an agonist with the substance). A typical medication protocol involves administration of sufficient doses to suppress the acute withdrawal syndrome, often by a slight intoxication. The dose is gradually tapered to produce a milder, controlled, relatively asymptomatic withdrawal. Usually, long-acting medication provides built-in self-tapering effects. The amount of medication used to prevent withdrawal depends on the dose being abused, the characteristic half-life of the drug of abuse, the medication used to treat the withdrawal syndrome, and the patient's ability to metabolize both the drug and medication used to prevent withdrawal symptoms. Standard instruments that aid in quantifying signs and symptoms of withdrawal, such as the Clinical Institute Withdrawal Assessment Scale for Alcohol Revised (CIWA-AR Scale) (Sullivan, Sykora, & Schneiderman, 1989), can guide the physician toward optimal medication management. The physician needs to be alert to the possibility that more than one substance is being abused (polysubstance abuse) and that several medications may have to be used to prevent withdrawal symptoms from medications of different classes.

Alcohol/Benzodiazepines/ Sedative-Hypnotic Withdrawal

Benzodiazepines are the medications of choice for treatment of alcohol and benzodiazepine withdrawal, because they have a wide margin of safety. Long-acting benzodiazepines, such as chlordiazepoxide (Librium), diazepam (Valium), and clonazepam (Klonopin), tend to be favored, because of their long, slow, self-tapering effects. Short-acting benzodiazepines, like oxazepine (Serax) or lorazepam (Ativan), can be used when the patient has impaired liver function, because metabolism of these drugs does not depend on oxidation in the liver. Withdrawal from sedatives/hypnotics is usually accomplished either by the acute use of a short-acting barbiturate such as pentobarbital (Nembutal) followed by phenobarbital detoxification or by phenobarbital detoxification alone.

Opiates Withdrawal

Methadone, buprenorphine (Buprenx), and clonidine (Catapres) are used for opiate withdrawal or detoxification. Methadone, a cross-tolerant opiate agonist, is very effective in the treatment of withdrawal but promotes drug-seeking behavior itself. Clonidine is not a cross-tolerant opiate, but does reduce the intensity of certain symptoms, such as craving, tachycardia, diarrhea, and anxiety. Buprenorphine is a partial opiate agonist, which is used in patients who have failed detoxification with methadone or clonidine. Buprenorphine's advantage over methadone is that it is not widely abused.

Maintenance of Abstinence

The psychosocial focus of treatment for substance abuse is on long-term rehabilitation or relapse prevention. However, pharmacological treatment also has a place and follows three basic approaches:

- Substitution of the abused substance with a cross-tolerant drug (safer than the abused substance) can facilitate a decrease in drug-seeking behaviors. The most commonly used substitution treatments are methadone maintenance for opiate dependence and the nicotine patch or replacement for nicotine dependence.
- Use of an antagonist drug that blocks the psychoactive effect of the abused substance to facilitate abstinence. Treatment of opiate dependence and alcohol craving with the opiate antagonist naltrexone is common. Naltrexone blocks the pleasurable mood-altering effect of opiates and is the only drug that decreases alcohol craving.
- The use of a medication that makes the use of an abused substance aversive rather than rewarding. For example, disulfiram (Antabuse) for the treatment of alcohol abuse makes patients sick when they drink. This drug is the only approved drug that has this effect.

Methadone maintenance is an effective treatment for opiate abuse, particularly intravenous use of heroin, because of its high potency, long duration of action, oral administration, absence of side effects, and ability to block the high of heroin. Methadone can be orally administered once a day in a clinic where the patient can also receive counseling. The rationale for use is that dependence without the drug lifestyle—stealing, crime, and risk of intravenous use diseases (e.g., HIV and hepatitis)—is better than the life and risk of street drug use. Methadone is also used for patients who protect themselves from these complications but have demonstrated they cannot discontinue the use of opiates. People on methadone maintenance frequently show improved psychosocial functioning, including the ability to hold a job.

Naltrexone is used to prevent the opiate high and is effective in highly motivated people who will take the medication regularly. Naltrexone is also effective at reducing alcohol craving in patients who are no longer dependent on alcohol but wish to reduce the risk of relapse.

Nicotine substitution therapy, either by oral or transdermal patch, is used to ameliorate the symptoms of nicotine withdrawal in people attempting to discontinue tobacco use. Despite its superiority over placebos in studies, long-term (6- to 12-month) abstinence rates for nicotine tend to be low, particularly when this treatment is not used in conjunction with a cognitive/behavioral program.

Although controlled clinical trials have failed to demonstrate superiority of disulfiram over placebos for problem drinkers, there is a place for this treatment in well-motivated, stable patients who repeatedly relapse. The benefit of its use as part of a structured program is that the decision not to drink has to be made only once a day (at the time of taking the medication). Once the disulfiram is taken (because of its long duration of action), drinking within the next 5 to 7 days will result in the patient becoming physically sick and unable to drink anymore.

REFERENCES

American Psychiatric Association. (1994). *Diagnostic and statistical manual of mental disorders* (4th ed.). Washington, DC: Author.

Brown, R. L. (1992). Identification and office management of alcohol and drug disorders. In M. F. Fleming & K. L. Barry (Eds.), *Addictive disorders*, p. 28. St. Louis: Mosby Year Book.

Engel, G. L. (1980). The clinical application of the biopsychosocial model. *American Journal of Psychiatry* (May), 535–540.

Fleming, M. F., Barry, K. L., Manwell, K. J., & London, R. (1997). Brief physician advice for problem drinkers: A randomized controlled trial in community-based primary care practices. *Journal of the American Medical Association, 277*, 1039–1045.

Hyman, S. E., & Tesar, G. E. (1994). *Manual of psychiatric emergencies* (3rd ed.). Boston: Little, Brown.

Khantzian, E. J. (1985). The self-medication hypothesis of addictive disorders: Focus on heroin and cocaine dependence. *American Journal of Psychiatry, 142*, 1259–1264.

Mayo-Smith, M. F. (1997). Pharmacological management of alcohol withdrawal: A meta-analysis and evidence-based practice guideline. *Journal of the American Medical Association, 278*, 144–151.

Miller, W. R., & Rollnick, S. (1991). *Motivational interviewing*. New York: Guilford Press.

Saunder, J. B., Aasland, O. G., & Babor, T. F. (1993). The development of the Alcohol Use Disorders Identification Test (AUDIT): World Health Organization collaborative project on detection of persons with Alcohol Consumption II. *Addiction, 88*, 791–804.

Shader, R. I. (1994). *Manual of psychiatric therapeutics* (2nd ed.). Boston: Little, Brown.

Sullivan, J. T., Sykora, K., & Schneiderman, J. (1989). Assessment of alcohol withdrawal: The revised clinical institute withdrawal assessment for alcohol scale (CIWA-AR). *British Journal of Addiction, 84*, 1353–1357.

Vaillant, G. (1995). *The natural history of alcoholism revisited*. Cambridge, MA: Harvard University Press.

CHAPTER 5

Psychiatric Symptoms Due to Medical Illness

Robert E. Feinstein

Primary care physicians are in the unique position to perform comprehensive evaluation and brief treatment of patients suffering from psychiatric disorders that are due to a medical illness. These heterogeneous disorders result from abnormalities in brain functioning and are not considered to be psychiatric in origin. Patients suffering from these disorders typically present with psychiatric symptoms or behavioral disturbances that are closely subserved by neuroanatomic, neurophysiologic, and neurochemical structures or processes.

Current clinical or medical technology can detect these disorders. This chapter will present a practical, clinical approach to evaluation, differential diagnosis, management, and brief office-based treatment of psychiatric disorders/syndromes that are caused by medical illnesses.

CLASSIFICATION OF COGNITIVE DISORDERS AND PSYCHIATRIC DISORDERS DUE TO A GENERAL MEDICAL CONDITION

Medical conditions that produce psychiatric presentations or symptoms were previously called "organic mental syndromes/disorders." However, with the advent of *DSM-IV* (1994), these disorders have a new nomenclature that eliminates the word *organic*. For example, what the *DSM III-R* (1987), third edition revised listed as "organic mental syndromes" was newly designated in *DSM-IV*, as "delirium, dementia, amnestic disorders, and cognitive disorders not otherwise specified." The International Disease Classification IDC 10 (see *DSM-IV*, 1994, 'Appendix H') has retained the organic classification schema.

CLINICAL SYNDROMES/DISORDERS

Delirium

The cardinal derangement of delirium has been variously described as the clouding of consciousness, confusion, global cognitive impairment, disorientation with memory disturbances, or deficit in attentional focus that impairs the ability to acquire new information. Delirious patients are often sleepy or agitated and have abnormal sleep patterns and perception or language difficulties. The following serve as diagnostic criteria for delirium if these symptoms are not better accounted for by a preexisting, established, or evolving dementia (*DSM-IV, 1994*):

- Disturbance of consciousness (decreased awareness, reduced ability to focus or to sustain or shift attention)
- Changes in cognition (memory deficits, disorientation, language, or perceptual disturbance)
- Development over a short time period (a matter of hours or days)
- A history, physical examination, or laboratory test that suggests a general medical condition as the cause

Neuropsychiatrically, delirium is caused by a disease process that produces a dysfunction of the reticular activating system (RAS) at the brain stem level. *DSM-IV* (1994) fourth edition subclassifies deliriums as (1) delirium caused by a general medical condition, (2) substance-induced delirium, (3) delirium due to multiple etiologies, and (4) delirium not otherwise specified.

Most forms of delirium are clinically indistinguishable from each other. Although their etiologies are diverse, electroencephalogram (EEG) changes always accompany delirious states. Patients with an EEG showing diffuse alpha-wave slowing typically have a somnolent, anergic, retarded clinical presentation (Engel & Romano, 1959). Delirious patients who are clinically hyperactive, hyperaroused, or agitated display an EEG pattern of low-voltage, fast-activity theta waves. As a patient passes from delirium into coma, the EEG may progress to high-voltage delta activity in either a bilateral synchronous or random pattern. When using EEGs to diagnose delirium, a clinician needs to obtain two or more to improve the chances that the EEG will be recorded during a period of the patient's confusion and not during a normal period. It is often the comparison and differences between two different EEGs that confirm the diagnosis of delirium. Alternatively, newer computer-assisted EEGs have a large database for comparison, making a single EEG sufficient to conclusively make the diagnosis of delirium.

Deliriums can be etiologically classified as "urgent life-threatening delirium" or "immediate-attention delirium" (Wise & Brandt, 1992). Urgent, life-threatening deliriums are medical conditions that, if not rapidly diagnosed and treated, can result in irreversible brain damage within seconds to minutes. The most commonly seen are intracranial bleeds, subdural hematoma, hypertensive encephalopathy, bacterial or viral meningitis, decreased cerebral perfusion secondary to cardiac or lung failure, Wernicke's encephalopathy, delirium tremens, and acute barbiturate withdrawal.

Immediate-attention deliriums are medical conditions that require recognition and treatment within hours to days. They can also be subclassified according to the six basic causes of all diseases: (1) central nervous system/structural diseases, (2) infections, (3) metabolic/nutritional disorders, (4) neoplastic conditions, (5) autoimmune diseases, and (6) drug abuse/poisoning. Common immediate-attention deliriums are those caused by seizures, stroke, brain tumors, multiple sclerosis, HIV and other central nervous system (CNS) infections, fluid and electrolyte abnormalities, thyroid disorders, diabetes, vitamin deficiencies, systemic lupus erythematosus, and drug- or poison-induced deliriums.

Dementia

Clinical Presentation

The cardinal feature of dementia is a slow, progressive cognitive decline in the absence of delirium. Common initial symptoms may include memory lapses, such as poor name recall, forgetting to turn off the lights, or getting lost. Cognitive changes are typically insidious in onset and are therefore often first recognized by the patient's family, friends, or coworkers. Diagnostic criteria for dementia (*DSM-IV*, 1994) include:

- Multiple cognitive deficits: memory impairment, cognitive impairment (aphasia, apraxia, agnosia, defects in executive functions)
- Deficits that cause significant impairments or a decline in social/occupational functions
- Deficits not caused by delirium

Patients suffering with dementia may conceal or not wish to acknowledge any cognitive deficits or their own emotional or behavioral changes. They gradually reveal a cognitive decline, which may be manifested as an inability to calculate, difficulty in balancing a checkbook, or problems with word finding, spelling, or perseveration of speech. Some patients show an alteration or increased rigidity of their personality traits. For example, a neat woman becomes compulsively orderly. As the cognitive decline progresses, patients may appear apathetic, dull, or depressed. Those patients with severe frontal-lobe pathology may present with fluctuating labile moods, disinhibitions, or a loss of social graces, including lewdness. Some patients with early dementia develop new checking rituals, such as door-lock checking. Often, behavioral, affective, and personality changes herald increasing cognitive decline. Memory is eroded from an initial sporadic loss of recall, followed by short-term memory deficits. In general, intermediate and long-term memory remain intact until very late in the illness.

Severely demented patients are typically calm yet easily startled when suddenly disturbed. This can result in exaggerated emotional expressions or, occasionally, unpredictable behavior. At the end stages of dementia, memory and cognitive capacities may decline to complete disorientation and an inability to carry out activities of daily living. Many patients become bedbound.

Etiologies of Common Dementias

Dementias can be caused by primary diseases of the nervous system or by secondary involvement of the CNS from a systemic disease. They can be classified according to six etiologies: (1) CNS disease/structural damage, (2) infectious agents, (3) metabolic/nutritional disorders, (4) neoplastic diseases, (5) autoimmune diseases, and (6) drugs/poisons. The major causes of dementia are listed in Table 5.1. It is very important to determine, if possible, the specific etiology of the dementia so that treatment can be specific to the diagnosis. The characteristic features of some common dementias are described below.

Alzheimer's Disease

Clinical Presentation

Alzheimer's disease is typical of many dementias that have an insidious onset with a slow, steady downward progression in functioning (Cummings, 1992). It is of heterogeneous etiology, probably caused by at least seven possible mutations of the amyloid precursor on chromosome numbers 14, 19, and 21. Cognitive deficits in this illness may be caused by dysfunction of the cholinergic, muscarinic, or nicotinic receptors, and in women, by menopausal loss of estrogens. Histopathology shows senile plaques, neurofibrillary tangles, and/or cerebral atrophy in the association area with relative sparing of the motor, visual, and somatosensory cerebral cortex.

Epidemiology

Alzheimer's disease is the fourth most common cause of death in the United States, accounting for 100,000 deaths per year and representing approximately 50% of all the dementias. It afflicts approximately 1.5 million to 2 million people. The mean survival time from onset of the disease to death is approximately 7 years.

Risk Factors

The prevalence of Alzheimer's disease from age 70 onwards doubles every 5 years so that by the age of 90 years, the prevalence rate is almost 50%. A family history increases the risk of developing the disease threefold or fourfold. A history of head trauma, Down's syndrome, or a deficit of the E4 allele of apolipoprotein E predisposes to Alzheimer's disease

Treatment

There is no specifically effective treatment for this illness. Cholinesterase inhibitors (tacrine and donepezil), vitamin E, selegiline, ergoloid mesylates, and, in women, estrogen replacement are the best pharmacotherapeutic interventions available now or expected to be available in the near future. Psychosocial interventions are extremely helpful.

Table 5.1 Etiologies of Dementia

Structural CNS Diseases	**Infectious Diseases**
Alzheimer's type Vascular dementia (Multi-infarct dementia) Parkinson's disease Huntington's chorea Pick's disease Multiple sclerosis Progressive supra-nuclear palsy Normal pressure hydrocephalus Traumatic brain injury Concussions, subdurals Seizure disorders Amyotrophic lateral sclerosis (ALS) Cerebellum dementias Olivopontocerebellar atrophy Friedreich's ataxia	HIV dementia Jakob-Creutzfeldt disease Chronic tuberculous meningitis Tertiary syphilis Chronic cryptococcus meningitis Brain abscess Virus (herpes, rabies, etc.) Lyme disease (CNS)
Metabolic/Deficiency Diseases	**Neoplastic Diseases**
Hypothyroidism Hypocortisolism Hyper/hypoparathyroidism Hyperinsulinism Wernicke-Korsakoff syndrome Niacin deficiency Vitamin B12 deficiency Folic acid deficiency Wilson's disease	Primary malignant brain tumors (gliomas, astrocytomas, glioblastomas) Benign meningiomas Metastatic lung, breast, kidney, and GI cancer Metastatic melanoma
Autoimmune Diseases	**Drugs/Poisons**
Systemic lupus erythematosus Rheumatoid arthritis (rarely) Polyarteritis nodosa, etc.	Alcoholic dementia Glue-sniffing dementia Phencyclidine Heavy metals (lead, mercury, arsenic, thallium, etc.) Organophosphates (pesticides) Organic solvent (alcohols, glycols, hydrocarbons, ketones, etc.) Biological toxins

Vascular Dementia/Multi-Infarct Dementia

Clinical Presentation

Vascular dementia (VD) has the signs and symptoms of all dementias, but it often follows a stuttering course with stable deficits for years and a stepwise deterioration with new brain infarcts. The volume and location of cortical damage determines symptoms. All patients with greater than 100 ml loss of brain tissue will show cognitive deficits. Multi-infarct dementia is produced by the occlusion of small cerebral vessels, which leads to focal or lacunar strokes. Patients may have dementia with frontal release signs or focal neurological deficits. It is not uncommon to have a mixed VD and Alzheimer's disease picture. CAT scan or MRI can reveal infarcts.

Epidemiology

Vascular dementia is the second most common form of dementia, representing approximately 10% of all dementias. It typically presents at an earlier age than Alzheimer's disease and is more common in men than women.

Risk Factors

VD is associated with cardiovascular risk factors, such as hypertension, abnormal lipid profiles, and smoking.

Treatment

There is no specific treatment for this condition. Prevention can be geared toward controlling hypertension and other cardiovascular risk factors. Psychosocial interventions are a helpful part of the management strategy.

HIV Dementia

Clinical Presentation

HIV dementia includes primary dementia caused by direct HIV brain infection, dementia caused by the secondary effects of immune suppression, or dementia secondary to HIV drug treatment. All dementias associated with HIV disease appear clinically similar to other dementias. They can best be differentiated by medical and laboratory testing.

HIV dementias may occur when HIV directly infects the brain, shortly after a serum conversion to HIV positive. In the early course of HIV disease, subclinical meningoencephalitis can produce a mild delirium. Later in the course, HIV can produce a subcortical dementia through an autoimmune reaction.

The earliest symptoms of HIV dementia include memory loss, depressive symptoms, decreased flexibility in thinking, personality changes, or difficulty with complex actions. Secondary causes of HIV dementia are either side effects of drugs, such as AZT, used to treat HIV infection or opportunistic illnesses caused by immune-system suppression, including brain lymphomas, Kaposi's sarcoma, toxoplasmosis, cryptococcus, cytomegalovirus, and herpes.

Epidemiology

There are no specific prevalence rates for HIV dementia in the total AIDS population, although the number of cases of HIV dementia should continue to rise with the rising incidence of AIDS.

Risk Factors

Specific risk factors for HIV dementia as opposed to delirium are not known. Risk factors for HIV infection include exposure to the virus via blood-to-blood contact through sexual activity, blood transfusions, and needle sharing during drug use.

Treatment

Treatment is geared toward preventing infection, improving immune status via lifestyle changes, anti-HIV medications, and treatment of specific opportunistic diseases. Psychosocial interventions are helpful in the long-term management of this chronic disease.

Parkinson's Disease with Dementia/Depression

Clinical Presentation

Patients with Parkinson's disease present with signs of a pill-rolling tremor, rigidity, festination (accelerated gait), and bradykinesia (slow volitional movements). The autonomic dysfunction of the disease can produce postural hypotension, urinary or bowel dysfunction, temperature regulatory problems, and excessive salivation.

Parkinson's dementia presents as a subcortical dementia, and unlike Alzheimer's disease and vascular dementias, often manifests with memory loss and apathy but with a relative preservation of intellectual ability. Aphasia, agnosia, and apraxia are infrequently present. Although the rigidity and bradykinesia associated with the disease often gives those afflicted with it the appearance of having a severe dementia, the dementia is in fact typically mild. Parkinson's appears to be an acquired disease, with associated depression and dementia mediated through neurotransmitter effects.

Clinical Depression

Depression can be the first sign of Parkinson's disease and is thought to be caused by neurotransmitter changes resulting from the disease itself, not as a psychological reaction to having the illness. This depression is usually mild and presents with vegetative signs. Suicidal ideation is rare. It is often extremely difficult to discriminate the psychomotor retardation, slowed mentation, and decreased concentration of depression from the rigidity and bradykinesia of Parkinson's disease. Response to use of various medications can often help make this differentiation.

Epidemiology

Parkinson's disease has a prevalence rate of 200/100,000, with males and females equally affected. Onset occurs between the ages of 50 and 65. Approximately 20% of patients present with depression as the first sign of the illness, and approximately 33% may suffer with depression at some point during this illness. Parkinson's dementia occurs in approximately 25% of patients with the disease, usually during its end stages.

Risk Factors

In the United States, Whites have a greater risk of contracting Parkinson's disease than do Blacks, males greater than females, residents of northern latitudes greater than those of southern latitudes, and residents of rural areas greater than those of urban areas. These risk factors suggest some environmental causes for the disease, such as chemicals or drinking water. Genetic studies have suggested increased risk in relatives of Parkinson's disease victims and autosomal dominance with reduced penetrance in some families.

Treatment

Specific treatment of the movement disorder associated with Parkinson's disease involves use of drugs such as levodopa/carbidopa, amantadine, anticholinergics, and L-deprenyl. However, drug treatment of the movement disorder does not seem to affect the development, course, or progression of the disease to dementia. Drug treatment can in itself exacerbate or produce a depression or create a psychosis with paranoia or hallucinations. Depression associated with Parkinson's disease can be treated with antidepressant drugs or by changes in the movement-disorder drugs that may be producing the depression. There is no specific treatment for the dementia of Parkinson's.

Pseudodementia (Dpression) in the Elderly

Pseudodementia is a common variant of depression in the elderly and has clinical signs and symptoms that can sometimes be differentiated from dementia. Patients with pseudodementia typically highlight their deficits and actively seek help. They often complain bitterly or dramatically about an acute onset of symptoms, which may include a fluctuating depressive mood, a patchy memory loss, or fluctuating intellectual deficits. On formal mental status questioning, they often do not show consistent and reproducible brain deficits. Acute symptoms are often triggered by a loss in patients who also have a preexisting personality disorder. See chapter 3, Depression, for a comparison with the presentation of classic vegetative depression.

Amnestic Disorder

Amnestic disorder is a syndrome of immediate memory deficits that create an inability to acquire or learn new information. This disorder is often caused by structural brain damage, especially in the area of the mammillary bodies. Long-term memories and cognitive capacities are typically preserved. *DSM-IV* (1994) subclassifies amnestic disorder as (1) amnestic disorder due to a general medical condition, (2) substance-induced amnestic disorder, and (3) amnestic disorder not otherwise specified. Amnestic disorder is common in special populations, such as in head trauma victims or in those patients suffering with thiamine deficiency. *DSM-IV* criteria for amnestic disorder are as follows:

- Memory impairment manifested by an inability to learn new information and an inability to recall previously learned knowledge
- Memory deficits that cause significant impairment in social or occupational functioning
- Disturbance that does not occur exclusively during the course of delirium or dementia
- Memory impairment cased by a general medical condition

Traumatic Brain Injury

Traumatic brain injury is a common structural CNS cause of amnestic disorder. The leading causes are head trauma from motorcycle/motor vehicle accidents, falls, or violence. These traumatic brain injuries are typically coup/contra coup lesions (e.g., posterior head injury produces traumatic injury to the frontal/temporal lobes). Structural anatomic damage to deep brain structures, especially the amygdala, produces the immediate memory deficit.

Epidemiology

In the United States, automobile accidents are the most common cause of death in people under the age of 35. Approximately 70% of automobile deaths are from head trauma. The incidence of traumatic brain injury is 370/100,000; however, the incidence of amnestic disorder in head trauma patients has not been reported.

Risk Factors

In patients who have amnestic disorder, 50% of cases result from motor vehicle accidents, 21% from falls, 12% from violence, 10% from sports and recreational head trauma, and 7% from other injuries.

Treatment

When possible, surgery is recommended. Otherwise the patient should receive supportive, medical/rehabilitative, and psychosocial care.

Thiamine Deficiency

Thiamine deficiency can also cause an amnestic syndrome, which is sometimes referred to as Korsakoff's disease or substance-induced, persisting amnestic disorder. It is a short-term memory deficit disorder produced by alcohol-related thiamine deficiency, which produces CNS mammillary body damage.

Epidemiology

Thiamine deficiency produces memory deficits in approximately 3% of alcoholics. Amnestic memory deficits often occur as a sequelae of the neurologic presentation called Wernicke's encephalopathy. Patients who present with the Wernicke's triad of ophthalmoplegia, ataxia, and nystagmus have a 17% mortality rate.

Risk Factors

Alcoholism, poor nutrition, and head trauma increase the risk of this memory disturbance.

Treatment

Wernicke's encephalopathy and Korsakoff's disease can often be prevented by early treatment of this vitamin deficiency disease with thiamine 100 mg, followed by an oral daily dose of 100 mg for 3 to 7 days.

Other causes of amnestic disorder include structural damage to the central nervous system from partial complex seizures or Alzheimer's disease, infections such as herpes encephalitis, neoplastic conditions affecting the deep brain memory structures, drugs such as phencyclidine, and autoimmune vasculitis affecting the posterior cerebral artery.

Psychiatric Disorders Due to a General Medical Condition

Certain medical conditions can give rise to psychiatric symptoms. These medical conditions can be clinically indistinguishable from their psychiatric counterparts. Differentiation between a medical condition causing psychiatric symptoms and a psychiatric illness can only be confirmed by laboratory testing or other special diagnostic tests such as a CAT scan. Medical conditions can sometimes produce psychotic disorders, mood disorders, anxiety disorders, and personality changes. The general *DSM- IV* criteria applicable to psychiatric disorders due to a general medical condition are as follows:

- Manifests with psychiatric signs and symptoms
- Shows evidence from medical history, physical examination, or laboratory tests of a medical condition judged to be etiologically related to the psychiatric signs and symptoms
- Does not occur with delirium and is generally excluded if dementia is present
- Is not better accounted for by another mental syndrome
- May cause significant distress or impairment in social or occupational functioning

Psychotic Disorders Due to a General Medical Condition

Patients with certain medical conditions can suffer from psychotic disorders that manifest themselves as delusions, hallucinations, or other schizophreniform symptoms, such as loose associations or bizarre affects. These schizophrenic-like illnesses can be diagnosed only in the absence of a delirium or dementia. To make the diagnosis, a specific medical etiology for the psychosis has to be suspected or determined. Patients can present with paranoia, delusions, isolated hallucinations, or with a mixed picture. The most common medical causes are substance-induced psychotic disorders, seizures, and brain lesions to the posterior nondominant cerebral hemisphere. The most common medical causes of hallucinations are alcoholic hallucinosis and sensory-deprivation-release hallucinations. Less common causes include systemic lupus cerebritis, multiple sclerosis, Alzheimer's disease, vitamin B12 deficiency, and porphyria.

Substance-Induced Psychotic Disorders

Substance-induced psychotic disorders are caused by stimulants such as cocaine, amphetamines, and phencyclidine. These drugs can commonly produce an acute psychosis that can be clinically indistinguishable from acute paranoid schizophrenia. Standard treatment for drug-induced psychosis is supportive care and/or neuroleptics, such as haloperidol. Chronic high-dose stimulant abuse from "crack" cocaine may produce a brain-kindling phenomenon, which presents as a persistent chronic psychosis and is caused by subclinical brain damage. Anticonvulsant treatment of stimulant psychosis may be superior to traditional neuroleptic treatment.

Partial-Complex Seizures and Psychoses

Partial-complex seizures and psychoses are caused by focal cerebral firings leading to automatisms, altered consciousness, flashbacks, and déjà vu and often present with a clear sensorium. When psychotic, patients with partial-complex seizures may have symptoms of paranoia, grandiosity, and systematized delusions that cannot be distinguished from schizophrenia except by EEG. Psychotic symptoms can appear between seizure episodes. Focal seizure activity can produce olfactory hallucinations or visual/perceptual changes that can distort the shape or size of images. Partial-complex or focal seizures are 90% temporal lobe and 10% frontal lobe in origin and are more common when the seizure foci are bilateral in the temporal lobes. To eliminate hallucinations, patients often require combination treatment with anticonvulsants and neuroleptics.

Hallucinosis

Hallucinosis is persecutory, auditory, and/or visual hallucinations that appear in the presence of a clear sensorium. It is most commonly caused by acute withdrawal from alcohol, benzodiazepines, or barbiturates. Hallucinosis can appear 6 to 24 hours after the cessation of heavy use of these substances and usually remits in a matter of days.

Alcohol hallucinosis is common in patients who have been drinking continuously for more than 5 years. Hallucinations can be treated acutely with neuroleptics, such as haloperidol. Some chronic alcoholics develop persistent alcohol-induced auditory hallucinations, which can be readily confused with schizophrenia. Chronic hallucinations can last for more than 6 months after the cessation of heavy drinking; most hallucinations gradually resolve.

Sensory Deprivation Hallucinations

These hallucinations may occur in patients who are living in sensory-deprived environments, such as an intensive care unit or solitary confinement. Diseases such as cataracts and otosclerosis can also radically reduce visual and auditory sensory input and thus can also cause sensory deprivation hallucinations. The treatment of choice is to restore sensory input.

Mood Disorders Due to a General Medical Condition

DSM-IV (1994) classifies mood disorders due to a general medical condition as (1) having manic episodes or features, (2) having major depressive episodes or features, or (3) having mixed features. Patients suffering from the vast majority of mood disorders caused by a general medical condition present with depressive symptoms. Commonly reported symptoms are a sad mood, feelings of hopelessness and helplessness, crying, sleep disturbances, and suicidal thoughts. Manic symptoms such as euphoria, talkativeness, irritability, increased energy, and grandiose plans or assertions are also common. Mixtures of depressed and manic symptoms are frequently present.

Medically induced mood disorders often go unrecognized because they can be mild or iatrogenically induced. The leading medical causes of depression are the endocrinopathies and drugs. Antidepressant medications and steroids can cause mania.

Endocrine disorders often present with mood or anxiety syndromes. Often, the hyper/hypo states have similar neuropsychiatric symptoms but can be distinguished by their different physical signs and symptoms.

Hyperthyroidism

Hyperthyroidism typically presents with fatigue, weight loss, sweating, heat intolerance, scant menstruation, tachycardia, tremor, and bulging eyes (proptosis). Frequent neuropsychiatric manifestations are insomnia, crying episodes that are easily confused with depression, and anxiety symptoms. The most common causes of hyperthyroidism are Graves' disease, inflammatory thyroiditis, excessive thyroid hormone replacement therapy, and, rarely, thyroid or ovarian cancers. The diagnosis is made clinically and confirmed by thyroid function tests and Thyroid Stimulating Hormone (TSH) levels. Antithyroid hormone treatment is recommended.

Hypothyroidism

Hypothyroidism often presents with fatigue, weight gain, constipation, cold intolerance, menorrhagia, goiter, reflex delay, and myxedema (dryness, hair loss, edema, hoarseness, and muscle weakness). Patients with mild cases of hypothyroidism may present with depression, suicidal ideation, or psychosis. When the disease is long-standing, it commonly presents as dementia. Hypothyroidism is often caused by overzealous treatment of hyperthyroidism with surgery or radiation, autoimmune thyroid disease, or pituitary or hypothalamic disease. It is sometimes a side effect of lithium treatment. Hypothyroidism can be confirmed by abnormally low readings from thyroid function tests and high TSH levels. Treatment with thyroid hormone replacement is indicated.

Drug-induced Mood Disorders From Prescribed Medication

Prescribed medications can sometimes produce depressive or manic symptoms, particularly in individuals who have a predisposition toward affective illness. The most common offenders producing depression are antihypertensive drugs: (1) CNS antihypertensives (e.g., methyldopa), (2) beta blockers (e.g., propranolol), (3) adrenergic stimulants (e.g., clonidine), (4) diuretics (e.g., hydrochlorothiazide or furosemide, although these are less likely to cause depressive symptoms), (5) peripheral-acting drugs (e.g., prazosin or terazosin hydrochloride and calcium channel blockers; of these, verapamil or nifedipine are the least likely to cause depression), and (6) angiotensin converting enzyme (ACE) inhibitors (captopril or benazepril probably do not cause depression). Other drugs that may produce depression are cimetidine, disulfiram, and steroids when they are being tapered. Drugs that may produce mania as a side effect include antidepressants, monamine oxidase inhibitors, stimulants, and baclofen.

Substance Abuse Mood Disorders

Patients with alcohol, opioid, phencyclidine, sedative, or hypnotic intoxication or in withdrawal states from stimulants or alcohol may present with depressive symptoms. It is common for patients acutely intoxicated with stimulants such as cocaine, amphetamines, methylphenidate, or such appetite suppressants as phenmetrazine or diethylpropion to present with manic symptoms. Additional drugs that can produce manic features during intoxication include phencyclidine, marijuana, hallucinogens, caffeine, inhalants, alcohol, anabolic steroids, and corticosteroids.

Anxiety Disorders Due to a General Medical Condition

Patients with anxiety disorders that result from a medical condition may present with generalized anxiety, panic attacks, social or other phobias, or agoraphobic symptoms. Obsessive-compulsive symptoms also may be seen in association with medical conditions and include repetitive worries, fears of diseases, and compulsive behaviors such as excessive hand washing. Following is a review of the most common.

Cardiac conditions, such as myocardial infarction and arrhythmias, can produce chest pain, shortness of breath, diaphoresis, and palpitations, all of which are easily confused with panic/anxiety. Crushing chest pain or pain radiating to the jaw or neck is typical in cardiac patients and is rarely described by patients having a panic attack. Panic patients often describe palpitations, chest discomfort, and sweating. Ultimately, an electrocardiogram and cardiac enzymes are definitive in this differential diagnosis. There is a controversial link between mitral valve prolapse and panic disorder.

Drug-induced anxiety disorders are caused by excessive caffeine intake and nicotine withdrawal.

Caffeine consumption of two to three cups of coffee per day can produce caffeine intoxication and symptoms of an anxiety disorder. Psychiatric symptoms include anxiety, panic, and, occasionally, depression. Physical symptoms include insomnia, tremor, restlessness, abdominal pain, increased heart rate, palpitations, and a flushed face. This disorder is easily treated by tapering caffeine consumption. Abrupt cessation is not recommended, as it can lead to fatigue, decreased attention span, irritability, and caffeine-withdrawal headaches.

Nicotine withdrawal produces a craving accompanied by psychiatric symptoms of a generalized anxiety disorder with complaints of nervousness, irritability, restlessness, frustration, poor concentration, and poor cognitive performance. Physical symptoms of withdrawal may include headaches, sleep disturbances, increased appetite, and weight gain. Tapering cigarette consumption or use of nicotine replacement medications can prevent nicotine withdrawal symptoms.

Cocaine intoxication or withdrawal, marijuana abuse, and alcohol and opiate withdrawal are common causes for substance-induced general anxiety and panic disorder. Chronic high-dose cocaine and stimulant abuse can produce an obsessive desire for sex and compulsive masturbation. Prolonged cocaine abuse can lead to physiologic impotence.

Pheochromocytoma is a catecholamine-secreting tumor of the adrenal medulla or other abdominal paraganglionic sites that can produce panic symptoms and, rarely, agoraphobia. Physical signs and symptoms include malignant hypertensive episodes, headaches, and/or severe abdominal, back, or pelvic pain. This disorder is diagnosed by testing a 24-hour urine specimen for high levels of catecholamines. Surgical treatment usually is required for removal of the tumor.

Personality Change Due to a General Medical Condition

Medical conditions can cause an exaggeration of existing personality traits or can lead to the development of a different personality style. For example, a shy person may become a recluse. A medical condition can cause a profound alteration in thinking, emotional expression, or behavior. When intellectual decline accompanies a personality change, the diagnosis should be dementia. The presence of delirium excludes the personality change diagnosis. Approximately 90% of patients with frontal lobe pathology have personality changes, which present as three commonly described frontal lobe syndromes: disinhibited (pseudo-antisocial), apathetic (pseudodepressed), and akinetic (pseudopsychomotor-retarded depression). More diffusely located brain pathology causes labile, aggressive, and paranoid personality changes. Medical disorders that commonly cause personality changes include multiple sclerosis, brain tumors, traumatic brain injury, drugs (phencyclidine, glue sniffing, lead poisoning) and partial complex seizures. *DSM-IV* lists specific types of personality changes.

Personality change from partial-complex seizures is characterized by a deepening of emotions and a preoccupation with moral or religious issues. The interictal personality change appears as a viscous communication style that is tedious, didactic, verbose, and circumstantial; men also report a decreased libido, whereas women may report an increase. The personality change is not caused by the seizure itself but rather the progression of the brain lesion(s) that produced the seizure disorder. Whether the personality changes are caused by all seizures or just partial-complex seizures is controversial.

THE INTERVIEW

Patients with psychiatric symptoms caused by a general medical condition are all suffering from some brain deficit. The manifestations of this deficit may be as subtle as inattention, poor concentration, a comprehension problem, or a minor memory deficit, or as obvious as fluctuating levels of consciousness, impairments in speech, hearing, and vision, or an intellectual decline. When evaluating patients with brain deficits, sensitivity and a willingness to modify the typical interviewing style are important. Table 5.2 provides a brief overview of interviewing techniques for this patient population.

Family interviews can be especially helpful when assessing the effects of a support system on a neuropsychiatric patient. These interviews follow the same basic pattern described in Table 5.2 but should be expanded to include observation of interactions between the patient and different family members. Does the family understand the patient's illness? Does the

Table 5.2 Interviewing Tips: 10 Steps

1. Adjust your interview style to account for the patient's deficits so the patient can see, hear, touch, and learn from you.
2. Be aware of common clinician countertransference, as the patient may appear brain damaged. The clinician's feelings of hopelessness can lead to pessimism about treatment, a decrease in appropriate referral, or an inability to consider alternative therapies.
3. Maintain a calm environment, privacy, and confidentiality.
4. Begin the interview with open-ended questions to establish rapport and observe the patient's deficits.
5. Move the interview to close-ended questions to assist the patient with difficult answers or to gather vital information quickly.
6. Help modulate the patient's anxiety. Avoid long silences.
7. Bolster the patient's self-esteem with realistic reassurance. Be sensitive to the patient's shame over his or her deficits.
8. Avoid catastrophic reactions by minimizing the test atmosphere. Tell the patient he or she cannot fail a mental status examination.
9. Try to develop a biopsychosocial differential diagnosis.
10. Interview the patient's family for information to assess members' emotional state and ability to assist in the patient's treatment.

patient highlight or conceal his or her deficits in the presence of the family? Can the husband, wife, and children help the identified patient and/or each other? Are some family members frightened, whereas others are good observers who are capable of helping? Does the family fight in nonhelpful ways? The physician can incorporate the family into the patient's medical care if the family is interested, available, and competent to help the patient. When families are overwhelmed, they may need the outside support of a professional, agency, hospital, or other social institution.

MEDICAL AND PSYCHIATRIC EXAMINATION

A comprehensive examination of a patient includes a history, a focal review of systems, observation of vital signs, detailed neurological and physical examinations, mental status/neuro-behavioral evaluation, and laboratory testing. Using this office-based approach, the physician can diagnose the vast majority of general medical conditions that manifest as psychiatric symptoms. Frequently, the causes can be determined and treatment initiated.

History

It is vital to elicit a detailed medical history from both the identified patient and the family. The medical history should include risk factors, mode of onset, the duration of the signs and symptoms, their progression, and an assessment of the patient's typical baseline level of functioning. It should also include a detailed psychological and social history, with special emphasis on the current living situation. This initial history should be geared toward the first step in differential diagnosis: determining whether the patient has a medical/neurological brain illness with psychiatric symptoms or is suffering from a psychiatric condition.

To make this first step in diagnosis, physicians should look for four clinical features: age of onset, acute onset of symptoms, new psychiatric symptoms without a prior psychiatric history, and drug-use history.

Age of Onset

Patients over 40 who present with new psychiatric symptoms should be suspected of having a general medical illness. Most psychiatric illnesses, such as schizophrenia, bipolar disorder, anxiety, and somatoform disorders, typically present before the age of 40. In addition, most medical conditions such as Alzheimer's disease, Vascular dementia, and Parkinson's disease typically present in an older age group. There are some exceptions to this general rule. For example, HIV dementia commonly presents in patients under 40, and new-onset depression is common in patients over 40.

Acute Onset of Symptoms

Acute onset of a brain illness, within hours to days, is a medical condition until proven otherwise. Brain deficits caused by anatomic disruptions will generally result in acute signs and symptoms. On the other hand, almost all the major psychiatric illnesses follow an insidious onset over weeks, months, or years. There are exceptions to this general principle. For example, patients with Alzheimer's disease present with a slow onset, whereas a brief reactive psychosis and a dissociative state may manifest acutely after a catastrophic psychological trauma.

New Psychiatric Symptoms Without a Prior Psychiatric History

New psychiatric symptoms in a patient with no prior psychiatric history should prompt an evaluation for a general medical condition. New symptoms include disturbances in thinking, affect, or behavior, or subtle neurological symptoms, such as tremors or tics. Although comprehensive medical evaluations are expensive and often prove negative, the expense of these evaluations may be justified to avoid the dire consequences of incorrectly prescribing a psychiatric or social treatment when a general medical condition is causing the psychiatric symptoms. Many psychiatrists recommend a complete medical/neurological evaluation for patients who are newly diagnosed with a major psychiatric illness. The medical evaluation includes a physical examination, blood work, CAT scan, MRI, EEG, lumbar puncture, or other sophisticated laboratory testing as indicated.

Drug Abuse

Drug abuse is probably the most common medical condition that causes psychiatric symptoms. In evaluating a patient with psychiatric symptoms, the physician must review all drugs of abuse, over-the-counter preparations, and physician-prescribed medications that the patient is using. The frequency of drug ingestion, typical daily doses, and the time of the last ingestion of each drug are helpful in developing management strategies.

Drugs are the great imitators of psychiatric illness, producing a wide array of deliriums and a myriad of syndromes that can be indistinguishable from psychiatric disorders. For example, cocaine-induced panic attacks or mania are indistinguishable from panic disorder or bipolar illness unrelated to drug-use history. The family of a suspected drug user can often provide the information necessary to confirm the diagnosis. Urine drug screens are helpful but can be misleading. For example, a negative drug screen will not rule out drug withdrawal, nor does it mean that a patient has not abused drugs. Incorrect labeling of a substance abuse disorder as a psychiatric condition readily leads to prescribing a misdirected management and treatment strategy for the patient.

Review of Systems: Medical, Neurological, and Physical Examination

A neurological review of systems as well as a focal review of other systems related to the patient's psychiatric complaints can aid in differential diagnosis. For example, panic should elicit a review of cardiac systems, and delirium should elicit a metabolic review. The measurement of vital signs often provides the earliest objective evidence for a known medical condition and can offer important clues. A detailed neurological examination should also be performed. The focal neurological examination should be completed, progressing to soft neurological and frontal release signs. Soft neurological signs include left/right confusion, mixed dominance, drift, overflow, incoordination, and learning disabilities. Frontal release signs suggestive of pyramidal tract disease suggest dementia. Frontal release signs include myoclonus, Babinski's sign, grasp reflex, root reflex, Hoffman's sign, palm-chin reflex, and blinking in response to a glabellar tap. A complete physical examination should also be performed to investigate other complaints.

Mental Status Testing

A formal mental status examination to differentiate psychiatric disorder from a general medical condition should be performed on all patients who show any changes in behavior, thinking, or affect. Mental status testing for nonpsychiatric brain deficits includes assessment of the level of consciousness, orientation, memory, and general cognitive functioning and specialized bedside testing, such as a set test or clock test. See Table 5.3 for details of mental status testing. Standardized and scored mental status tests can also be used to detect psychiatric disorders arising from a general medical condition. Folstein's Mini-Mental State Examination Scale is one commonly used option (Folstein, Folstein, & McHugh, 1975). Other more complicated research scales are the Brief Cognitive Rating Scale, Alzheimer's Disease Assessment Scale, and the Wechsler Adult Intelligence Scale.

Neurobehavioral Assessment

If there are abnormal findings on the clinical mental status examination, a clinician can attempt to localize the deficit using a simple neurobehavioral assessment (Smith & Craft, 1984). The three neurobehavioral brain axes are the vertical axis (brainstem, subcortical to cortical structures), lateral axis (hemispheric localization), and horizontal axis (divided by the rolandic fissure).

The vertical brain axis runs from the brainstem, to subcortical structures, to cortical structures. The basic function of the vertical axis is

Table 5.3 Checklist for Assessing Mental Status for Nonpsychiatric Brain Deficits

LEVEL OF CONSCIOUSNESS

Fluctuations in consciousness? Alert and awake? Can the patient sustain attention, focus, and process and/or acquire new information?

ORIENTATION

Time: Date, time of day, day of week, month, year, season.

Place: Institution, city, state, country, continent.

Person: Do you know who you are? Your name?

If the disorder is organic, the patient will tend to lose time orientation first, place orientation second, and person orientation last.

MEMORY

Immediate recall: Recall the physician's name or a 7-number digit span.

Short term memory : Repeat names of 3 objects. Recall at 5 min. (auditory testing).

- If recall is <3/3 at 5 min., ask for recognition memory. Give a new list of 3 objects. Ask the patient to select the forgotten item(s) from the new list.

Follow-up short term memory testing:

- Repeat & show 3 objects; recall at 5 min. (auditory & visual input).
- Repeat, show, touch 3 objects; recall at 5 min.(auditory, visual, & tactile input).
- If the patient continues to have memory deficits with this testing, the likelihood of an organic problem increases.

Intermediate memory: Current events or yesterday's weather.

Long-term memory: Past presidents from present on backwards. Ask for birth date, home address, and phone, only if this information can be objectively verified.

- If organic, the patient will tend to lose memory in the sequence of immediate or short term recall first, intermediate next, long term last.

COGNITIVE FUNCTION

Determine educational level and begin with simple math (addition, subtraction, multiplication, or division) to lower anxiety and build the patient's confidence. Alternatively, use money calculations or spell "world" backwards.

SPECIALIZED BEDSIDE TESTING

Clock test:† Clock drawing, setting, and reading

- Clock drawing: Draw a clock indicating all numbers in the correct locations.
- Clock setting: Draw clocks with hands at 1:00, 11:10, 3:00, 9:15, and 7:30.
- Clock reading: Read the time on several different clocks (use times above).
- Deficits on two or more componets is 93% accurate at differentiating Alzheimer's from normal elderly.

Word intrusion test:* 3 sets of 10 objects: Name 10 foods, 10 cities, 10 colors.

- Scoring: >25/30 = normal: 15–25/30 = equivocal: >15/ 30 = abnormal.
- A word intrusion is mixing categories, e.g., while naming 10 cities, food and colors are mixed in with the city list. Scores >15/30 with intrusions increase the likelihood of Alzheimer's by 10–20%.
- Scores >15/30 with no intrusions suggests a non-Alzheimer's dementia.

†From: Tuokko, H., Hadjistavropoulos, T., Miller, J. A. (1992). The clock test: A sensitive measure to differentiate normal elderly from those with Alzheimer's disease. *Journal of the American Geriatrics Society, 40*, 579–584.

*From: P. A. Fuld, (1983). Word intrusion as a diagnostic sign in Alzheimer's disease. *Geriatric Medicine Today, 2*, 33–41.

arousal, short-term memory, attention, and the ability to process new information. The reticular activating system controls these functions and can be alerting; fluctuating, which appears as a delirium; or barely functioning, which may appear clinically as semicoma. Deficits in vertical axis functioning may appear as fluctuating levels of consciousness, inattention, disorientation, memory deficits, and delay in speed and flexibility of cognitive tasks.

Lateral brain axis refers to the functioning of the dominant/nondominant cerebral hemispheres. The dominant cerebral hemisphere primarily controls language and is the left brain cortex in 97% of right-handed and 50% of left-handed patients. Hemispheric function can be screened by naming, repeating, and performing a bidirectional complex action across the hemispheric midline. If a patient can name an object (e.g., ask the patient to name a pen from your pocket), then Broca's area is grossly intact. If a patient can repeat a simple phrase, read, write, and do simple math, then Wernicke's area is intact. A complex action across the midline indicates that interhemispheric connections are intact. Deficits in dominant hemispheric functioning may appear as disturbances in language and comprehension.

Nondominant hemispheric function is responsible for spatial relations and pattern recognition and awareness of the contralateral side of the body. Deficits in spatial relations can be elicited by having a patient copy a square, triangle, or other geometric shape. Pattern recognition can be tested by having the patient recognize the faces of famous people from magazines, by tapping out the beat of a tune with one's hand, or by drawing a clock. Deficits in nondominant hemispheric functions may also appear as neglect of the contralateral side of the body.

The horizontal axis refers to an arbitrary division of the cortex, with the rolandic fissure as a dividing line. Deficits of structures anterior to this fissure may manifest themselves as frontal release signs; frontal lobe syndrome with distortions in affects, thoughts, or behaviors; or problems in planning or organization. The clinician can screen for organizational ability by asking a patient to describe how to plan a party. Deficits in structures posterior to this fissure (parietal and occipital cortex) often present with intellectual decline as manifested by problems in reading, writing, and comprehension. Visual field testing can also elicit postrolandic deficits and visual field deficits.

Laboratory Testing

Table 5.4 reviews laboratory screening tests that may help diagnose a general medical condition producing psychiatric symptoms. Specialized technological testing should be reserved to confirm unusual presentations.

Differential Diagnosis

There are three important levels of differential diagnosis in evaluating psychiatric symptoms due to general medical conditions.

- Level 1 diagnosis helps differentiate psychiatric symptoms due to medical conditions from psychiatric disorders.
- Level 2 diagnosis is the classification by syndrome such as delirium, dementia, amnestic disorder, and other cognitive disorders; psychotic, mood, and anxiety disorders; personality changes due to a general medical condition; or substance-induced psychiatric symptoms.
- Level 3 diagnosis is determination of the specific etiology of the medical condition that is producing psychiatric symptoms. The etiologic diagnosis is the most important for selecting a specific medical treatment.

TREATMENT

The treatment of psychiatric symptoms due to a general medical condition begins with the diagnosis of the medical condition that is responsible for producing the psychiatric disorder. Helping a patient involves the integration of diagnosis and treatment of the medical and psychiatric conditions. Medical treatments routinely involve the use of medications and surgery or other health-promoting measures, such as improvement in diet and sleep, increased exercise, reduced stress, smoking cessation, and weight reduction.

The biopsychosocial treatment of patients with medical brain deficits is often neglected. Clinicians may incompletely treat these disorders due to their countertransference which leaves them unduly pessimistic about a patient's capacity to benefit from psychiatric treatment. Realistically, brain damage may not be curable, but psychiatric treatment can often restore the

Table 5.4 Diagnostic Medical Testing

Routine Laboratory Testing
Complete Blood Count with differential.
Electrolytes: Na, Cl, K, HC03, Ca, Mg.
Glucose and or albumin.
Bun/creatinine.
Liver function tests.
Thyroid function tests.
Erythrocyte sedimentation rate.
Venereal Disease Research Laboratory Test (VDRL).
Urinalysis.
Arterial blood gas.
Specialized Laboratory Testing
EKG or chest X-rays as indicated.
Lumbar puncture.
Immunological testing: ANA, RF, HIV, CD4.
Hormonal levels.
Drug or toxicological screening.
Viral titers (e.g., Lyme disease and herpes).
Vitamin levels.
Ceruloplasmin.
Other.
Technological Testing
Serial EEGs or computer-assisted EEGs.
CAT scan.
MRI scan.
PET scan/SPECT scan if available or indicated.

patient to optimal brain functioning and improve quality of life. The major forms of treatment available include psychotherapy, behavioral treatment, family therapy, and psychopharmacological management.

Psychotherapy

Supportive psychotherapy (Forrest, 1987) is designed to create a therapeutic relationship geared toward understanding the patient's deficits and improving the patient's adaptation to his or her illness. This can be accomplished by offering a caring, emotionally supportive, and safe environment in which a patient can talk about his or her deficits, feelings, stresses, and attempts at adaptation. The clinician can answer a patient's questions, discuss the patient's realistic capacities and limitations, and plan specific interventions. The clinician also can help mobilize medical support services, help a patient recognize marital stresses and financial concerns, and uncover other problems of daily living. These efforts will often improve the patient's functioning and decrease his or her vulnerability.

While conducting supportive psychotherapy, it is important to recognize that a patient's brain deficits may require specific adaptations in psychiatric techniques. For example, a clinician can improve a patient's brain-based inattention by eliminating all sensory distractions from the office and by speaking with clear, evocative language and simple syntax. A clinician can also encourage a patient by praising any efforts the patient makes toward recovery or adaptation to illness.

Supportive psychotherapy can be further improved if the clinician is able to differentiate brain/cortical deficits from psychological defense mechanisms. For example, a neurological/cortical deficit such as neglect can easily be misinterpreted as psychological denial. Pathological neurocortical defenses are better treated with education or environmental manipulation. Psychological denial can be treated via an exploratory or interpretative approach.

Behavioral Treatments

The traditional behavioral approach to psychosocial disorders looks at the sequence of events leading to a specific maladaptive behavior and the consequences of that behavior. Planned alterations in the events prior to the manifestation of the maladaptive behavior as well as a change in the consequences of the behavior can alter the behavior itself. For example, a behavioral treatment was applied to a patient with Alzheimer's disease who developed violent outbursts whenever his wife tried to comb his hair. Analysis of the postviolence consequence revealed that the patient's spouse would then leave in disgust and be replaced by the patient's favorite nurse. A behavioral treatment of these violent outbursts was devised. His wife stopped grooming him (this removed the negative reinforcer of violence) and instead began each meeting by bringing his favorite food (a positive reinforcer of nonviolence). The nurse agreed to perform regularly scheduled grooming (using the nurse as a positive reinforcer of nonviolent behavior). This behavioral intervention reduced the frequency of violent episodes.

A social learning treatment is appropriate for neurologically impaired patients who can learn to correct their maladaptive behaviors by modeling new behaviors after others whose behaviors are socially appropriate. For example, a social skills group can retrain some patients to groom themselves, improve their manners, or reestablish their social graces. These groups rely heavily on modeling, role playing, and positive reinforcements.

A cognitive-behavioral treatment (see chapter 19, Behavioral Counseling and Medical Adherence), focuses on an individual's distorted thought processes that affect the patient's mood and behavior. Cognitive therapy may help a stroke victim who feels useless, who sees himself or herself as a burden to the family, and who is unable to meet his own expectations for recovery. His negative view of himself, defeatist attitude, sense of hopelessness, and perception of himself as a burden are part of a distorted, automatic, pathological thought process. In cognitive treatment, a therapist would challenge all of these negative views. The patient would be asked to record his negative attitudes toward himself and moods. He would be encouraged to test reality to see if his family finds the patient to be a burden. The patient would be asked to utilize and test all of his capacities. Repeated confrontation of cognitive distortions can lead to an improvement in the perception of reality and a decrease in maladaptive behaviors.

There are many cognitive rehabilitative techniques that may be helpful in the treatment of specific brain deficits. Deficits in memory, orientation, attention, language, or visual-spatial relationships can be remedied. For example, memory can be assisted by techniques such as reminders, cueing, the use of mnemonics, list writing, and a memory book, or by the assistance of a pocket computer. Problems of orientation may be ameliorated by having the caretaker repeat the day, date, time, and place. Patients can also be taught to orient themselves through the use of a calendar, newspaper, or watch. Language deficits can be improved by speech therapy, cognitive retraining, and comprehension exercises. Some intellectual deficits can be compensated for by a reeducation process that breaks down the components of an intellectual task into small, manageable steps. Each step can then be relearned with alternative brain capacities. These techniques can be used to teach a patient to drive, do math problems, or read in a different way.

Family Therapy

Family therapy (see chapter 18) is a powerful and effective form of treatment. Family structure often is dramatically changed when one member is incapacitated by a brain syndrome. Most patients lose prestige and power and experience a radical change in their functioning within the family. As a result, new family members assume leadership and others undertake different roles.

Patterns of family communications may also be radically altered when one member of a family becomes neurologically disabled. Communication problems can readily occur between the patient and family members as a result of the patient's deficits in communication. Alternatively, the general patterns of communication within the entire family, or between dyads within the family, may also be altered. If family patterns of communication are not successfully negotiated, problems can develop, which will decrease a family's cohesiveness and capacity to solve problems.

Families need help in order to understand the signs and symptoms of the illness and its stages of deterioration. They need a description of the progression of the illness, the chances of remission or cure, help with daily routines, information about available treatment, the long-term prognosis, and, when necessary, preparation for dying and death. A clinician can teach family members about the patient's deficits and behaviors so as to help them differentiate deficits from willful acts of defiance. The clinician should focus on realistic changes that will increase hope and foster new family coping strategies.

After sharing educational information, it is generally imperative to help all family members deal with the grief caused by the losses related to the patient's impairment. The stages of grief include denial, anger, bargaining, mourning, and grief resolution.

Organization collapse and family conflict often arise. Family treatment for these problems follows a structural or strategic family approach, which is described in chapter 18. Physicians should be comfortable referring families for therapy when they recognize emerging family strain.

Psychopharmacological Therapy

Medication can be an important adjunct for treatment of psychiatric symptoms such as depression, anxiety, behavioral disturbances, and memory loss. When prescribing for patients with brain syndromes, it is important to remember the following guidelines: (1) Try to prescribe a specific drug known to work for the specific condition (e.g., tacrine or donepezil for

Alzheimer's disease). (2) Begin with low doses of all medications, because elderly or debilitated patients may have a slowed liver or renal clearance and/or an increased sensitivity to medications. (3) Medication should be chosen for either a specific desired effect or to avoid certain side effects. (4) Interactions with other medications need to be carefully considered. (5) Avoid polypharmacy whenever possible. Patients requiring more than three psychoactive medications are probably not being optimally managed. Their medication should be reevaluated for a simplified regimen. Drugs that can be used for specific syndromes or diagnoses are summarized in Table 5.5.

Table 5.5 Pharmacologic Treatment of Psychiatric Conditions Due to Medical Conditions

Disorder	Preferred Drug	Doses	Avoid
Acute delirium	haloperidol	1–5mg po/im; max*. 30 mg or 1–5 mg bolus IV+ drip.	anticholinergics
	lorazepam alone or alternate haloperidol	1–2mg/ po/im max. 30 mg.	
	droperidol	2.5 mg (1ml)/50 lb. max. dose 45 mg	
Chronic delirium	haloperidol	1 mg bid	anticholinergics
	risperidone?	0.5–1 mg bid; 8–15 mg max.	
	olanzapine?	5 mg od; 10–15 mg max.	
Alzheimer's dementia	tacrine	10 mg/qid initial; 160 mg/day max.	anticholinergics cimetidine
	donepezil	5 mg/day initial; 10 mg/day max.	theophylline
Dementia with depression or pseudodementia	bupropion	75 mg bid; max. 400 mg	anticholinergic
	SSRIs	variable with each drug	+/-tricyclics
	trazodone/nefazodone	50 mg hs; max. 600 mg	
	venflaxine	75–225 mg/day in bid doses	

* max. = maximum dose/24 hrs.

Disorder	Preferred Drug	Doses	Avoid
Vascular dementia or strokes with depression	SSRIs nortriptyline trazodone/ nefazodone methylphenidate tricyclics	variable with each drug 20–150 mg od 50–600 mg/day 5–40 mg/day 25–400 mg/day	bupropion maprotiline venflaxine?
Movement disorder with depression (Parkinson's, etc.)	nortriptyline anticholinergic TCAs bupropion	25–150 mg od 25–400 mg/day 75 mg bid; max. 450 mg	amoxapine MAOI SSRI?
Psychotic disorder due to a general medical condition	haloperidol risperidone olanzapine neuroleptics	1–5 mg od max. 30 mg 0.5–1 mg bid; 8–15 mg max. 5 mg od; 10–15 mg max. variable	antidepressants alone
Anxiety disorder due to a general medical condition	Buspirone (GAD) SSRIs (panic, OCD, and social phobia) Alprazolam (panic) clonazepam (panic) MAOIs (social phobia)	5 mg tid: max; 20 mg tid variable with each drug and disorder 0.25–3 mg tid 0.25–2 mg bid 10 mg–60 mg od	
Mood disorder due to a general medical condition	**Depression** SSRIs paroxetine fluoxetine sertraline fluvoxamine	 5–40 mg od 5–80 mg od 25–200 mg in bid doses 50–440 mg in bid doses	

* max. = maximum dose/24 hrs.

(continued)

Table 5.5 *(continued)*

Disorder	Preferred Drug	Doses	Avoid
	venflaxine	25–350 mg in bid doses	
	bupropion	75 mg bid; max. 450 mg	
	trazodone/nefazodone	50–600 od	
	tricyclics	25–450 mg od	
	MAOIs (phenelzine)	15–30 mg tid	
	Mania		
	clonazepam	0.25–2 mg bid	If a manic Hx, avoid antidepressants alone
	lithium	300–900 mg tid	
	carbamazepine	250–400 mg tid	
	valproate	250–750 mg tid	
Personality change disorder due to a general medical condition	antidepressants	as needed	
	anti-anxiety	as needed	
	testosterone antagonist	for lewdness	
	lithium		

* max. = maximum dose/24 hrs.

REFERENCES

American Psychiatric Association. (1994). *Diagnostic and statistical manual of mental disorders* (4th ed.). Washington, DC: Author.

Cummings, J. L. (1992). Neuropsychiatric aspects of Alzheimer's disease and other dementing illnesses. In S. C. Yudofsky & R. E. Hales (Eds.), *The American Psychiatric Press textbook of neuropsychiatry* (2nd ed., pp. 605–620). Washington, DC: American Psychiatric Press.

Engel, G. L., & Romano, J. (1959). Delirium: A syndrome of cerebral insufficiency. *Journal of Chronic Diseases, 9*, 260–277.

Folstein, M. F., Folstein, S. E., & McHugh, P. R. (1975). "Mini-mental state": A practical method for grading the cognitive state of patients. *Clinical Journal of Psychiatric Research, 12*, 189–198.

Forrest, D. V. (1987). Psychosocial treatment in neuropsychiatry. In S. C. Yudofsky & R. E. Hales (Eds.), *The American Psychiatric Press textbook of neuropsychiatry* (pp. 387–409). Washington, DC: American Psychiatric Press.

Fuld, P. A. (1983). Word intrusion as a diagnostic sign in Alzheimer's disease. *Geriatric Medicine Today; 2*, 33–41.

Smith, D. B., & Craft, R. (1984). Sudden behavioral change: Guide to initial evaluation. In J. B. Green (Ed)., *Symposium of the borderland between neurology and psychiatry. Neurologic Clinics, 2*, 3–74.

Tuokko, H., Hadjistavropoulos, T., & Miller, J. A. (1992). The clock test: A sensitive measure to differentiate normal elderly from those with Alzheimer's disease. *Journal of the American Geriatrics Society, 40*, 579–584.

Wise, M. G., & Brandt, G. T. (1992). Delirium. In S. C. Yudofsky & R. E. Hales (Eds.), *The American Psychiatric Press textbook of neuropsychiatry* (2nd ed., pp. 291–310). Washington, DC: American Psychiatric Press.

CHAPTER 6

Somatoform Disorders

Brian A. Fallon

Patients with unexplained physical symptoms and irrational fears of illness plague the primary care physician. The symptoms trouble the patient despite a doctor's careful examination and reassurance that nothing is physically wrong. At times these patients have been referred to as "crocks" or "the worried well." Not more than a decade ago very little was known about how to diagnose and treat these problem patients. However, recent advances in biometrics and the development of novel pharmacologic agents have provided a basis for a doctor's attitude to shift from traditional therapeutic nihilism toward a more optimistic hope that these patients can in fact be helped. This chapter will focus on three somatoform disorders: hypochondriasis, body dysmorphic disorder, and somatization disorder. A better understanding of patients with these disorders will enhance their well-being and bring greater satisfaction to the treating physician.

HYPOCHONDRIASIS

The essence of hypochondriasis is the irrational fear or belief that one has a serious illness based on a misinterpretation of physical signs and symptoms. A thorough examination by the physician and reassurance that no serious illness is present may be temporarily reassuring to the patient, but often the reassurance lasts only a few days or weeks. Gradually, the fear returns. New bodily sensations bring new fears. Head throbbing signifies an expanding brain tumor on one day, whereas fatigue the next day most certainly indicates previously undetected AIDS. Although not often recognized, medically ill patients can be hypochondriacal as well. If one has a stable illness about which one worries excessively, then it is most likely that hypochondriasis is present.

Signs and Symptoms

Pilowsky (1967) identified three central aspects of hypochondria: fear of illness, disease conviction, and bodily preoccupation. These three aspects may occur in any combination such that one aspect may dominate over the other two and give the patient a distinctly different clinical profile. For example, a patient with a high degree of illness fear may actually avoid going to see a doctor, fearing that the doctor will confirm that the patient does indeed have the dreaded disease. Such patients often have good insight into the irrationality of their fears when they are not in the midst of a hypochondriacal attack. On the other hand, a patient with high disease conviction and lower fear often has continuously poor insight and may pursue a diagnosis with relentless persistence, berating doctors who fail to repeat a full battery of tests and becoming enraged by medical science's inability to help. A patient with high bodily preoccupation but lesser conviction may present to the physician with a variety of inexplicable physical complaints and appear to have somatization disorder. Only when the physician asks for the patient's fears regarding the significance of the bodily symptoms does it become clear that the patient suffers from hypochondriasis, the irrational fear or belief that one is seriously ill. It appears that there is a spectrum of insight into the unreasonableness of illness fears, represented at one end by complete recognition and at the other end by delusional conviction.

Course of Illness

Concerns about illness are reasonable when a person develops a new physical symptom. It is when worry persists even after a doctor's reassurance that a patient can aptly be described as having the symptom of hypochondriasis. In some cases, the fear is only mildly distressing and not associated with functional impairment. When the distress is more severe or when functional impairment occurs, then the disorder hypochondriasis exists.

The term *transient hypochondriasis* is employed to describe people who have illness fears that last weeks or months but that do not become the chronic problem characteristic of true hypochondriasis. Student nurses or doctors often develop transient hypochondriasis after learning about a new horrific disease. Transient hypochondriasis may abate on its own or persist in a milder episodic state for many years. To meet the criteria for the disorder of chronic hypochondriasis, the disease fears or convictions have to be persistent and present for at least 6 months. Hypochondriasis as defined in *DSM-IV* (1994) is unlikely to spontaneously remit, although its course may wax and wane in severity, exacerbated by the stressors in the patient's life. See Table 6.1 for criteria for the diagnosis of hypochondriasis.

Epidemiology

The prevalence of hypochondriasis in the general community is not known. However, one study conducted in Vermont among 325 households found that fears of illness and injury are among the most common phobic symptoms and that illness fears are an intense preoccupation in about 3.3% of the general population (Agras, 1969). In the medical setting, the prevalence of hypochondriasis is higher: 5% among 193 newly referred medical patients in the Netherlands (Van Hemert, 1993) and 4.2 to 6.3% among 1,389 general medical clinic patients in Boston (Barsky, Wyshak, Klerman, & Latham, 1990). Of patients identified in psychiatric clinics or medical settings, women are more commonly identified as hypochondriacal than men, at a ratio of 3:1 to 4:1. The typical age of onset is the early 20s, and many patients have suffered with hypochondriasis for more than a decade before seeking treatment (Fallon et al., 1993).

Clinical Interview

Hypochondriacs will not identify themselves as hypochondriacal. Their fear, after all, is that they have a serious, unrecognized physical illness. How does the physician recognize these patients? What questions should one ask? Clinical clues to spot hypochondriasis can be found in how the patient behaves and in how the physician feels in response to the patient.

The Patient's Reaction

Hypochondriacal patients often exhibit excessive fear, repetitive questioning during the office visit or contacts by phone after the session is over, and a failure to be reassured. There may be evidence of nonhypochondriacal obsessional traits. Patients may also have a personal or family history of excessive worrying. Common features include the following:

FEAR. Excessive fear may be manifested by reluctance to talk about symptoms, tearfulness, or elevated pulse and blood pressure during the initial exam that normalizes by the end of the examination.

PATHOLOGIC DOUBT. When patients ask the same question over and over again, in slightly different ways, they are exhibiting anxiety and pathologic doubt. Patients with pathologic doubt often cannot be certain that they conveyed their symptoms thoroughly enough, that enough tests were done, or that they understood the doctor correctly. Typically, these patients will ask, "But doctor, how do I know . . . ?" or "Doctor, how can you be certain . . . ?" Although major advances in medical science have occurred, the art of medicine requires the clinician's judgment to reconcile the inevitable uncertainties inherent in good medical care. Hypochondriacs, plagued by the tyranny of doubt, cannot accept uncertainty.

CONVICTION. Patients may be so certain that they are dying that either they do not seek help or they fail to be able to accept the doctor's reassurance for even a brief period. Many of these patients will be in the throes of a concurrent major depression in which they feel nothing but despair. They know that they are ill regardless of what the doctor says. Such conviction can reach delusional proportions and place the patient at a significant risk of suicide. If a patient comes to the office complaining of abdominal pain and fears pancreatic cancer, for example, that patient should be reassured when the physical exam and blood tests come back normal. Failure to be reassured should alert the clinician to probe more carefully for suicidality, underlying depression, or a delusional disorder.

OTHER OBSESSIONAL FEATURES. Other obsessional traits may be present currently or in the hypochondriac's past and include a fear that terrible harm might come to loved ones; intrusive, horrific images; obsessive thoughts about dirt or germs; an anxiety-driven need for perfection, order, or symmetry; troubling sexual images; and scrupulous moral or religious concerns. Common compulsions include excessive checking, cleaning, and counting.

PERSONAL AND FAMILY HISTORY. Hypochondriacal patients often know that they are overly concerned about illness. Typically, these patients are

Table 6.1 Critical Pathway, Somatoform Disorders

Disorder	DSM IV criteria	Associated Features	Physician Checklist	Differential Diagnosis	Treatments	Interviews or Screening	Physician Education Self-help
Hypo-chondria*	a. Fear of having a serious disease based on symptom misinterpretation b. Failure to be reassured despite a good medical evaluation c. Not delusional d. Marked distress or impaired functioning e. Lasts >6 months f. Not better accounted for by other psychiatric diagnoses (e.g., panic)	a. Pathologic doubt b. OCD features c. Symptom amplification d. Depression	a. Thorough medical evaluation? b. Recent onset of stress? c. Masked depression/ panic? d. Family Hx of anxiety/ depression? e. Culturally syntonic?	Exclude medical causes such as: a. Fibromyalgia b. Chronic fatigue syndrome c. Multiple sclerosis d. Chronic Lyme disease e. Comorbid psychiatric Dx	a. Education b. Reassurance c. Cognitive behavior therapy d. Psychiatric medication, such as OCD-dosage range of serotonin reuptake inhibitors	Whiteley Index of Hypochondria (Pilowsky 1983) Illness Attitude Scale (Kellner, 1987)	*Phantom Illness: shattering the myth of hypo-chondria (Cantor, 1996)*

Disorder	DSM IV Criteria	Associated Features	Physician Checklist	Differential Diagnosis	Treatments	Interviews or Screening	Physician Education Self-help
Body dysmorphic disorder*	a. Preoccupation with defect in bodily appearance b. Marked distress or functional impairment c. Preoccupation is not better accounted for by another mental disorder (e.g., anorexia nervosa)	a. Mirror checking or avoidance b. Excessive grooming c. Camouflaging of the "defect" d. Social isolation e. Reassurance seeking	a. Evaluate "defect" b. Distress? c. Checking or avoidance? d. Suicidal? e. Prior medical or surgical procedures?	Exclude as primary: a. Physical deformity b. Anorexia nervosa c. Gender identity disorder d. Major depression e. Social phobia f. OCD	a. Reassurance after appropriate evaluation b. Medicate with SSRIs c. Psychotherapy for suicidal feelings and social isolation	BDD Exam (Rosen, 1996) BDD Obsessive -Compulsive Scale (Phillips, 1996)	*The Broken Mirror Under-standing and Treating BDD* (Phillips, 1996)
Somatization disorder*	a. Many physical complaints <age 30 occur over several years and result in medical treatment or functional impairment b. All four of the following at any time of the illness: 1. Four pain symptoms 2. Two gastrointestinal symptoms	a. Consultation with several physicians concurrently b. Dramatic symptom description in multiple organ systems c. Chaotic interpersonal life	a. Review medical treatments/Hx of hospitali-zations b. Early age of onset without known cause? c. Review records from diagnostic w-ups.	Exclude medical Dx: a. Endocrino-pathies b. Porphyria c. Multiple sclerosis d. Systemic lupus e. Chronic Lyme disease	a. Reassurance after medical evaluation b. Treat comorbid anxiety or depression with pharma-cotherapy	PRIME-MD (Spitzer, 1994)	*Phantom Illness* (Cantor, 1996) *Abnormal illness and behavior* (Pilowsky, 1983)

continued

Table 6.1 *(continued)*

Disorder	DSM IV criteria	Associated features	Physician checklist	Differential diagnosis	Treatments	Interviews or screening	Physician education self-help
Somatization disorder* *(continued)*	3. One sexual symptom 4. One pseudoneurological symptoms c. Either 1 or 2: 1. Physical symptom can't be explained by a known medical condition or effects of substance abuse 2. If symptom present and patient has a medical illness, the impairment is excessive d. Symptoms are not intentionally produced or feigned	d. Comorbid substance abuse, anxiety or depression e. Antisocial behavior in male relatives	Were they thorough? d. Inquire about family history of somatization, substance abuse, antisocial personality	f. Other conditions with multiple symptoms Exclude primary anxiety and mood disorders. Note: Onset of multiple physical symptoms after age 30 is almost always due to general medical condition.	c. Educate about stress and symptom formation d. Schedule regular office visits e. Refer for group psychotherapy f. Relaxation techniques g. Couples/ family therapy, if indicated		*Somatization and Hypochondriasis* (Kellner, 1986)

*DSM-IV abridged criteria. 1994.

Reprinted with permission from the Diagnostic and Statistical Manual of Mental Disorder, Fourth Edition. Copyright 1994 American Psychiatric Association.

told by family members and friends that they are chronic worriers. There may also be a family history of an anxiety or depressive disorder.

The Physician's Reaction

Physicians often find hypochondriacal patients to be frustrating in that they are quite demanding but also reject help. The experience of frustration itself can alert the clinician to examine the patient for the presence of hypochondriacal fears and obsessive worries. Rather than experiencing frustration and wanting to rush the patient out of the office as quickly as possible, the inquiring clinician may take note of the frustration and then take a few extra minutes to probe further, looking for hypochondriasis in the patient's interpretation of the physical symptoms, a personality disorder as evident in their interpersonal relationships, or other comorbid Axis I psychiatric disorders.

Questions to ask include the following:

- Is the patient excessively fearful of an imagined illness or of a stable illness?
- Is the hypochondriasis of recent onset? If so, can a stressor be identified that may have triggered it?
- Has a thorough medical work-up been conducted?
- Are there other concurrent psychiatric disorders that can be readily treated?
- Is hypochondriasis a culturally syntonic mode of affect expression?
- Is there a family history of anxiety or depression that might suggest that the patient's hypochondriasis is biologically driven?

Differential Diagnosis

The diagnosis of all somatoform disorders is a diagnosis of exclusion. All other reasonable medical causes for the patient's physical symptoms need to be ruled out before the diagnosis can be made. In a recent review of 10 patients referred to the author by medical doctors for the treatment of hypochondriasis, 4 of the 10 did not have a somatoform disorder. One believed he had had a heart attack because he had been hospitalized to rule out myocardial infarction; his cardiologist had not successfully conveyed to this man that not only had a heart attack been ruled out but his heart was normal. Two patients suffered from the residual symptoms commonly seen in Lyme disease. One patient had probable chronic fatigue syndrome. Finally, it is worth noting that one of the patients who had been a hypochondriac for at least three decades came with the chief complaint of abdominal pain, which he interpreted as a sign of enlarging renal cysts. This abdominal complaint was hypochondriacal; however, this man's speech was worsening—a problem that was evolving and not being addressed. Within a few months, he became unable to talk and to swallow, and a work-up revealed amyotrophic lateral sclerosis. It appears that his increasing preoccupation with his abdomen was a displacement of anxiety about his real problem, the worsening speech. Hypochondriacs get sick too. This point is made in the joke often told by hypochondriacs: "They'll write on my tombstone, 'He thought he was sick.' "

It is not uncommon for patients to be told they are hypochondriacal if they suffer from a disease for which there are no adequate diagnostic tests to mark its presence. Paradigmatic medical disorders include such conditions as fibromyalgia, chronic fatigue syndrome, Lyme disease, and irritable bowel. Working with patients who have these conditions can be frustrating, because their course may be relapsing and recurrent despite the physician's best efforts. One study noted that the single greatest factor that led a physician to consider a patient hypochondriacal was the degree of frustration in treating that patient (Barsky, 1991). Although frustration is a clue, it is not a diagnostic criterion for hypochondriasis. First and foremost, the presence of a medical disorder needs to be acknowledged and treated or ruled out. Other medical conditions that need to be considered in the differential diagnosis include the early stages of neurological conditions (e.g., multiple sclerosis and myasthenia gravis), endocrinopathies (e.g., thyroid and parathyroid diseases), multisystem diseases (e.g., systemic lupus erythematosus), and occult malignancies.

The differential diagnosis of hypochondriasis also needs to include other psychiatric disorders. Most importantly, common conditions that might have a hypochondriacal presentation include panic disorder, major depression, generalized anxiety disorder, and obsessive compulsive disorder. The term *hypochondriasis* should be used only if the patient's symptoms are not best described by one of these other disorders.

Remarkable similarities exist between hypochondriasis and obsessive compulsive disorder. In hypochondriasis, the patient has intrusive thoughts about illness, fear of impending harm, and compulsions to check his or her body or to seek reassurance from medical texts or health professionals. In obsessive-compulsive disorder (OCD), the patient may have intrusive obsessional thoughts about germs, fear of impending harm, somatic preoccupations, and compulsions to hand wash, check, or repeat behaviors. The essential difference is that the hypochondriac fears having an illness, whereas the OCD patient fears getting an illness. The OCD patient must also have nonhypochondriacal obsessions. The similarities between hypochondriasis and OCD have important treatment implications because current research suggests that the methods of treating OCD are also effective for hypochondriasis.

Etiology

The etiology of hypochondriasis is unclear but undoubtedly includes psychological, cultural, and biological components. Psychologically, hypochondriacal anxiety may serve as a window into unresolved emotional issues or earlier developmental conflicts. For example, a 26-year-old woman presented with unexplained chest pain and terrifying fears of a heart attack. She knew that her symptoms began shortly after her mother's death, but she was unaware that her chest pain was directly linked to unresolved grief over her mother's death from a heart attack 1 year earlier. Culturally, hypochondriacal and bodily concerns may be an acceptable mode of expressing emotional stress; this is particularly common in certain Hispanic groups. One popular current theory emphasizes that hypochondriacs have a tendency to amplify, augment, and misinterpret normal bodily sensations, experiencing interoceptive cues as more intense and noxious.

With respect to a biologic etiology, recent research (Gramling, Clawson, & McDonald, 1996) demonstrated that hypochondriacs compared to nonhypochondriacs are more reactive in the physiological domain. For instance, hypochondriacs show a greater increase in heart rate to a cold water bath as well as a significant drop in hand temperature compared to nonhypochondriacs. Although this could have occurred as a result of an acquired response learned via modeling or classical conditioning, these physiological differences might also reflect constitutional differences. The neurochemical underpinnings of these constitutional differences in the hypochondriacal patient may be similar to the predominantly serotonergic imbalance seen in obsessive-compulsive disorder, or it may be more reflective of the noradrenergic imbalances seen in panic disorder. Studies to answer these questions have yet to be done.

Treatment

A patient with acute hypochondriacal concerns may respond to the physician's reassurance. When the concerns persist, the primary care physician should ask about recent stressors or the death or loss of a loved one. Simply identifying the stressor and its relationship to the hypochondriacal symptom may enable the patient to begin to relieve some of the conflict through words rather than physical pain. In these situations, the primary care physician may help to heal the patient by listening. If the stressors are severe or the patient is unstable, referral to a psychotherapist is warranted. Patients may accept the referral once the link with the stressor is identified.

If comorbid psychiatric disorders are present, the physician should assess whether the disorder is severe or moderate. If severe, referral to a psychiatrist is recommended for combined psychotherapy and pharmacotherapy. If moderate, the patient may respond well to the administration of appropriate pharmacotherapy for that particular disorder. For example, major depression might remit after 6 to 8 weeks of a tricyclic or serotonergic antidepressant. Obsessive-compulsive disorder might substantially improve after 6 to 12 weeks of treatment with clomipramine, fluoxetine, or fluvoxamine. With panic disorder, alprazolam or clonazepam might bring rapid relief, whereas imipramine might require 6 to 8 weeks of treatment before improvement is seen, using a very gradual dosage titration upwards from 10 mg/day to 125 to 150 mg/day.

What should the physician do when faced with a hypochondriacal patient who does not have a comorbid psychiatric disorder and who has not been recently stressed? The first task is to convince the patient that treatment might be indicated. Hypochondriacs hate the term *hypochondriac*. The term implies that nothing is physically wrong with the patient. In fact, something *is* physically wrong. In our studies of these patients, we use the term *heightened illness concern*, because the term itself is more accurate and less pejorative. Hypochondriacs are known to have an increased sensitivity to bodily sensations and an inability to let go of the accompanying intrusive illness fears. Just like an obsessive-compulsive patient who scans his or her external environment for signs of germs or dirt, the hypochondriac scans his or her internal environment—his or her body—for signs of disease. The hypervigilance, need for certainty, and heightened state of arousal characteristic of OCD patients presumably reflect the activation of a central alarm mechanism heavily influenced by serotonergic neurons. This may also be true for the hypochondriac. Telling the hypochondriac about this hypothesized serotonergic imbalance lends validity to the hypochondriac's condition and also provides a biological model to explain the uncontrollable fear so characteristic of his or her clinical experience.

Recent work with patients who have primary hypochondriasis has focused on two areas: cognitive behavior therapy and pharmacotherapy. Cognitive behavior therapy is best given by a therapist trained in this technique who will educate the patient about the contribution of cognitive distortions, symptom amplification, and mood to his or her problem. In addition, the patient will learn through experience that repetitive reassurance seeking is actually counterproductive, because it increases the intensity of fear in the long run. Pharmacotherapy can be given by the primary care physician. Work at Columbia University and the New York State Psychiatric Institute demonstrated in an open trial that 70% of patients treated with fluoxetine at doses ranging from 20 to 80 mg/day were much improved or very improved after a 12-week course of treatment (Fallon et al., 1993). Some patients did not respond until 6 to 12 weeks of medication. Therefore, the physician should start low (10 or 20 mg) and build up every 2 weeks by 20 mg to a maximum dose of 80 mg. Given the success of fluoxetine with OCD, it is not surprising that hypochondriasis (an obsessive-compulsive spectrum disorder) might similarly respond. Other medications effective for OCD might also be effective for hypochondriasis, including fluvoxamine (increasing to 300 mg/day), sertraline (increasing to 200 mg/day), and clomipramine (increasing to 250 mg/day).

Optimal treatment may consist of a combined approach in which pharmacotherapy, psychodynamic psychotherapy, and cognitive-behavioral therapy are provided simultaneously.

Finally, some patients will not respond to any of the above treatments. In these cases, empathic support by the primary care physician accompanied by regularly scheduled (not more than once every 2 months) visits can provide valuable connection and reassurance.

BODY DYSMORPHIC DISORDER

Body dysmorphic disorder (BDD) was first recognized as a separate clinical problem in 1987 with its inclusion in *DSM-III-R* (1987). Table 6.1 provides criteria for this disorder. The primary care clinician will be puzzled by patients presenting with this disorder who worry about a defect in bodily appearance that is either imagined or a gross magnification of a minor physical anomaly. These patients may focus on such features as the slope of their nose, thinning hair, acne, scars, swelling, and facial asymmetry. These preoccupations seem absurd to the outside observer, but to the patient the worries are so tormenting that he or she may seek plastic surgery to correct the defect. Patients suffering with this disorder may seek help only from the primary care physician and not from a psychiatrist. In a report on 100 subjects with BDD, 72% sought medical treatment to correct their imagined problem (Phillips, McElroy, & Keck, 1994). It therefore behooves the primary care clinician to be aware of the manifestations of this disorder. Like hypochondriasis, BDD is considered an obsessive-compulsive spectrum disorder because of the endless obsessions and bodily checking associated with it.

Signs and Symptoms

To meet *DSM-IV* criteria for BDD, the patient must have a preoccupation with a defect in appearance that is excessive, distressing, or impairing and not better accounted for by another disorder, such as anorexia nervosa, in which the concern is about body shape and size. These concerns commonly involve the face or head, for example, imagined defects in nose, eyes, eyelids, ears, mouth, or lips. Any other bodily part may also be a focus of concern, such as breasts, thighs, hips, or in men, body build. Patients with this disorder may request a urologic consult because of a small penis, an endocrine consult because of excessive facial hair, or a dermatologic consult because of skin lesions or hair thinning. The preoccupation may consume 3 to 8 hours daily. Patients often have ideas or delusions of reference in that they suspect or are convinced that other people are talking about the imagined defect. This leads them to avoid socializing and functioning in society. Typical compulsive behaviors include comparing one's features to others, mirror checking, camouflaging with a hat or cosmetics, reassurance seeking, excessive grooming, and skin picking.

The degree of distress among BDD patients is considerable; in one study, 70% considered suicide and 22% actually made a suicide attempt (Phillips, Gunderson, McElroy, Mallya, & Carter, 1995).

Course of Illness

BDD usually begins during adolescence but does not come to medical attention until years later. This is because patients with this problem are reluctant to discuss the problem with others due to embarrassment. The course of the disorder is usually continuous, although the intensity of symptoms wax and wane with time. Patients may remain totally fixated on one body part or change preoccupation from one area to another.

Epidemiology

No community studies of BDD have been conducted. In one study of patients requesting cosmetic plastic surgery, 2% were diagnosed as having BDD (Aronowitz, Hollander, Simeon, & Cohen, 1995). The sex ratio for BDD is 1:1 in a psychiatric clinic. Among patients suffering from BDD, women are more likely to have lifetime bulimia, and men are more likely to have lifetime alcohol abuse or dependence.

Clinical Interview

If a person comes into the clinician's office inordinately distressed about a defect in appearance, the clinician usually examines the area and reassures the patient that nothing is wrong. The patient with BDD is not convinced. Although empathizing with absurd preoccupations can be difficult, failure to empathize will lead the patient to leave the office in greater despair and in search of another physician. The alert clinician who suspects BDD and understands the torment can proceed with a set of questions that will provide considerable comfort to the patient. Because these patients are so embarrassed by their appearance and their behaviors, a set of targeted questions from the clinician will enable the patient to talk about the problem and enable the clinician to demonstrate empathy with the patient's distress.

Questions to ask include:

- How distressing is your concern?
- Can you control the preoccupations?
- How many hours a day do you worry about it?
- Do you avoid work or social situations?
- Do you check in the mirror or other reflecting surfaces (e.g., store windows and framed glass)?
- Do you groom excessively? Avoid mirrors?
- Have you felt so despairing that you have contemplated suicide?
- Have you had prior medical, dental, or surgical treatments to correct the defect?

A patient who is asked these questions for the first time will be surprised and relieved and may then inquire about treatments for BDD.

Differential Diagnosis

BDD should not be diagnosed if the focus of concern is restricted to body shape or size, as in anorexia nervosa, or primary/secondary sex characteristics, as in gender identity disorder. Although patients with social phobia or avoidant personality disorder will also avoid social situations, their reason relates to a fundamental discomfort with social interactions, not a fear that others will be talking or noticing an imagined bodily defect. As in hypochondriasis, a separate diagnosis of OCD is only given if non-appearance-related obsessions and compulsions are present.

Etiology

The etiology of BDD is poorly understood but undoubtedly multifactorial. Psychologically, a focus on poorly shaped breasts may emerge after an interpersonal rejection, suggesting that the somatic preoccupation is a displacement of anxiety over interpersonal loss. Or a young adult obsessed with the appearance of his or her face might have had a long history of interpersonal teasing in childhood as a result of minor acne, resulting in the face as a fixation point for any subsequent stress.

Cultural components may also play a part, as in Southeast Asia, where Koro has been described. Koro refers to a preoccupation that the penis is shrinking and will disappear into the abdomen, causing death. Unlike BDD, Koro usually has a short duration, an excellent response to reassurance, and may occur in an epidemic fashion. Biological factors may also contribute, particularly considering the unshakable delusional fixation in some patients, the response to pharmacotherapy, and the similarities between BDD and OCD. Given the abnormally increased frontal lobe radiotracer uptake commonly seen in single photon emission computed tomography (SPECT) and positron emission tomography (PET) studies of OCD, and the abnormalities known to exist in the serotonergic and dopaminergic neurotransmitter functioning in OCD, it is reasonable to speculate that patients with BDD might also have similar biological abnormalities. Supporting an overlap between BDD and OCD are comorbidity studies, such as that done during the *DSM-IV* field trial of 442 OCD patients, in which 12% were found to have a lifetime comorbid diagnosis of BDD (Simeon, Hollander, Stein, Cohen, &Aronowitz, 1995).

Treatment

There have been no well-controlled treatment trials of BDD. In one retrospective report, insight-oriented psychotherapy was not helpful for any of the 24 treated patients. Pharmacotherapy with serotonin reuptake inhibitors was helpful, with more than half of the therapeutic trials resulting in clinical improvement with either fluoxetine (at least 60 mg/day for 4 weeks) or clomipramine (at least 200 mg/day for 4 weeks) (Phillips, McElroy, & Keck, 1993). In another study (Hollander, Simeon, Cohen, & Aronowitz, 1995), clinical trials with the SSRIs (clomipramine, fluoxetine, and fluvoxamine) resulted in much improvement in BDD severity, whereas following administration of tricyclics, BDD severity was unchanged.

Case Study

A handsome 20-year-old singer comes for treatment because of profound distress over a scar on his cheek. The scar is not visible to the examining physician, but the imagined defect causes such distress to the young man that he can no longer socialize or practice his profession. There was a past history of moderate obsessive-compulsive symptoms, such as hand washing and counting. Fluvoxamine was prescribed, starting at 50 mg po qhs, increasing by 50 mg increments every week to 300 mg/day in bid dosing. By the fourth week of treatment, the preoccupation with his face started to diminish, and by the sixth week, this young man was free of bodily preoccupations and had started to socialize again. The remarkable effectiveness of this treatment surprised and pleased the patient. This treatment was continued for 6 months, then gradually tapered to see if the clinical improvement was sustained.

SOMATIZATION DISORDER

Patients with somatization disorder demonstrate a pattern of recurrent, troubling, unexplained physical complaints that begin before age 30 and occur over a period of years, resulting in the taking of medication or in significant impairment in their interpersonal or work life. These physical complaints cannot be fully explained by a known general medical condition. If a medical problem is present, the distress or disability caused by the physical symptom is in excess of the expected.

Signs and Symptoms

To meet *DSM-IV* diagnostic criteria for somatization disorder (see Table 6.1), there must be a history of each of the following: pain related to at least four different sites (e.g., head, back, rectum) or functions (e.g., sexual intercourse, urination, menstruation), at least two gastrointestinal symptoms other than pain (e.g., nausea, abdominal bloating, diarrhea), at least one sexual or reproductive symptom other than pain (e.g., irregular menses or ejaculatory dysfunction), and at least one nonpain pseudoneurological symptom (e.g., impaired balance, paralysis, numbness, amnesia).

Although hypochondriacs in general tend to be obsessional, somatization patients tend to be more dramatic and histrionic. Rather than presenting with a well-organized list of symptoms, somatization patients confront the physician with a long, disorganized list of physical symptoms and a history of seeing many physicians at the same time. These patients urgently want relief from their physical distress, whereas hypochondriacs want relief from their fear of illness. The interpersonal life of the somatization patient is often chaotic, accompanied by marital discord, suicide attempts, substance abuse, and/or antisocial behavior.

The persistent physical symptoms and "doctor shopping" that characterize somatization disorders often result in fragmented patient care, unnecessary repetitive tests, and costly, potentially dangerous surgeries. Physical examination and laboratory results are often unremarkable.

Course of Illness

Somatization generally starts in the teenage years, and the full criteria for the disorder are met by the mid-20s. The course is a chronic one, with a waxing and waning pattern. Somatization disorder patients get caught in a damaging spiral of health-seeking behavior. The physician runs a gamut of tests to try to identify the underlying cause, but these tests prove unhelpful. The patient seeks answers for the distress and pain and is not satisfied with the lack of a diagnosis. The physician in turn is frustrated by the patient's apparent lack of progress and persistent illness. A referral is made to a specialist, who orders more tests, until once again no diagnosis is made. Because of the large number of serologic tests or X-rays ordered, a false-positive result may then occur, further confusing the diagnostic picture and leading to several more rounds of tests and procedures. Frustration rises, and new doctors are sought. Inappropriate diagnosis and treatment may result, along with excessive use of the health care system.

Epidemiology

Although the tendency to somatize is not rare, the full syndrome of somatization disorder is uncommon in the general community. Epidemiological studies have reported prevalence rates of somatization disorder of roughly 2 to 3 per 1,000 of the general population (Robins et al., 1984). Estimates of the prevalence of somatization disorder in the general medical setting are higher, ranging from 8% to 9% of all patients (deGruy, 1987; van Hemert, 1993). If even only 5% of primary care patients do have somatization disorder, then somatization disorder is a common problem in the medical setting, as common as diabetes mellitus and urinary tract infections.

Women are more frequently affected than men, with a female-to-male ratio of 10:1 in the community and 5:1 in the primary care setting.

The criteria for somatization disorder are restrictive. For example, patients who have only four unexplained symptoms would not meet criteria. To estimate the prevalence of subthreshhold "somatizers" in the general population, Escobar and colleagues (Escobar, Rubio-Stipec, Canino, & Karno, 1989) created a diagnostic category that required patients to have only six unexplained symptoms for women or four for men . Using these criteria, the prevalence of somatizers in the general population is 4% to 12%.

Family studies have shown that 10% to 20% of female first-degree biological relatives of women with somatization disorder will also have the disorder. The male relatives of women with somatization disorder have a greater risk for antisocial personality disorder and/or substance abuse. Adoption studies have shown that genetic and environmental factors contribute to the risk. Having a parent with somatization disorder, substance-related disorder, or antisocial personality markedly increases the likelihood that the child will experience any one of these disorders, including somatization disorder.

Clinical Interview

Physicians faced with a somatizing patient are often thrown off guard by the exclusively somatic complaints. Clinicians who would in other circumstances rapidly recognize and treat depression or anxiety are led by the somatizing patient on a fruitless search for the phantom diagnosis. In one study of 685 primary care patients, Kirmayer and colleagues (Kirmayer, Robbins, Dworkind, & Yaffe, 1993) demonstrated that over 75% of patients with depression presented somatically. Among patients with either major depression or an anxiety disorder, a somatic presentation reduced physician recognition of a mental illness from 77% among those who reported life stressors to 22% among those who reported only physical symptoms.

In the office interview, asking about the symptoms of depression or anxiety can be very helpful and relatively quick. Does the patient have a disturbance in sleep, a change in appetite, increased fatigue, poor concentration, decreased interest in hobbies or work, or feelings of hopelessness? Does the patient have abrupt but brief attacks of physical symptoms, with many of the symptoms of panic disorder, such as dizziness, chest pain, shortness of breath, and tremors? Many patients with panic disorder are initially unaware that this psychiatric disorder's primary presentation is unprovoked by stressors and predominantly physical. How is the person's work life, marriage, or relationship with his or her children? In most patients who present with only two or three symptoms, the presenting physical symptom is a sign of interpersonal distress and an acceptable way for the patient to gain access to further care.

Key to the diagnosis of somatization disorder is the presence of many unexplained symptoms over a long period of time beginning prior to the age of 30. Therefore, if a 40-year-old patient comes into the office with multiple unexplained symptoms that have existed for only 2 to 3 years, the diagnosis of somatization disorder is by definition excluded. The most likely cause is an underlying anxiety or depression or an as yet unidentified primary medical condition.

Differential Diagnosis

Ruling out a general medical disorder is essential. Clues to the diagnosis of somatization disorder include the absence of physical signs or structural abnormalities, a lack of response to prior treatments, multisystemic symptoms, neurologic complaints that do not follow expected nerve pathways, the absence of lab abnormalities for conditions in which reliable and sensitive lab assays exist, and early onset and chronic course.

Although these clues are helpful in diagnosing somatization disorder, the physician still needs to rule out medical conditions with vague presentations or for which no clear laboratory test yet exists. These include disorders such as Lyme disease, acute intermittent porphyria, multiple sclerosis, chronic fatigue syndrome, and irritable bowel syndrome.

By definition, patients with somatization disorder complain of pain, sexual problems, and pseudoneurological symptoms. Although hypochondriasis and somatization disorder are often confused, there are often clear differences. The focus in somatization disorder is on the sensation, whereas in hypochondria the focus is on the meaning of the sensation. The somatization disorder patient wants to get rid of the symptom and discomfort, whereas the hypochondriac wants to be told that the symptom does not signify a serious dreaded illness. In somatization disorder the physical symptoms predominate, whereas in hypochondriasis the cognitive interpretation of the symptoms creates the problem.

Another common error is to confuse somatization disorder with factitious disorders, such as Munchausen syndrome. Unlike malingers who manipulate society by taking on the sick role or Munchausen patients who manipulate health professionals in order to be treated as a patient, somatization disorder patients genuinely experience their symptoms.

Patients with schizophrenia may have multiple somatic delusions, but in these patients the significance of the somatic complaints is maintained with a delusional intensity.

Patients with panic disorder have multiple somatic complaints, but these occur primarily during brief panic attacks. Patients with generalized anxiety disorder also may have numerous physical symptoms, but their worry is not limited to the domain of physical health. Patients with depression may present solely with somatic complaints, yet a careful history reveals that these symptoms were not present prior to the onset of the depression. A key feature that distinguishes somatized anxiety and depression from somatization disorder is the absence of a lifetime history of multiple, unexplained somatic symptoms.

Etiology

The etiology of somatization disorder is unknown. Stress is known to exacerbate somatic complaints in somatizing individuals, resulting in either new symptoms or increased health care–seeking behavior. These patients experience their health as being very poor. Based on self-report measures, when the health of patients with somatization disorder was compared to that of patients with chronic medical conditions (e.g., hypertension, rheumatoid arthritis, and chronic obstructive pulmonary disease) somatization disorder patients reported their physical status as much worse (Smith, Monson, & Ray, 1986). Genetic and environmental factors may also contribute to the development of somatization disorder, as suggested by studies that show considerable overlap in families of somatic patients between somatization, substance-related disorders, and antisocial behavior.

Treatment

There are no well-established treatments for somatization disorder; however, there is abundant evidence that many patients with somatization disorder have comorbid anxiety or depression. Treatment of the comorbid condition may result in a marked diminution in symptom amplification and distress. The most common comorbid conditions include major depression in approximately 55% of patients, generalized anxiety disorder in 34% of patients, and panic disorder in 26% of patients.

Some patients with somatization disorder may perceive their emotional reactions as unacceptable and therefore have difficulty labeling their feelings. Instead, they speak of their emotion through the metaphor of physical symptoms. This preoccupation with physical symptoms makes the verbal art of psychotherapy difficult. Because these patients often have such a hostile relationship with their own bodies, therapeutic techniques that emphasize developing a less stress-filled awareness of the body may be particularly helpful. These therapies include yoga, relaxation therapies, and meditation.

Although there is no great hope for the treatment of somatization disorder per se, some studies demonstrate that specific functional somatic symptoms may in fact diminish with a targeted treatment. In one study of short-term psychotherapy (Benson, Hanson, & Matarazzo, 1959), improvement occurred in approximately half of the women with pelvic pain in whom no organic pathology could be found. Patients with irritable bowel syndrome benefited from group psychotherapy in one study, and this benefit was sustained in 1-month follow-up (Wise, Cooper, & Ahmed, 1982).

Group psychotherapy may be particularly helpful for somatization disorder patients. In one recently reported randomized controlled study, patients who received group therapy reported significantly better physical and mental health than patients who did not receive therapy (Kashner, Rost, Cohen, Anderson, & Smith, 1995).

Controlled double-blind drug trials demonstrate that benzodiazepines are more effective than placebos in reducing somatic symptoms in anxious patients (Glass, Uhlenhuth, & Kellner, 1987). Similarly, controlled studies demonstrate that antidepressants such as imipramine (a tricyclic antidepressant) or phenelzine (an MAOI) can be very effective in reducing physical symptoms in anxious patients (Sheehan, Ballenger, & Jacobsen, 1980).

When using imipramine in somatizing patients, the physician should make sure the patient does not have a cardiac conduction delay. Start at a very low dose and gradually increase. The following schedule is often well tolerated: 10 mg × 1 day, 20 mg × 1 day, 30 mg × 1 day, 40 mg × 1 day, 50 mg × 4 days, 75 mg × 4 days, 100 mg × 1 week, 125 mg × 1 week, then 150 mg po qhs. Patients may need the higher dosages of 200 to 300 mg po qhs that are typically used to treat depression. Imipramine has the advantage of being sedating and thus helping a person with insomnia, but the disadvantage of causing anticholinergic side effects such as constipation and dry mouth. Because somatizing patients are so somatically preoccupied, the serotonin reuptake inhibitors may be better tolerated because of their generally more favorable side-effect profile. Controlled studies of these agents in somatization disorder patients have not yet been conducted. The MAOIs are not often used by physicians because of the need for the patient to maintain a strict tyramine-restricted diet. Failure to maintain the diet can result in severe blood pressure elevations and possibly death. MAOIs, however, can be very effective for anxious and somatizing patients and should be used in the compliant patient when other safer antidepressants have failed to help.

Because no treatments have yet been identified that "cure" patients with somatization disorder, most clinicians focus on how better to manage the problems presented. Research studies suggest that these strategies result in either improved or maintained perceived health status, decreased utilization of health services, and increased patient satisfaction with care (Kashner et al., 1995). A typical program incorporates the following elements. First, make the family doctor the patient's primary and preferably only physician; this enables a trusting relationship to be established. Second, schedule brief but regular outpatient visits (15 minutes q4 to 6 weeks); this will allow the patient to come to see the doctor without having to have a new symptom to get an appointment. Third, on subsequent office visits, the physician should conduct an abbreviated physical exam with the focus on the presenting symptom; this enables the physician to rule out the development of a new, legitimate medical problem while at the same time reassuring the patient that his or her symptoms were heard. Fourth, never disqualify the patient's experience of pain; pain as a symptom is real, and failure to respect the patient's experience will create major problems in the management of the somatizing patient. Fifth, after an empathic doctor-patient relationship is established, attempt to educate the patient about the role of stress in exacerbating physical symptoms; the patient may then be more amenable to a referral to a mental health professional.

Finally, when working with the somatizing patient, one should be compassionate and ready to acknowledge the limitations of our medical understanding of unexplained physical symptoms. It is worth remembering Sir William Osler's statement: "The greater the ignorance, the greater the dogmatism."

The somatoform disorders by definition require that no organic cause exist to account for the severity of the discomfort, distress, or pain associated with a particular symptom. Given the subjective nature of sensation and symptom reporting, it is often not possible to prove that no organic cause exists for a particular symptom. Therefore, physicians will need to rely primarily on their clinical judgment rather than on laboratory tests and radiological procedures.

This chapter has presented in detail a clinical "feel" for the patient with each of the three disorders so as to give the physician greater confidence and tools with which to make diagnostic and treatment decisions.

The art of clinical medicine is best tested on the battlefield where ambiguity exists. Armed with empathy, respect, and a knowledge of the complexity of soma-psyche relationships and the limitations of medical science, the clinician can engage the somatoform patient in collaboration rather than confrontation, resulting in reduced somatization and increased patient-physician satisfaction.

REFERENCES

Agras S. (1969). The epidemiology of common fears and phobia. *Comprehensive Psychiatry, 10*, 151–156.

American Psychiatric Association. (1994). *Diagnostic and statistical manual of mental disorders* (4th ed.). Washington, DC.: Author.

Aronowitz, B., Hollander, E., Simeon, D., & Cohen, L. J. (1995). A survey of plastic surgery patients. *Proceedings of the 148th Annual Meeting of the American Psychiatric Association, 33*, pp. 74–75. Washington, DC: American Psychiatric Association.

Barsky, A. J., Wyshak, G., Klerman, G. L., & Latham, K. S. (1990). The prevalence of hypochondriasis in medical outpatients. *Social Psychiatry Psychiatric Epidemiology, 25*, 89–94.

Barsky, A. J. (1991). Hypochondriacal patients, their physicians, and their medical care. *Journal of General Internal Medicine, 6*, 413–419.

Benson, R. C., Hanson, K. H., & Matarazzo, J. D. (1959). Atypical pelvic pain in women: Gynecologic-psychiatric considerations. *American Journal of Obstetrics and Gynecology, 77*, 806–825.

Cantor, C., & Fallon, B. A. (1996). *Phantom illness: Shattering the myth of hypochondria*. Boston: Houghton Mifflin.

deGruy F. (1987). Somatization disorder in a university hospital. *Journal of Family Practice, 25*, 579–584.

Escobar, J. I., Rubio-Stipec, M., Canino, G., & Karno, M. (1989). Somatic symptom index (SSI): A new and abridged somatization construct. *Journal of Nervous and Mental Disease, 177*, 140–146.

Fallon, B. A., Liebowitz M. R., Salman, E., Schneier, F. R., Jusino, C., Hollander, E., & Klein, D. F. (1993). Fluoxetine for hypochondriacal patients without major depression. *Journal of Clinical Psychopharmacology, 13*, 438–441.

Glass, R., Uhlenhuth, E. H., & Kellner, R. (1987). The value of self-report assessment in studies of anxiety disorders. *Journal of Clinical Psychopharmacology, 7*, 74–75

Gramling, S. E., Clawson, E. P., & McDonald, K. (1996). *Perceptual and cognitive abnormality model of hypochondriasis: Amplification and physiological reactivity in women. Psychosomatic Medicine, 58*, 423–431.

Hollander, E., Simeon, D., Cohen, L. J., & Aronowitz, B. (1995). Overview and psychopharmacology of body dysmorphic disorder. *Proceedings of the 148th Annual Meeting of the American Psychiatric Association, 33*, p. 74. Washington, DC: American Psychiatric Association.

Kashner, T. M., Rost, K., Cohen, B., Anderson, M., & Smith, G. R., Jr. (1995). Enhancing the health of somatization disorder patients. *Psychosomatics, 36*, 462–470.

Kellner, R. (1986). *Somatization and hypochondriasis.* New York: Praeger.

———. (1987). *Abridged manual of the illness attitude scales.* Albuquerque: Author. This publication is available free of charge from the Department of Psychiatry, School of Medicine, 2400 Tucker NE, Albuquerque, NM 87131.

Kirmayer, L. J., Robbins, J. M., Dworkind, M., & Yaffe, M. J. (1993). Somatization and the recognition of depression and anxiety in primary care. *American Journal of Psychiatry, 150*, 734–741.

Phillips, K. A. (1996). *The broken mirror: Understanding and treating body dysmorphic disorder.* New York: Oxford University Press.

Phillips, K. A., Gunderson, C. G., McElroy, S. L., Mallya, G. K., & Carter, W. P. (1995). A comparison study of Body Dysmorphic Disorder and OCD (New Research Abstract No. 374). *Proceedings of the 148th Annual Meeting of the American Psychiatric Association, 33*, 156–157. Washington, DC: American Psychiatric Association.

Phillips, K. A., McElroy, S. L., & Keck, P. E. (1993). Body dysmorphic disorder: 30 cases of imagined ugliness. *American Journal Psychiatry, 150*, 302–308.

———. (1994). A comparison of delusional and nondelusional body dysmorphic disorder in 100 cases. *Psychopharmacology Bulletin, 30*, 179–186.

Pilowsky, I. (1967). Dimensions of hypochondriasis. *British Journal of Psychiatry, 113*, 89–93.

Pilowsky, I., & Spence, N. D. (1983). *Manual for the illness behavior questionnaire (IBQ)* (2nd ed.). Adelaide, Australia: Author. Available from Professor I. Pilowsky, University of Adelaide, Department of Psychiatry, Adelaide, Australia 5000.

Robins, L. N., Helzer, J. E., Weissman, M. M., Orvaschel, H., Gruenberg, E., Burke, J. D., Jr., & Regier, D. A. (1984). Lifetime prevalence of specific psychiatric disorders in three sites. *Archives of General Psychiatry, 41*, 949–958.

Rosen, J. C., & Reiter, J. (1996). Development of the body dysmorphic disorder examination. *Behavior Research and Therapy, 34*, 755–766.

Sheehan, D. V., Ballenger, J., & Jacobsen, G. (1980). Treatment of endogenous anxiety with phobic, hysterical, and hypochondriacal symptoms. *Archives of General Psychiatry, 37*, 51–59.

Simeon, D., Hollander, E., Stein, D. J., Cohen, L. J., & Aronowitz, B. (1996). Body dysmorphic disorder in the *DSM-IV* OCD field trial. *Proceedings of the 148th Annual Meeting of the American Psychiatric Association, 33*, 74. Washington, DC: American Psychiatric Association.

Smith, G. R., Monson, R. A., & Ray, D. C. (1986). Psychiatric consultation in somatization disorders: A randomized controlled study. *New England Journal of Medicine, 314*, 1407–1413.

Spitzer, R. L. Williams, J. B. W., Kroenke, K., Linzer, M., & deGruy, F. V. (1994). Utility of a new procedure for diagnosing mental disorders in primary care: The PRIME-MD 1000 Study. *Journal of the American Medical Association, 272*, 1749–1756.

van Hemert, A. M. (1993). Psychiatric disorders in relation to medical illness among patients of a general medical out-patient clinic. *Psychological Medicine, 23*, 167–173.

Wise, T. N., Cooper, J. N., & Ahmed, S. (1982). The efficacy of group therapy for patients with irritable bowel syndrome. *Psychosomatics, 23*, 465–469.

CHAPTER 7

Violence and Suicide

Robert E. Feinstein

Patients exhibiting violent or suicidal behavior suffer with dangerous psychiatric symptoms expressed as feelings, thoughts, fantasies, or destructive behaviors. These symptoms do not arise from a specific physical disease, although they may arise from feelings of depression or hopelessness associated with serious illness. The intensity of violent or suicidal symptoms and behaviors varies along a spectrum of risk ranging from minimal to potentially fatal.

Clinical work with high-risk patients is often anxiety-provoking and extremely challenging. To recognize violent and suicidal patients and to understand, manage, and briefly treat them, the primary care clinician needs a specific biopsychosocial approach that assesses dangers, avoids harmful or fatal consequences, and organizes effective treatment.

DEFINITIONS OF VIOLENCE AND SUICIDE

Violence can be defined operationally as the use of verbal threat or actual physical force with the intent of causing intimidation, harm, injury, or death to individuals or causing property damage. Violence may be considered worthy of medical/psychiatric treatment when it is clearly related to biological or genetic factors, to psychiatric illnesses, or to social problems such as domestic abuse. Violence as a focus of medical/psychiatric intervention and treatment should be distinguished from crime, homicides, or institutionalized violence such as war or terrorism that are undertaken as a matter of rational choice.

Suicidal ideation is clinically defined as the conscious thought or unconscious wish to kill oneself as a solution to life's pain or problems. Although there is a popular euthanasia or "a rational decision to die" movement, 95% of suicidal patients have some form of psychiatric illness (Robbins, Murphy, & Wilkinson, 1959). Compared to suicidal ideation from psychiatric illness, the rational decision to die is a very infrequent occurrence. Understanding the psychodynamics of suicidal thoughts, feelings, and behaviors is crucial for assessing suicide risk, preventing suicide, and facilitating treatment of suicidal symptoms.

EPIDEMIOLOGY

Violence and suicide are major public health problems whose true magnitude may be impossible to estimate. Incidence and prevalence data vary widely because violent and suicidal behaviors are often defined differently in different contexts. Law enforcement, for example, reports violence differently than the medical community. Even if accurate figures with the same definitions were available, the true magnitude of these problems would probably still be underestimated. This is because many episodes of violence and suicide are never reported and because deaths reported as accidents may be covert suicides or homicides. In assessing the incidence and prevalence of these symptoms, the clinician should be aware of these limitations in the data.

Epidemiology of Violence

Over six million Americans are the victims of violent crime every year, and statistics on the nature and incidence of this violence are generally available from police and health care sources. Police crime statistics, which are forwarded to and compiled by the Federal Bureau of Investigation, are the most accurate and detailed.

Epidemiology of Suicide

Suicide is the eighth leading cause of death in the United States, with approximately 12 suicides/100,000 population. This totals approximately

30,000 successful suicides annually. Suicide is the second leading cause of death in people under the age of 35. There is a 10:1 ratio of suicide attempts versus completed suicides, with men completing suicide three times as often as women and women attempting suicide 10 times as frequently as men.

Suicide occurs in all age groups. The incidence of suicide peaks for both sexes between the ages of 15 and 19, and thereafter, rates return to baseline for both sexes. Suicide rates in women remain at baseline until they rise to a second, greater peak between ages 45 to 55, after which rates return to baseline. Men show a steady increase in suicide rates from ages 45 to 80, after which the rate starts to decline.

ASSESSING AND PREVENTING RISK OF IMMEDIATE HARM

In most instances, clinicians evaluate patients for risk of violent and suicidal behavior only after they have either expressed homicidal or suicidal ideation, have committed a violent act, are a victim of domestic violence, or have made a suicidal gesture. However, whenever possible, all contacts with a patient should involve behavioral observations to protect both the patient and the clinician from acute risk and immediate harm.

The risk of encountering a violent or otherwise dangerous patient exists in many primary care settings, including medical emergency rooms, intensive care units, general hospital floors, nursing homes, public health clinics, and urban practice setting where substance abuse and crime are prevalent. Physicians should make a special effort, as should other personnel in the practice, to observe patients at their point of entry or in an open waiting area to limit the risk of encountering a violent patient in a closed office space.

Identifying risk factors for violence is always a primary care issue. Patients can be observed for hygiene, signs of obvious trauma, intoxication, agitation, social interactions, and their level of physical activity. There are generally five levels of activity that patients display that indicate increasing risk of acute danger to others or themselves. These are the calm phase, the psychomotor agitation phase, the verbal phase, the acting-out phase, and the post-acting-out phase. The primary care clinician and the office staff should be alert to these behaviors for their own protection and that of the patient.

Calm Phase

Patients are at the lowest level of immediate risk for dangerous behaviors when they appear calm, maintain a level of good self-care, are alert and fully conscious, have no visible signs of physical trauma, and engage in normal social interactions. These patients typically sit quietly and comfortably in the waiting area and appear at ease, perhaps reading a magazine or engaged in normal waiting room conversations.

Psychomotor Agitation Phase

Patients are at a slightly greater risk for violent or suicidal actions as their level of physical movement increases. Psychomotor agitation is characterized by an increase in such physical activity as tapping the feet, leafing rapidly through a magazine, compulsive smoking, pacing, and so forth. Physically hyperactive patients may also be psychologically agitated. Such patients often experience anxiety, diffuse uneasiness, increased tension, or confusion.

Patients in the psychomotor agitation phase should be approached with a supportive attitude. Remarks such as "How can I help?" "You seem a bit upset," or "Is there some way I can help you?" may calm a patient so that the clinical interview can begin. Offering food or juice, when medically acceptable, may also be effective to prevent an escalation to a more dangerous phase.

Imminent Violence Risk

Patients prone to violence typically show approach-avoidance behavior similar to that of a lion preparing to attack. Patients may approach the office staff with a hypervigilant or paranoid glare and then walk away. Increases in the frequency and intensity of such behaviors are often the cardinal sign of imminent violence. To prevent possible violence, patients exhibiting such behavior should be searched for weapons with the assistance of security personnel or the police. These patients need constant observation, and some may need to have physical restraints applied. The patient may require antianxiety or antipsychotic medication to decrease agitation.

Imminent Suicidal Risk

Agitated patients who are imminently suicidal may give clues to impending suicidal actions. A sudden increase in impulsive behaviors, conflicting and ambivalent statements about suicide, a general evasiveness, or opposition to acute treatment recommendations should raise suspicion of suicidal intent. Additional nonverbal clues suggesting suicidal thoughts include appearing mute, sad, or depressed; avoiding eye contact; or sitting in an isolated location as if to shun other people. Alert clinicians will quickly pick up on these signals from the patient, avoid leaving the patient alone, and immediately escort the patient to a safe environment such as an emergency room.

Most suicidal patients will need observation for hours and should be searched for pills, razor blades, knives, and other weapons and have belts and shoes removed as part of an acute suicide prevention. Antianxiety or antipsychotic medication may be administered to decrease agitation. Sometimes, physical restraints are necessary to prevent wrist slashing or self-mutilation.

Verbal Phase

Violence Risk

Patients who progress from the psychomotor agitation to the verbal phase have an increased risk of imminent violence. The verbal phase begins as language is added to actions.

In the early verbal phase, patients may question authority and progress to demands. Typical questions may include "How much longer do I have to wait?" "What's taking so long?" and "Who's in charge?" The clinician often can manage these demands with a supportive, caring, interested attitude. Potentially violent patients can be directed to take a "time out," spending a few minutes of quiet time to think things over. Offers of cool liquids to drink or medication may assist in diffusing potential violence in the early verbal phase.

Some violent patients escalate into a later verbal phase, when they begin cursing and shouting and approach-avoidance behaviors markedly increase. These preattack behaviors are warning "If you don't do something quickly, I will go out of control." Intervening with such a patient should always have safety in mind. If a patient makes a clinician feel frightened or threatened, he or she should leave the area and return with both security personnel and additional psychiatric support staff, if necessary. Supportive verbal interventions generally are not effective at this late verbal stage; however, directive, short verbal statements may help establish control without posing a threat. For example, command "Calm down! Sit down! Tell me what is bothering you."

When speaking with a patient who is almost out of control, remain at a safe distance of at least one-and-a-half leg lengths. To appear less threatening, adopt a slumping posture and turn to the side with hands visible. In other circumstances, use of counterprojective statements can be very effective at diffusing violence. These are statements with three components: They focus a patient's intense affect, typically anger, "out there," away from the physician; they call attention to others not present who may have caused the patient's anger; and they express the patient's feelings about the problematic situation. For example, a physician could say to a patient in handcuffs who is cursing, "You're pissed off at the police, enraged, caged, and feeling helpless. Let's try to figure out this mess together. If you stay calm and talk with me, we will be able to remove the handcuffs." If agitation cannot be controlled by verbal means, it may be necessary to use a show of force, involuntary medication, or restraint.

Suicidal Risk

Patients who are imminently suicidal may or may not proceed through a verbal phase. Suicidal patients who are on drugs or who are suffering with agitated depression or a personality disorder may be talkative, loud, and threatening suicide. These patients are generally managed as described for the violent patient. There are, however, many suicidal patients who are quiet, withdrawn, or secretive about their suicidal feelings. A careful clinician who suspects a patient of suicidal ideation should ask directly, "Are you thinking of hurting or killing yourself?" Most patients will be reassured by this inquiry and may nod yes or begin to talk. If you are unsure of a patient's suicidal risk, it is safest to place the patient under the constant observation of family members while the patient obtains outpatient psychiatric treatment. If this is not possible or practical, the patient should be referred immediately for constant psychiatric observation in an emergency room or psychiatric facility.

Acting-Out Phase

The behavior of some patients continues to escalate into either impulsive violent episodes or suicidal acts. In such situations, it is usually imperative to use physical restraint protocols and pharmacological interventions. The therapeutic goal of a restraint is to help patients regain control of their aggressive impulses. Restraints are usually applied by specially trained personnel, optimally four staff members, who know how to use restraints and medication as part of a therapeutic encounter. However, anyone can apply restraints if the need arises and specially trained personnel are not available. Specific medication may be administered that targets the underlying cause of acting out, such as haloperidol for psychosis or lorazepam for anxiety or alcohol withdrawal.

Post-Acting-Out Phase

After a violent episode or a suicide attempt, most patients feel guilty about losing control, fear punishment or retaliation in the immediate future, or experience a loss of self-esteem. Patients may need to be reminded that restraint or medication was part of a therapeutic encounter used to help them regain self-control. Reassuring the patient that there will be no future punishment or retaliation alleviates the patient's fears and decreases the chance of a repeat episode. It also may prevent the patient from developing a grudge against the clinician or a particular staff member. Appropriately timed and graduated release from restraints helps restore dignity and improves self-esteem. It is extremely important to review the episode with the patient a few hours later, discuss the patient's embarrassment or shame about losing control, and make specific plans to prevent future episodes.

THE CLINICAL APPROACH

A patient with acute violent or suicidal impulses suffers with a turbulent emotional crisis that has left him or her fragile, volatile, and with a desire to take action. It is important to remind both yourself and the patient that the main purpose of the interview is to understand what is driving the patient to desperation. This inquiry can only begin after acute harm prevention has established a safe environment for both the frightened patient and the apprehensive clinician.

Once a safe environment has been established, the interview can begin by inquiring about acute precipitants of the violent or suicidal impulses. It is important to pay special attention to the meaning and sequence of events over the last 6 weeks that have led up to the present situation. Selected exploration of earlier life events may help deepen your understanding of the current problem.

A suicidal patient may feel that his or her situation is hopeless and that he or she is helpless to change it, or the patient may use suicide threats as a means of manipulating a situation he or she feels unable to change. Such a patient can elicit rescue fantasies in the physician or, conversely, feelings of anger at the patient and even the wish that the patient will die or succeed in a suicide attempt.

A violent patient is often irritable, angry, and impatient and may use threats of violence to gain control. Common physician countertransferences with such a patient include a desire for revenge, excessive anger, hate, moralizing, or retaliation. In dealing with both suicidal and violent patients, the physician needs to avoid struggles over power, realizing that patients often feel weak, humiliated, or demeaned. The physician also should avoid the traps of moralizing or hating these patients, seeking revenge or the urge to punish. While maintaining a safe physical distance, the physician should try to form an alliance with the part of the patient that is looking for help in regulating and working through his or her anger and violent or suicidal potential. Helpful patient management strategies can be directing the patient to calm down, asking for time out, using medication as necessary, or using counterprojective statements.

If this individual approach is not helpful, it may be useful to interview the patient's family or support network. The crisis and family approaches are described in chapters 17 and 18, respectively.

RISK ASSESSMENT

It is not possible to predict over a long period of time when, where, how, or with whom future dangerous events may occur. However, researchers can predict short-term probability, from hours to weeks, in special populations. Collective clinical wisdom suggests that there are many variables that can be evaluated to assess danger over a short time span. Table 7.1 is a validated published version of the Violence and Suicide Assessment (VASA) scale. The major components of safe management of violent and suicidal symptoms are the variables enumerated in the VASA scale and additional clinical factors, such as psychiatric diagnosis, neurological and medical evaluations, and psychodynamic considerations.

Ideation

Violent or suicidal ideation can be conceptualized as a spectrum of probability of danger ranging from higher to lower risk.

Spectrum of Homicidal Ideation

An intense desire to kill or hurt a specific person is the highest risk violent ideation and suggests a high probability of imminent violence. For example, a high-risk patient is a spouse abuser who wishes to intimidate his wife or a drug dealer who seeks revenge against another dealer. Patients with command hallucinations ("voices"), delusions about killing or hurting someone, or impulsive thoughts of violence are also experiencing high-risk violent ideation.

On the spectrum, lower risk violent ideation may be a nonspecific wish to hurt or kill. For example, a patient who wants to kill all homosexuals or AIDS patients may be at moderate risk of violence. Ambivalent wishes to hurt someone or damage objects or nonspecific feelings of hostility may carry lesser risks. Patients who have no thoughts of violence or homicide have the lowest risk of short-term violence.

Spectrum of Suicidal Ideation

The wish to hurt or kill oneself can be deliberate and planned, ambivalent, or have the character of fleeting thoughts or fantasies. An intense wish to kill oneself as a specific solution to a specific problem suggests high risk. An example of a patient with high-risk ideation is one who has the means (e.g., a gun) and a plan to kill himself or herself in order to get out of serious debt and leave his or her family with life insurance. Patients who are suicidal, psychotic, or delusional and are responding to command hallucinations (e.g., voices commanding him or her to "die") are at the highest risk. Patients without plans who are ambivalent about hurting themselves may have a smaller risk. There is a low risk of suicide when a patient expresses no suicidal thoughts or fantasies.

History

When a patient's thoughts about violence or suicide progress to actions, the risk of loss of life increases. The clinician should examine recent events—those actions or events that have occurred within weeks—that may predispose a patient to future risk of suicide.

Recent Violent Behaviors

Violent behaviors may be impulsive or they may be deliberately planned. These behaviors typically have a specific external trigger or internal pre-

Table 7.1 Violence and Suicide Assessment (VASA) Scale

Score	Item
Current violent thoughts (during the interview)	
4	Expresses an intense wish to kill someone specific
3	Reveals command hallucinations to injure someone
2	Expresses ambivalent wish to kill someone specific
1	Expresses nonspecific feelings of rage and belligerence
0	Reveals no homicidal ideas
Recent violent behaviors (during the past several weeks)	
4	Showed serious assaultive behavior (e.g., tried to strangle, stab, or shoot someone)
3	Beat up someone badly (e.g., broke bones or required hospitalization)
2	Slapped or pushed or punched someone (no serious outcomes)
1	Broke things in the house or elsewhere
0	Showed good control over his or her behavior
Past history of violent/antisocial/disruptive behaviors (lifetime history)	
4	Has committed violent acts in the past (e.g., has beaten up people)
4	Has been arrested for assaultive behavior
3	Carries weapons (e.g., knife, gun, chain, razor)
3	Has access to weapons
2	Has been arrested for automobile infractions
2	Has a criminal record
2	Chronic problems with authority (e.g., truancy, running away from home, family fights)
2	Has a history of impulsive/unpredictable behavior (e.g., loses temper, overeats, promiscuity)
2	Frequent changes in living situation as a child
0	Has no past history of violence
Current suicidal thoughts (during interview)	
4	Expresses an intense will to kill self and has made a plan
4	Reveals psychotic or delusional ideation or hallucinations to kill or injure self
3	Expresses an intense wish to kill self but has made no plan
2	Expresses ambivalent wishes to kill self
0	Reveals no suicidal ideas
Recent suicidal behaviors (during the past several weeks)	
4	Made a serious suicide attempt (e.g., tried to kill self by gunshot, ingestion, hanging, or jumping)
3	Made a suicidal gesture (e.g., superficially cut wrist or ingested two pills)
3	Made a specific suicide plan
3	Attempt made with little chance of discovery by others
2	Had no interest or hope for the future
0	Has no suicidal plans or attempts

Past history of suicide (lifetime history)

4 Mother, father, or sibling has committed suicide or made a suicide attempt
3 Has or had a diagnosis of major affective disorder or psychosis
3 Has made one or more previous suicide attempts
2 Current attempt is an "anniversary" reaction
2 Has a serious medical illness or disability
0 Has no past history of suicidal ideas or attempts

Support systems/stresses

3 No family, friends, social agency, or psychiatrist available
2 Has tenuous connection with family, friends, social agency, or psychiatrist
2 Has had many recent life stresses (e.g., job, family, children, health)
1 Has a family that is marginally willing or able to help
0 Has a family strongly committed and able to help

Ability to cooperate

3 Refuses to cooperate with interview and treatment plan
2 Unable to cooperate with interview and treatment plan
1 Wants help but motivation weak
0 Actively seeks treatment; willing and able to cooperate

Substance abuse

3 Is intoxicated
3 Is in withdrawal
3 Is a compulsive long-term drug abuser (includes alcohol or other drugs)
2 Is an occasional drug abuser (alcohol or other drugs)
0 No abuse of any drugs

Reactions during interview

4 Assaultive behavior against a person (or object) in the environment
3 Challenges authority (e.g., curses, yells, screams)
2 Shows approach-avoidance behavior toward interviewer
1 Shows motoric activity (e.g., pacing, smoking, fidgeting)
1 Seems very impatient
0 Calm, seated, responsive to questions.

Scoring: >11 consider admission or extensive outpatient plan
<11 considered less risk, outpatient treatment recommended

Souce: Reprinted with permission. Feinstein, R., & Plutchik, R. (1990) Suicide and violence risk assessment in the psychiatric emergency room. *Comprehensive Psychiatry, 31*(4), p. 339. W. B. Saunders.

cipitant. An example of an external trigger could be a woman's failure to immediately attend to her partner's needs, which may trigger an episode of domestic abuse. An internal precipitant could be an angry thought or fantasy. Assessment of recent violence involves uncovering a specific pattern or sequence of events that culminate in violence.

> Patrick was chronically suspicious that his wife was having an affair. When he saw his wife talking to a neighbor, he accused her of inviting the neighbor into the house. When she denied this, he beat her and said, "Does it give you that much pleasure to humiliate me?"

Recognizing a pattern of domestic abuse or the sequence of events that precipitate episodic violence can help prevent future violence.

The nature and specific kind of recent violent behaviors can also be conceptualized as a spectrum of events, from higher to lower probability, for repeated violence within the next several weeks. Those patients who have committed a recent impulsive or planned assault with weapons have the highest risk for imminent, lethal violence. Patients who are impulsive, who demonstrate a pattern of domestic violence, or who have committed a planned physical assault without weapons that have caused physical injuries also have a very high probability for new outbreaks of violence. Recent impulsive, nonphysically damaging assaults, such as slapping, pushing, or hitting, probably carry a moderate risk for future violence. Patients who have damaged property but have never hurt a person have less of a probability for future violence against others. Those patients who are verbally abusive or use threatening language, because they have not yet crossed the boundary from words to actions, may have less risk for future physical violence. If a patient is not impulsive and shows normal social interactions, there is less risk of imminent violence.

Suicidal Behavior

There is a spectrum of recent suicidal events or behaviors that correlate with the degree of imminent danger. For example, a spectrum of suicidal behaviors from highest risk to a lower future probability of suicide might include (1) a serious suicide attempt by lethal means (e.g., gunshot, ingestion, hanging, jumping, or a specific suicide plan); (2) a suicide attempt made with little chance of discovery; (3) a suicidal gesture (e.g., superficial cutting of the wrists or minor ingestion of small amounts of pills) with a great likelihood of being discovered; (4) suicide notes or nonverbal suicide messages, such as writing a will, giving away prized possessions, or purchasing a hand gun; or (5) changing attitudes toward life and death, such as a sudden change in religious practices or beliefs.

While there may be a spectrum of recent behaviors and events that pose a greater risk for suicide than others, from a clinical point of view, all suicidal behavior should be taken seriously and receive prompt evaluation and treatment.

Past History

Past history may be the best single predictor of imminent dangerous acts. However, past events offer little information about the timing of a future episode.

Lifetime Patterns of Violent Behaviors or Events

A detailed history of a patient's lifetime pattern of violence is essential for the understanding and treatment of imminent violence. The precipitants of past violent episodes and the intensity, frequency, nature, and context of the violence deserve special inquiry. Patients who have learned to use violence as a method of coping will continue to use violence to solve problems in the future.

> George would begin cursing, threatening, and beating his wife whenever she did not respond quickly to satisfy all of his wishes. The terror in this home allowed him to dominate his wife and control his children.

Past history that is associated with future violence includes a history of past arrests, a criminal record, automobile infractions, and involvement in frequent legal proceedings. A childhood history of disruptive changes in caretakers, child abuse, domestic violence, cruelty to animals, or an adolescent history of problems with authority (e.g., truancy, running away, or losing one's temper), sexual promiscuity, premenstrual syndromes, and overeating are also associated with increased risk for imminent violence.

Lifetime Patterns of Suicidal Behaviors or Events

An understanding of the past precipitants, lethality, means, motives, frequency, timing, and the nature and context of prior suicide attempts will help the clinician assess short-term suicidal risk. Additional past history that may also be associated with future suicidal risk includes depression, alcoholism, prior suicide attempts, anniversary reactions, previous psychiatric admissions, loss history (e.g., losses from deaths, divorce, separations, or finances), severe physical impairment, disability, serious chronic medical illness, or a family history of suicidal behaviors.

Support Systems

A support system comprises the social network in which a patient lives. It consists of family, relatives, friends, religious groups, community organizations, and the health care and social welfare systems. In general, the larger, more stable, and helpful a support system, the greater the buffers it provides against stresses that produce violent or suicidal symptoms. The strongest of social networks, such as closely knit families or religious communities, can be so helpful that no member of the group is ever suicidal or violent. In contrast, a patient without a network of family or friends is at higher risk for violent or suicidal behavior.

When evaluating the strength of a patient's network, the physician should assess the competence, interest, and availability of the support system. A *competent* support network can help the patient directly in the resolution of violent or suicidal symptoms. This help could be emotional, psychological, intellectual, legal, or financial. An *interested* network has a personal investment in the patient's welfare. Sometimes family members feel used up or are angry at the patient and are not willing to help. If they cannot be enlisted in treatment, a different support network must be sought.

Support networks must also be *available*. Sometimes, family work schedules or child care demands make the family practically unavailable to help a patient. It is vital that a family be continually available if they are to serve as a network for a suicide watch or as a buffer against violence. When the patient's network has problems with either competence, interest, or availability, the patient is at increased risk for recurring suicidal or violent behavior. Under these circumstances, a new support system such as a crisis service, social service agency, or hospital must be sought to facilitate safe treatment.

Medical and Neurological Evaluation

Every suicidal or violent patient or victim of domestic abuse should undergo a medical and neurological evaluation to determine if there are medical illnesses that are contributing to, exacerbating, or causing the symptoms. Medical illness associated with increased risk of suicide includes chronic diseases such as diabetes, renal dialysis, AIDS, or chronic obstructive pulmonary disease. Medical illnesses causing depression, such as thyroid disease and drug abuse, also increase the risk of suicide. Common medical illnesses that may be associated with violence include mental retardation, traumatic brain injury, delirium, dementia, seizures, and drug abuse.

Psychiatric Differential Diagnosis

Violence

The potential for violence is greatest when the patient is either intoxicated or in withdrawal from alcohol or other drugs. Alcohol reduces inhibitions and is strongly associated with all forms of violence. Cocaine intoxication frequently leads to impulsiveness, paranoia, and grandiose delusions with poor judgment and an increased potential for violence. Use of phencyclidine (PCP/angel dust) is associated both with aggression and retrograde amnesia for the violent events. Withdrawal syndromes such as alcohol delirium tremens and opiate or nicotine withdrawal can lead to uncharacteristic expressions of anger and belligerence.

Disorders causing brain damage are commonly associated with violence. Each year in the United States there are approximately 1 million cases of new brain injury caused by trauma, strokes, and tumors. Approximately 70% of people with traumatic brain injury develop irritability and aggressiveness within months of their injury. Twenty-five percent of all nursing home patients are agitated or aggressive in association with dementias such as Alzheimer's disease and multi-infarct dementias. Mentally retarded patients also show an increased chance of violence compared to patients with other psychiatric diagnoses. In addition, some authors report an association between partial-complex seizures and violence.

Patients suffering from manic behavior are the most likely to become assaultive because of their tendency to be irritable, labile, and impulsive. Psychotic patients who have paranoid symptoms or delusions or psychotic command hallucinations are also at risk for violence. In addition, patients suffering from posttraumatic stress disorder or from antisocial or borderline personality disorders have an increased likelihood of becoming aggressive than the general population.

Suicide

The causes of suicidal ideation and behavior are multifactorial; however, they are frequently associated with psychiatric conditions. The most common diagnosis associated with suicidal ideation or behaviors is depressed mood or depression. Depression and feelings of hopelessness are major risk factors for completed suicide, and the greatest risk of suicide occurs when a patient is recovering from depression.

Recent work indicates that patients suffering from major depression in conjunction with other psychiatric disorders are at increased risk of suicidal behavior. Anxiety or panic disorder, in combination with depression and substance abuse, has been reported to increase the likelihood of suicidal behaviors (Henriksson et al., 1996). Ten percent to 25% of patients with significant suicidal risk also carry a diagnosis of alcohol abuse, intoxication, or withdrawal. Ten percent to 20% of patients who have suicidal risk carry a diagnosis of schizophrenia. Less frequent diagnoses associated with suicide risk include borderline, histrionic, and antisocial personality disorders. Patients who have multiple diagnoses associated with suicide, such as a severe personality disorder and substance abuse, have the very highest risk for suicidal behaviors.

Ability to Cooperate With Treatment

In working with patients at high risk for violence or suicide, it is important to attempt to assess the patient's motivation and ability to cooperate with treatment and to adhere to a treatment plan. Those patients who either refuse or are unable to cooperate with treatment often need to be hospitalized. Violent and suicidal patients should be asked to demonstrate their ability and willingness to cooperate with treatment. For example, a clinician can ask such a patient to take the first dose of a medication or to call to arrange a psychiatric appointment while in the clinician's presence. Violent or suicidal patients who do not demonstrate high motivation and ability to adhere to treatment should be managed conservatively with consultation for an acute voluntary hospitalization, or when indicated, commitment.

Role of Substance Abuse

The association between drug abuse and all forms of violent and suicidal behavior is exceedingly high. The U.S. Department of Justice estimates that 33% of prisoners were under the influence of drugs at the time of their violent offense. Substance abuse can act as a trigger for suicide and is the most frequent comorbid condition associated with suicide completions and attempts (Moscicki, 1997). Some experts on incest believe that many acts of father-daughter incest are committed while the father is intoxicated with alcohol (Van der Kolk, 1987).

Drug abuse produces violent or suicidal behaviors because of pharmacologically induced changes in a patient's physiological, cognitive, and emotional state. Patients at acute risk for violence or suicide who are actively abusing drugs must be managed with extreme caution. Intoxicated patients or patients who are showing any signs of drug withdrawal should be held in a medical setting until the intoxication or withdrawal symptoms have completely resolved. It is also likely that compulsive drug abusers are at greater risk for violence and suicide than intermittent or recreational drug abusers. Although abuse of any drug probably increases the risk of violence or suicide, drugs such as PCP, cocaine, narcotics, and alcohol are more likely to produce dangerous behaviors than are other abused drugs, such as marijuana and diazepam.

Subjective Experiences During the Interview

When interviewing violent or suicidal patients, the clinician may sense that the patient is in imminent danger of harming himself or herself or others. Such subjective, nonspecific reactions in the clinician are typically elicited by patient behaviors, such as an increase in the patient's physical activity level, frustration or impatience, challenges to the clinician's authority, or approach-avoidance behaviors. These subjective reactions of the clinician are clinically important and should serve as prompts that an evaluation needs to be performed before the patient can be safely discharged.

Psychodynamic Variables

Problems in reality testing are manifested as hallucinations, delusions, depersonalization, derealizations, mini-psychotic breaks, or massive confusion. Patients who have these problems in reality testing, and those with certain defensive styles and maladaptive coping mechanisms, may be predisposed to an increased risk for violent or suicidal behavior. Patients who are intoxicated or who have severe personality disorders may also suffer a loss of reality. Deficits in the perception of reality increase the likelihood for suicidal or violent symptoms.

Apter and colleagues (1989) have suggested that the defense mechanisms of projection and displacement are associated with violence, whereas repression and regression are associated with suicidal tendencies. Many psychoanalysts believe that the primitive defenses of acting out, denial, splitting defenses, and projective identification can also contribute to both violent and suicidal tendencies. Patients who extensively use these defenses are probably at greater risk for suicidal or homicidal impulses.

Violent or suicidal symptoms also appear when a habitual coping style fails and a patient feels that he or she has no alternative way to cope with an overwhelming problem. Also, suicidal or violent behaviors can become a pathological coping style in patients with severe psychopathology, as is commonly seen in domestic abusers.

ETIOLOGY

Violent and suicidal symptoms are seen across all levels of psychopathology and are reported in all cultures. They are often associated with a psychiatric diagnosis but may emerge under many different life circumstances.

Neurobiological research into violent and suicidal symptoms has focused on measurements of the metabolites of serotonin (either 5-hydroxytryptamine [5-HT] or its metabolite, 5-hydroxyindoleacetic acid [5-HIAA]) in the blood, in cerebrospinal fluid, or by measuring low 5-HT receptors or an increase in 5-HT2 receptors on platelets or in brain tissue. Measurements at many different sites often identify a relative serotonin deficiency as the biological underpinning for violent and suicidal impulses.

Violent and suicidal symptoms also can result from the interplay between the following psychosocial factors: (1) multilayered psychological conflicts often involving low self-esteem, a sense of powerlessness, and a lack of reality-based options; (2) current repetition of previous life traumas; (3) breaks in reality testing that are leading the patient toward psychosis; (4) pathological defenses and coping style for dealing with difficult life circumstances; and (5) symptoms within the family context that may signal a pathological form of communication or are the clue to deeper and more troubling family problems.

Violent and suicidal symptoms are exacerbated in patients from poorer socioeconomic classes and appear with greater frequency during economic prosperity or economic collapse. These symptoms are also influenced by cultural norms that support or condemn the use of violence or suicide as part of the common value system. Another controversial factor exacerbating such symptoms is the media's glamorizing of violence or suicide.

LEGAL ISSUES

The most important legal considerations when working with violent or suicidal patients are involuntary hospitalization (commitment), confidentiality, and "duty to warn" responsibilities. Laws may differ from state to state, although the basic legal concepts are similar.

Commitment

Patients can be involuntarily hospitalized when a physician or court finds that a patient meets two criteria: (1) a patient has a mental disorder, and (2) the patient is dangerous to himself or herself or others. Clinically, a patient can be committed if he or she has a psychiatric disorder and has attempted or is threatening violence or suicide. Many states have a broad definition of "dangerous" that also includes those who have a mental illness and impaired judgment such that they do not perceive the need for psychiatric treatment. This broad approach to dangerousness is applied to chronically ill individuals (e.g., patients with schizophrenia or manic depressive illness) who are psychotic and refusing help. A patient can be so mentally disabled that he or she cannot take care of such life-sustaining functions as eating, getting medical treatment, and avoiding freezing to death during cold weather. In most states, any physician can involuntarily detain a patient in an emergency room or by admission to a psychiatric facility. Patients can be held for days and sometimes weeks against their will.

Although it is common for "committed" patients to initially protest their involuntary hospitalization, most patients eventually appreciate the psychiatric help. Once committed, patients still retain all of their civil rights, including the right to manage their own money, the right to vote, and the right to make their own health care decisions. A committed patient can obtain a mental health lawyer at no charge and can request a court hearing if he or she disagrees with the need for involuntary hospitalization. At the court hearing, a judge decides on the release or continuation of the commitment.

After an involuntary acute hospital treatment of several days, most patients are no longer an immediate risk for dangerous behaviors. However, this does not always mean that the patient's illness has been sufficiently treated. This sometimes creates a bind for the physician, who legally may have to let the patient leave the hospital when in the physician's clinical judgment, the patient requires further treatment.

Confidentiality

In general, communications between a psychiatric patient and his or her therapist are confidential. This includes the psychiatric record and all communications about treatment. There are significant exceptions to this general rule that apply to patients who are violent or suicidal.

Violent or Homicidal Patients and the "Duty to Warn"

Physicians are generally excepted from confidentiality requirements when a patient is potentially violent or is threatening to commit violence or homicide. State laws in this area vary widely; however, California's Tarasoff Decision has become a national clinical standard in relationship to duty to warn.

The original case, *Tarasoff* v. *Regent of University of California*, resulted in a 1974 California Supreme Court decision that was revised by a 1976 ruling. In this case, a former lover of Tatania Tarasoff murdered her after confiding his intention to kill her to his University of California therapist. The court held the university and therapist guilty of "failure to warn" Tarasoff or her family that her life had been threatened by her former suitor. This case established a therapist's duty to warn a potential victim that his or her life is being threatened or endangered by a homicidal patient.

The 1976 ruling broadened the options available to clinicians for clinically managing the homicidal patient. Under this ruling, a clinician can warn potential victims but is not required to do so if he or she "uses reasonable care to protect the intended victim against danger." "Reasonable care" is interpreted to mean that a clinician must take action to prevent potential violence. Practically, this means a physician can hospitalize a violent patient or prescribe outpatient day hospital treatment, crisis intervention, or other intensive outpatient treatment. The clinician can warn all intended victims, suggest an order of protection to intended victims, involuntarily hospitalize the homicidal patient, or vigorously treat the patient in a day hospital. Whatever the planned intervention, it should be designed to decrease the potential for violence. The court's 1976 ruling about confidentiality with homicidal patients can be summarized as "Protective confidential privilege ends where the public peril begins."

Although *Tarasoff* v. *Regent of University of California* is a precedent-setting case, many states have no legal requirements or obligations for a duty to warn. Despite this, experienced clinicians tend to follow the Tarasoff guidelines, as they offer a safe clinical practice of warning and protecting others.

Confidentiality Exceptions With Suicidal Patients

A patient who is suicidal may attempt to put a clinician in a confidentiality bind by asking the clinician, prior to revealing suicidal feeling or intentions, "Are our conversations completely confidential?" This question should alert the clinician to the fact that the patient is probably suicidal and is trying to bind the physician, by a legalistic use of confidentiality, not to reveal suicidal intentions to family or friends. Because a physician may not be able to provide safe optimal care while maintaining confidentiality, a wise clinician might answer, "Our communications are generally confidential unless there is a danger to you or to someone you know. Under these circumstances, I cannot keep your intentions secret, because my first responsibility is to try to keep you and others alive." This will usually reassure most patients. It also frees the clinician to take whatever steps are necessary, including disclosing the suicidal intentions to family, friends, physicians, or others.

In most states, the law recognizes that a breach in confidentiality that reveals the suicidal or violent intentions of a patient may keep a patient alive. In these circumstances, protecting the life of the patient takes precedence over confidentiality.

TREATMENT

The treatment of violent or suicidal symptoms involves several factors. For example, the patient and clinician will need to make decisions about hospitalization versus outpatient care. The patient may need to be examined and medical illness ruled out as a cause of symptoms. Clinician and patient must consider acute pharmacological interventions and treatment that often integrate crisis intervention, systems theory, family treatment, and individual therapy.

Hospitalization

Violent or suicidal patients may need to be hospitalized for their own protection and that of others. A psychiatrist is often the clinician who makes the decision to hospitalize, but in most states any physician can hospitalize a violent or suicidal patient.

The decision to hospitalize is based on an assessment of risk factors. In general, the greater the risk factors for violent or suicidal behavior, the greater the need for hospitalization. Patients scoring higher than 11 on the VASA scale (refer back to Table 7.1) should be considered for treatment as an inpatient, whereas those scoring under 11 can often be treated in an intensive outpatient setting.

Common reasons for hospitalization include situations in which the patient poses severe danger to himself or herself or to others; is acutely dangerous, disorganized, or unable to care for himself or herself; or has poor social supports. Patients are often hospitalized when outpatient treatment has failed.

Patients can voluntarily request or accept inpatient hospitalization. Those who do so are more motivated for inpatient treatment and are often more easily engaged in their treatment than those who are involuntarily committed. However, it is not uncommon for an involuntary hospitalization to allow some treatment-refractory patients to engage in productive therapy. Hospitalization allows interventions such as the use of one-on-one, continuous supervision of patients, seclusion, restraints, and involuntary pharmacotherapy if the patient becomes newly dangerous to himself or herself or others.

Hospitalized patients typically undergo an extensive biopsychosocial evaluation that includes a psychiatric diagnosis; medical/neurological evaluation; assessments and treatment of occupational, family, and social support systems; and individual psychotherapy. Acute hospital care rarely lasts for more than 3 weeks.

Outpatient Treatment

Intensive outpatient treatment of violent and suicidal patients is also possible in a partial hospital program but should only be attempted when a clinician is very certain that the patient wants help and that the patient has a support network available that is capable of preventing harm to all concerned. In such cases, a specific contract should be negotiated with the patient and members of his or her support network that includes a plan for prevention that anticipates acute reemergence of violent or suicidal symptoms. A crisis intervention approach (see chapter 17), individual counseling (see chapter 16), and family approaches (see chapter 18) will tend to maximize safe outpatient treatment. A crisis practitioner who is able to provide home visits and who has ready access to the police in case of a new life-threatening situation can conduct daily outpatient sessions. There should also be provision for rapid, accessible psychiatric hospitalization should outpatient treatment fail (Table 7.2).

Acute Pharmacotherapy

Acute pharmacological interventions with violent and suicidal patients are geared toward establishing safety and calm. This generally is accomplished in an emergency room, in a general hospital setting, or in an acute inpatient psychiatric service.

The goal of acute pharmacological interventions is to have the acutely dangerous patient lightly sedated yet easily aroused. When possible, the medication chosen should be directed at the immediate causes of the symptoms. In situations in which a patient is actively violent or suicidal and the clinician has little or no information about the patient, restraints should be applied first. Every hospital has a specific restraint protocol. Restraint provides immediate safety for all involved and allows time for information gathering and a thoughtful choice of medication. If immediate pharmacotherapy is required, patients usually can be medicated safely with either haloperidol or lorazepam. Haloperidol is given as 2 to 5 mg PO/IM every half hour, with a maximum dose no greater than 30 mg in a 24-hour period. Alternatively, lorazepam, 1 to 2 mg PO/IM, may be given every half hour, rarely exceeding 20 mg in 24 hours.

Some clinicians choose to alternate low doses of haloperidol and lorazepam. This has the advantage of permitting lower doses of the antipsychotic medications, thereby decreasing the likelihood of unwanted side effects. However, alternating doses of different medications has the disadvantage of introducing polypharmacy in a patient who may already be abusing drugs or may be using prescribed medications of which the clinician is unaware.

When necessary, other medications may be used to acutely treat a specific cause of violent or suicidal symptoms. For example, a patient who becomes violent from heroin withdrawal might be acutely treated with methadone and diazepam. Violence precipitated by a seizure might be

Table 7.2 Treatment of Mild Suicidal/Violent Symptoms

Crisis Treatment

1. Determine precipitants of the symptoms.
2. Develop the meanings of the acute violent or suicidal behaviors.
3. Develop a 6-week time line of events that have contributed to the problem.
4. Uncover a focal past history that is linked to acute risky ideation/behaviors.
5. Make a support network map and utilize the support network.
6. Formulate an understanding of "Why now?"
7. Develop a plan to address all causative or contributing factors.
8. Teach crisis resolution.

Psychotherapeutic Treatment

1. Focus on breaks/distortions in reality. Provide treatment/referral if the patient is psychotic.
2. Interpret pathological defenses such as splitting and projection with special attention to displacements, which can lead to violence, and regression/denial, which can lead to suicidal ideation or behaviors.
3. Try to understanding the patient's view of himself or herself as powerless, out of control, hopeless, helpless, or rooted in low self-esteem. Help the violent/suicidal patient feel empowered.
4. Try to correct the patient's distortions in his or her view of others. Are others as mad, angry, uncaring, unfeeling, or unavailable as they seem?

Family Treatment

1. Discover the problematic dyad that is involved in violence or suicide. Work to resolve the conflict between them.
2. Utilize the entire family to buffer against future harm and to help intervene with the dyad.
3. Work toward improving family communication, better delegation of roles and responsibilities within the family, and observe and comment on changes in the emotional climate of the family.
4. Utilize the healthiest part of the family to assist the patient directly.

treated with diazepam or phenytoin. A depressed alcoholic might be suicidal while in alcohol withdrawal and might be treated initially with antianxiety medications and, subsequently, with an antidepressant.

Long-term Pharmacotherapy

Optimal long-term pharmacotherapy for violent and suicidal symptoms has not yet been established. Recent interest has focused on treatment of the relative serotonin deficiency associated with these symptoms using SSRIs or buspirone. Pharmacological treatment of suicidal or violent symptoms often focuses on treating associated illnesses that may be producing or aggravating these symptoms. Antidepressants are used to treat depression associated with suicidal symptoms and may have some limited effectiveness in violent patients as well.

If violent or suicidal symptoms emerge from a psychosis, then treatment of the psychosis becomes paramount. In this situation, a patient may be treated with atypical neuroleptics such as risperidone, olanzapine, and clozapine or with traditional neuroleptics such as haloperidol.

Lithium and anticonvulsants may be used as primary treatment for affective disorders that are associated with an increased incidence of suicidal and violent symptoms. Violence linked to manic excitement or irritability is especially responsive to these drugs. These medications also may be used to reduce impulsivity associated with impulse control disorders and/or personality disorders. Decreasing impulsivity may reduce suicidal or violent symptoms. When used to treat suicidal or violent symptoms, standard doses are lithium 600 to 1,800 mg/day, carbamazepine 600 to 1,000 mg/day, and valproic acid 1,000 to 2,000 mg/day. These drugs require regular monitoring for therapeutic blood levels, efficacy, and side effects.

Antianxiety medications generally are contraindicated as primary drug therapy in depressed, suicidal, or violent patients. This is because such drugs may worsen depressed moods, increase suicidal risk, or cause a disinhibition that exacerbates impulsive behaviors, all of which can lead to an increase in violence or suicidal behaviors.

Recent reports suggest that patients who have a primary panic disorder have an increased risk for suicide. In this specific patient group, treatment of the panic disorder with alprazolam 1 to 6 mg/day, clonazepam, or standard antidepressants may decrease suicidal potential.

Buspirone is a distinctive antianxiety agent that is reported to increase serotonin levels. Clinical case reports suggest that some violent patients may be helped by buspirone 60 to 90 mg/day.

Anticonvulsants can be extremely effective when used to treat aggression related to partial-complex seizures. These medications may also be helpful in violent patients who have nonspecific abnormalities on their EEGs, traumatic brain injury, dementia, or an impulse-control disorder. Valproic acid 250 to 2,000 mg/day or carbamazepine 600 to 1,000 mg/day are commonly used.

Propranolol is probably helpful in the long-term management of aggression associated with traumatic brain injury or geriatric organic brain conditions such as Alzheimer's or multi-infarct dementia. It may also be helpful in nonpsychotic impulse-control disorders. Propranolol is used in higher-than-standard doses, typically in the range of 200 to 800 mg/day, with an onset of action in 4 to 6 weeks. A full response may take months.

Office-based Treatment Given by a Primary Care Physician

Most primary care physicians will refer violent or suicidal patients to a psychiatrist or mental health professional. Some physicians may try to treat patients with mild violent or suicidal symptoms. Treatment of these symptoms may best be attempted utilizing a crisis intervention approach (see chapter 17), a counseling approach (see chapter 16), a family approach (see chapter 18), or a combination of approaches.

PARTNER VIOLENCE

Violence between partners is a special class of domestic abuse that crosses all boundaries of social class, race, and age. It may be defined as a partner establishing coercive control of another partner through physical, psychological, or sexual abuse, or by denying resources for self-support such that the other partner is unable to leave.

Statistics regarding partner abuse describe the nature and extent of this significant social problem. Women are six times more likely to experience violence from an intimate partner than men. Seventeen percent of the nation's homicides occur within the family, and 50% of these are women murdered by their current or former partners (Feldhaus et al., 1997). National home surveys indicate that approximately 1 million women and 150,000 men are victims of partner abuse each year (Bachman & Saltzman 1995). The National Coalition Against Domestic Violence (1997) reports that 90% of women do not report abuse.

One out of 20 women seen in primary care settings have experienced some form of partner abuse in the last year. In this same population, the lifetime prevalence rate is 1/5. Partner violence is the leading cause of injury to women between the ages of 15 and 44 and is a more common cause of injury than muggings, automobile accidents, and cancer combined. Because of the high prevalence rates of partner abuse and its major health consequences, the American Medical Association Council on Ethical and Judicial Affairs has suggested that routine questions about partner abuse be incorporated into the routine medical history.

Screening for Partner Violence

The primary care clinician should routinely incorporate inquiries about partner abuse into history taking and should be alert to signs of abuse detected during physical examination. Patients who are battered often present with physical symptoms. Physicians should have a high index of suspicion for partner violence in patients who complain of any of the following: traumatic injuries, pelvic discomfort or pain, a high miscarriage rate, history of rape or incest, headaches, chronic pain, functional gastrointestinal disorders, a history of substance abuse in the patient or the partner of the patient, chronic complaints of stress, insomnia, suicide attempts, depression, or anxiety. Risk factors for domestic abuse are summarized in Table 7.3.

The most important help a physician can provide to a suspected victim of partner abuse is to ask the patient about these suspicions. Research has shown that patients overwhelmingly want to be asked about partner violence; however, only 7% of physicians incorporate domestic violence questions into their routine medical care (Gremillion & Kanoff, 1996).

Physicians can use a variety of methods to screen for domestic violence. The SAFE questions are a helpful tool: *S*: Are you *stressed* and/or do you feel *safe* in your relationships? *A*: Do you feel *afraid* or have you been *abused* by anyone? F: Are *friends* and *family* aware and/or can you tell them about it? *E*: Do you have an *emergency* plan? Can you get to an emergency room or a domestic violence shelter? Do you have friends to help you or access to a social worker who will assist you? (Neufeld, 1996).

In addition or as an alternative to SAFE questions, there are brief, standardized screening instruments that also can be used. The Partner Violence Screen (PVS, Feldhaus et al., 1997) asks three questions, one addressing physical violence and two assessing the patient's sense of safety. These questions are: (1) "Have you been hit, kicked, punched, or otherwise hit in

Table 7.3 Risk Factors for Partner Abuse

Risk Factors for Victims	Risk Factors for the Abuser
Female	Male
Ages 17 to 28	Any adult age
Low self-esteem/insecurity	Low self-esteem/insecurity
Family history of partner abuse	Family history of partner abuse
Corporal punishment as a child	Corporal punishment as a child
Abuse of alcohol/substance abuse	Abuse of alcohol/substance abuse
Lower socioeconomic status	Job loss
Pregnancy	Cerebral factors: seizures or Minimal Brain Dysfunction
Single > separated > divorced	Personality disorders

the last year? If so by whom?" (a yes answer to this question has the best correlation with partner violence); (2) "Do you feel safe in your current relationship?" and (3) "Is there a partner from a previous relationship who is making you feel unsafe?" Women who answer yes to any one of these three safety questions or are unsure are considered positive responders. This particular screening instrument requires less than 20 seconds to administer and will detect 71.4% of cases of partner abuse compared to the gold-standard screening instrument, the Conflict Tactics Scale Form N (CTS). Administering the CTS, a 19-item questionnaire, is time consuming and therefore not a practical tool in the primary care setting (Feldhaus et al., 1997).

Another brief system for screening for acute and prior partner violence are the following questions: (1) "Are you here today due to injuries from a partner?" (2) "Are you here today because of illness or stress related to threats, violent behavior, or fears related to a partner?" (3) "Have you ever been assaulted or injured severely enough to seek medical attention, or have you ever called the police for help with a dispute with an intimate partner?" A yes answer to 2 of these questions is considered positive for partner abuse (Feldhaus et al., 1997).

Phases of Partner Violence

The three phases of the partner abuse cycle have been described as (1) the verbal abuse and hostility phase, in which the abuser systematically isolates the victim and, by verbal attacks, gradually undermines the partner's self-esteem; (2) the violent stage, in which assault and battery occur; and (3) the honeymoon period, in which the offender is remorseful and promises that violence will never occur again. This entire cycle is too often repeated.

Physician Intervention in Partner Abuse

When attempting to intervene in partner abuse, a primary care physician has to consider seven clinical domains: (1) establishing an alliance with the patient; (2) providing urgent medical care; (3) reviewing treatment options with the patient; (4) developing an acute intervention plan and/or a specific exit plan; (5) understanding and advising the patient about legal options and ramifications; (6) documenting partner violence; and (7) arranging for follow-up visits and/or communications.

Establishing an Alliance

One effective way to establish an alliance with a victim of partner abuse is to listen carefully to everything the patient has to say about the partner involved in the violence. It is important to communicate intense concern without blame for the victim.

It is also important to understand that victims of partner abuse are often intensely ambivalent about their partners. It is not uncommon for a patient victimized by a partner to return to live with the abuser. In the interview, try to focus on the patient's ambivalence and confusion about the situation without making any judgments. Offer the abused partner immediate protection and assure him or her that you will be available in the future. In addition, try to foster the patient's independent thinking, decision-making ability, and healthy coping styles and ally with the patient by making contingency plans for dealing with new episodes of abuse.

Provide All Necessary Medical Care

Initially, the physician must attend to acute medical problems related to abuse, which are typically injuries and physical trauma, miscarriage, sexual abuse, and rape. If sexual violence or partner violence has occurred, it is very important to follow a standardized medical protocol for collecting evidence and providing necessary medical treatment.

Review Treatment Options With the Patient

Patients suffering from partner violence almost always need additional support. At a bare minimum, refer the patient to the National Domestic Violence Hotline (800-799-7233). Encourage the patient to seek additional treatment, such as that offered through special domestic violence treatment services, a victim's service program, a mental health clinic, or refer the patient to a private practitioner with special expertise in domestic violence. Some patients will benefit greatly from group treatment, and occasionally, patients can be helped in couples or family treatment with the abusing partner present.

Some patients, victimized by a partner, may suffer with comorbid psychiatric conditions such as depression, suicidal tendencies, substance abuse, anxiety, or PTSD. A primary care physician needs to be alert to these additional complexities and refer the patient for appropriate psychiatric evaluation and treatment.

Develop an Acute Intervention Plan and/or an Exit Plan

Try to help the patient formulate an immediate plan for dealing with partner abuse and/or a future exit plan. If the patient is asking for immediate protection and shelter, review with the patient options for staying with friends and/or extended family. Remember that the only safe location is one where the abusing partner cannot find the victim. You may recommend that the patient go immediately to the nearest domestic violence shelter for an immediate safe haven and call the shelter to arrange for the patient's admission. Alternatively, you can enlist the help of a social worker or other mental health professional to assist the patient in dealing with the abuse and finding shelter.

It is especially important that the clinician try to develop a future exit plan with patients who are not yet ready to leave their abusers. Ask the patient to establish a safe, secret place outside the home for vital documents such as a driver's license, health insurance information, green card, and social security card. Advise the patient to put aside an extra set of car or house keys, emergency money, and some clothing and to have available emergency phone numbers, including friends, family, a domestic violence hotline, and the physician's telephone number. Where possible, have the patient notify friends and/or family of the future possibility of violence and arrange in advance a secret hiding place should it become necessary for the patient to leave home.

Advise the Patient of His/Her Legal Rights

Patients often need to be reminded that domestic violence is against the law. Some patients may increase their personal safety and improve their psychological recovery if they press charges against their partners. Partners who commit violence can be arrested and will be charged with felony crimes. Inform patients suffering from domestic abuse about the process of obtaining an order of protection. Protective orders, often issued from a family court, can be a valuable deterrent for future partner violence. You can also suggest that the victim seek legal assistance with separation, divorce, child custody issues, or other civil litigation that can develop out of partner violence.

In some states, the physician may be required under law to report partner violence to local authorities or agencies. Be aware of state requirements for reporting, and follow the local laws.

Follow-up Plan

After the initial diagnosis and treatment of partner violence, it is important to arrange for a follow-up visit with the patient. Do not assume that someone else—a social service agency, domestic violence service, or other personnel—will follow up on these cases. Instead, arrange a follow-up visit within 1 week of the initial visit, and encourage liberal phone contact between you and the patient. Make plans in advance with the patient as to what you will do if the patient misses the follow-up appointment for any reason. Obtain at the initial visit the patient's phone numbers and those of several emergency contact persons. If the patient does not attend the follow-up meeting, attempt to contact him or her or call the emergency contact telephone numbers. If you are unable to reach the patient, notify the appropriate family members, friends the patient has designated, the appropriate social service agency, or the police.

Record Keeping

Physicians need to document records of patients presenting with symptoms of partner abuse, both in the context of a biopsychosocial history and as a comprehensive medical history and detailed physical examination. In addition, you should document plans for follow-up meetings and results of those meetings. Be aware that medical records in partner violence are often used as evidence in legal proceedings and can be subpoenaed. It is best to avoid legal language in the medical record, such as "the alleged beating." Instead, report the details of events with specific documentation of all physical findings and follow-ups. For example, it is preferable to write "The patient was beaten around the eyes and sustained multiple facial fractures" than to write a more generic note, such as, "The patient was assaulted several times."

REFERENCES

Apter, A., Plutchik, R., Sevy S., Korn, M., Brown, S., & van Praag, H. (1989). Defense mechanisms in risk of suicide and risk of violence. *American Journal of Psychiatry, 146*, 1027–1031.

Bachman, R., & Saltzman, L. E. (1995). *Violence against women: Estimate from the redesigned survey, Bureau of Justice Statistics special report* (No. NCJ-154348). Washington, DC: U.S. Department of Justice.

Feldhaus, K. M., Koziol-Mclain, J., Amsbury, H. L., Norton, I. M., Lowenstein, S. R., & Abbott, J. T. (1997). Accuracy of three brief screening questions for detecting partner violence in the emergency department. *Journal of the American Medical Association, 277*, 1357–1361.

Gremillion, D. H., & Kanof, E. P. (1996). Overcoming barriers to physician involvement in identifying domestic violence. *Annals of Emergency Medicine, 27*, 769–773.

Henriksson, M. M., Isometsa, E. T., Kuoppasalmi, K. I., Heikkinen, M. E., Marttunen, M. J. & Lonngvist, J. K. (1996). Panic disorder in completed suicide. *Journal of Clinical Psychiatry, 57*, 275–281.

Mosciki, E. K. (1997). Identification of suicide risk factors using epidemiologic studies. *Psychiatric Clinics of North America, 20*(3), 499–517.

National Coalition Against Domestic Violence. (1997). *National coalition against domestic violence (pamphlet).* Denver: Author.

Neufeld, B. (1996). SAFE questions: Overcoming barriers to the detection of domestic violence. *American Family Physician, 53*(8), 2575–2580.

Robins, E., Murphy, G., & Wilkinson, R. (1959). Some clinical considerations in the prevention of suicide based on a study of 134 successful suicides. *American Journal of Psychiatry, 115*, 724–733.

Van der Kolk, B. A. (1987). *Psychological trauma.* Washington, DC: American Psychiatric Association.

CHAPTER 8

Personality Disorders in Office Practice

Robert E. Feinstein and Susan Vanderberg

"'Hateful patients' are those whom most physicians dread" (Groves, 1978, p. 883). They are objectively difficult and can elicit hate in many doctors. They are not patients "with whom a physician may have an occasional personality clash" (Groves, 1978, p. 883). These difficult patients may mobilize intense feelings in a physician, which may ultimately determine the quality of care the patient receives. "Hateful patients" often make physicians feel inadequate or impotent, elicit anger that is not adequately understood, or are sexually stimulating or arousing. They often develop an intense, aggressive, dependent clinging that can be exhausting for the physician. Unconscious physician anger toward such a patient ultimately results in a breakdown of patient-physician trust. The patient feels frustrated, unheard, not consulted, or angry with the physician; and the physician often feels misunderstood, devalued, or dissatisfied with his or

Note to reader: This chapter is best utilized in combination with chapter 16, Consulting and Counseling in Primary Care. Together, these chapters describe the basic approach to management of personality disorders for the purpose of improving the delivery of necessary medical care.

Reprinted with permission from Feinstein, R. E., and Vanderberg, S. (1995). Personality disorders in office practice. In R. Rakel (Ed.), *Textbook of family practice.* (5th ed., pp. 1510–1522). Philadelphia: W. B. Saunders.

her work. A dysfunctional patient-physician relationship contributes significantly to the deterioration of the medical experience and to poor medical care.

There are many causes of the dysfunctional patient-physician relationship. A leading cause not frequently discussed is the patient (or physician) with a personality disorder. Personality disorders often go unrecognized, because those so afflicted may not verbalize or manifest the more typical psychiatric symptoms or complaints, despite the fact that they may suffer from significant personal distress. Commonly, personality disorders can be secondarily recognized and experienced through the complaints of family, friends, or others who have had extended contact with the patient. It is easy to recognize the "personality disorder" when the individual suffers severe impairment in social, interpersonal, or occupational functioning. Patients and physicians have felt many disturbing emotions toward each other that are caused by the dysfunctional interaction of the patient with a personality disorder.

DEFINITION: PERSONALITY STYLE VERSUS PERSONALITY DISORDER

A *personality style* is the lifelong habitual way one thinks, feels, and behaves. This definition implies that each individual has a unique, enduring, slowly evolving organization of his or her perceptions, a typical style of thinking and fantasy, a hierarchy of emotional needs, a value system, and ideals. Personality style also implies a characteristic way in which one relates to oneself and manages internal conflicts, a typical way in which one relates to others, and a usual way of interacting and adapting to external reality.

The distinction between personality style and a personality disorder is a matter of degree. Personality styles that become rigid, extreme, maladaptively damaging to oneself and/or others, or that lead to social or occupational impairment are called *personality disorders*. Although each person is unique, there seems to be a continuum of personality styles and disorders that are commonly encountered. We can recognize some personality disorders in characters from the movies: the hysteric in Scarlet O'Hara from *Gone With the Wind*, the obsessive-compulsive in Felix Unger from *The Odd Couple*, or the borderline portrayed by Glenn Close in the movie *Fatal Attraction*.

CLASSIFICATION

Personality disorders generally are classified using a categorical or dimensional approach. The categorical system describes individuals as having clusters of associated traits, symptoms, or behaviors that form discrete, separate personality disorders, called prototypes. *DSM-III-R* (1987) and *DSM-IV* (1994) use a prototypic personality disorder classification and outline diagnoses, such as obsessive-compulsive and histrionic personality disorders. Categorical approaches have the advantage of colorfully describing personality styles and have been the most popular approach to classification among physicians.

These two systems exhibit variations along common dimensions. For example, Siever and Davis (1991) have suggested a set of four personality dimensions: cognitive/perceptual, anxiety/inhibition, impulsivity/aggression, and affective/stability. With the dimensional approach, a patient is classified along each dimension, with gradations from high to low. This system accounts for a spectrum of personality traits that are observed in many patients who do not fit into the discrete prototypes.

Whereas the dimensional approach has promising biologic, research, and treatment links, the categorical approach follows the medical diagnostic thinking of physicians, which organizes diseases into categories of illness. For this reason, this chapter focuses on categorical approaches.

To be classified as a prototypic personality disorder, an individual must have a minimum number of traits. The primary care categorical approaches to personality disorders are exemplified by Groves (1978), Kahana and Bibring (1969), and *DSM-IV*. Groves described four categories of "hateful patients": dependent clingers, entitled demanders, manipulative help rejecters, and self-destructive deniers. Kahana and Bibring delineated seven categories of personality types and attitudes: (1) dependent overdemanding; (2) orderly, controlled; (3) dramatizing, emotionally involved, captivating; (4) long-suffering, self-sacrificing; (5) guarded, querulous; (6) those with feelings of superiority; and (7) patients who seem uninvolved and aloof.

The *DSM-IV* is psychiatry's contributions to the categorical classification of personality disorders. This multiaxial system encourages physicians to consider personality variables for every patient. *DSM-IV* divides the personality disorders into three clusters. An abridged, listing of these disorders appears in Table 8.1.

Table 8.1 Abridged Summary of DSM-IV

CLUSTER A (Odd or eccentric)

Paranoid: Expects exploitation/harm; questions loyalty/fidelity; bears grudges; easily slighted

Schizoid: Loner; aloof; indifferent to praise or criticism; social anxiety; constricted affect

Schizotypal: Odd/eccentric; social anxiety; magical thinking; suspicious/paranoid ideation

CLUSTER B (Dramatic/emotional/erratic)

Antisocial: Cruelty; problems with authority; unlawful behavior; dishonesty; irresponsibility; exploits others

Histrionic: Overly emotional; seductive/sexual; attention seeking; shallow/superficial

Borderline: Unstable, intense relationships, self-destructive/ suicidal; impulsive; affective instability; identity disturbances

Narcissistic: Grandiose; inflated self-importance; entitled; exploits others; lacks empathy; needs admiration; hypersensitive to criticism

Self-Defeating: (DSM-IV Appendix) Suffers; self-sacrificing; defeats others; self-destructive; cannot enjoy; easily hurt

CLUSTER C (Anxious or fearful)

Dependent: Indecisive; lacks initiative; submissive; helpless; dependent; fears abandonment

Passive-Aggressive: Procrastinates; scorns authority; resents suggestions; superficially compliant; obstructs

Obsessive-Compulsive: Perfectionist; inflexible; detail preoccupation; wish to control others; stingy; overly conscientious; Excessively moral or ethical

Avoidant: Easily hurt; timid/fearful; social discomfort; avoids interpersonal interactions

Reprinted with permission from the *Diagnostic and Statistical Manual of Mental Disorders*, Fourth Edition. Copyright 1994 American Psychiatric Association.

PHYSICIAN REACTIONS

Physicians working with patients who suffer from personality disorders seem to have specific, characteristic reactions to such patients that must be recognized, understood, and utilized for a patient's benefit. Typical subjective experiences and reactions to a patient should alert a physician to a possible diagnosis of a patient with a personality disorder. These experiences and reactions include intense feelings, uncharacteristic fantasies, and atypical behaviors by the physician.

Intense Feelings

Intense feelings may comprise hate, fury, and frustration toward a patient. Feelings of love, sexual arousal, wishes to rescue the patient or give "exceptionally" good care may alternate with a wish to avoid the patient, terminate the relationship, or transfer the patient to the care of a colleague.

Physician Fantasies

A physician may recognize that he or she is interacting with a difficult patient by his or her own fantasies. Such fantasies include excessive worrying about a patient after normal work hours, dreaming about a patient, or experiencing exaggerated and/or intrusive, angry, sexual, or curious fantasies about the patient during personal time.

Physician's Atypical Medical Behaviors

A physician may also notice medical behaviors with a specific patient that are atypical to his or her customary medical practice. These unusual physician behaviors should trigger self-examination by the physician and evaluation of the possibility that the patient may have a personality disorder. Frequently, patients with a personality disorder are capable of arousing unconscious reactions that lead to new noncustomary physician behaviors.

Common atypical medical behaviors aroused in the physician may include the following: ordering of tests to placate a patient; asking for more than the usual number of consults on a patient whose case does not seem medically complicated, suggesting the increase of aggressive diagnostic testing or procedures when the yield of these tests is likely to be low; repeatedly extending the time spent with a particular patient or family; offering free samples of drugs; and lowering the customary fee or offering free treatment. A list of common physician reactions associated with specific personality disordered patients are summarized at the end of this chapter in Table 8.4. Recognition by the physician of his or her own unconscious and unanalyzed feelings, fantasies, and behaviors may aid in the diagnosis of a personality disorder. More importantly, physicians who can recognize their own unusual reactions are better able to tolerate them, avert acting out their feelings with a patient, and thereby improve their medical decision making.

Patients' Psychological Fears

Most patients are afraid when consulting a physician. The patient with a personality disorder may have fears that are exaggerated in their intensity and idiosyncratic in their quality. These fears rooted in the patient's basic personality organization are readily activated during a routine visit to the physician or when they feel sick and vulnerable. The capacity to delineate and empathize with the patient's fear and distorted world allows the physician to tailor the medical interaction toward alleviating the patient's fears. This "tailoring" can dramatically improve interactions with a patient and thus improve the quality of medical care. For example, a patient with a paranoid personality is extremely mistrustful and expects to be deceived or harmed by a dangerous world. When ill, he or she may become increasingly angry, suspicious, and mistrustful. Empathizing with the patient's paranoid worldview, may help the physician to realize that the patient requires an openness and honesty in all communications. The patient may also be helped by a comprehensive explanation of the physician's future medical intentions.

Patients with a borderline personality disorder fear separation, loss, or abandonment. When ill, they may cling to the physician and react to a separation (such as the physician's vacation) with anger, manipulative attempts, devaluing attacks, or panic. By understanding the patient's fears, it is possible to prevent worsening of his or her condition while the physician is away. This can be done by empathizing and discussing the patient's fears of separation or loss. The patient can be reassured of the physician's realistic medical availability and limits. In an effort to prevent a crisis from separation, prior to the physician's departure a patient can be scheduled for a meeting with the colleague who will be providing coverage. It may also be helpful to explore with this patient what he or she can do to cope while the physician is away (refer to Table 8.4).

PSYCHOPATHOLOGICAL LEVEL OF PERSONALITY FUNCTIONING

A particularly useful model for describing the level of personality organization was introduced by Kernberg (1975, 1984) and simplified by Goldstein (1988). Kernberg assessed the psychopathological level of personality organization as functioning on neurotic, borderline, and psychotic levels. These levels of functioning are determined by assessing reality testing, defenses, and identity diffusion (see Table 8.2).

Neurotic Personality Organization

Patients with a neurotic personality organization have the capacity to differentiate what is real from what is not. When their reality testing is intact, patients can (1) differentiate their own thoughts from external sensory perceptions; (2) distinguish themselves from others; and (3) realistically evaluate how their own emotions, behaviors, and thoughts are perceived in relation to ordinary social norms. Neurotic patients typically use high-level defense mechanisms centered on repression. These include reaction formation, displacement, suppression, and inhibition. Such patients have stable, slowly evolving views of themselves and of others as having a mixture of both good and bad qualities.

Borderline Personality Organization

Patients with a borderline personality organization generally have intact reality testing; that is, they can differentiate reality from fantasy, ideas from perceptions, and so on. However, the stresses of an illness, extreme emotions, or drugs may precipitate transient breaks in reality that last seconds, minutes, or even hours. Breaks in reality often present as severe distortions of what the physician has said to them, transient misperceptions of reality events, feelings of unreality, depersonalization, and, in the extreme case, temporary hallucinations or changing delusions. Patients with borderline personality organization use defenses that are centered on splitting (all good or all bad thinking and feeling). Associated defenses include idealization, devaluation, and particular forms of projection. These patients suffer from an unstable identity (identity diffusion) that manifests as radically alternating and exaggerated views of self. For example, a patient may see himself or herself as a kind, caring, giving person who is

Table 8.2 Personality Organizations

Neurotic Personality Organization

1. Reality testing intact
2. Defenses: higher level; repression
3. Stable view of self and physician

Borderline Personality Organization

1. Reality testing generally preserved: loss of reality testing with stress
2. Defenses: splitting
3. Identity diffusion: changing views of self and physician

Psychotic Personality Organization

1. Reality testing lost
2. Defenses: splitting and primitive
3. Identity diffusion prominent: chaotic or changing views of self and physician

close to perfection. This perception oscillates within a brief time with a view of himself or herself as a selfish, demanding, or hateful person. Patients who manifest identity diffusion see themselves and others in extremes of good and bad. There is memory for these alternating states, but the apparent contradictions seem to have no emotional relevance to the patient (i.e., splitting).

Psychotic Personality Organization

Patients with a psychotic personality organization have a gross loss of reality testing that permits them to be differentiated from patients with borderline personality organization. They may have inappropriate or bizarre affect, behavior, and thought content; or they may suffer from hallucinations and delusions. They are frequently unable to empathize or clarify how others see them (Kernberg, 1984). They typically use primitive defenses (e.g., projection, incorporation, or denial of reality), and have confused, blurred, or generally chaotic views of themselves and others. For example, they may see themselves as God at one time and the devil the next, or they may feel that they have both male and female sexual organs.

Variability in Personality Organization

Personality organization levels generally are stable for each patient, although stress may cause a patient to vary within a limited range of personality organizations for each specific *DSM-IV* personality category. For example, patients with paranoid, schizotypal, or schizoid personality disorders generally function at a psychotic personality organization but, at their best, can function on a borderline level. Alternatively, patients with antisocial, histrionic, borderline, or narcissistic personality disorders typically function at a borderline level. With stress (such as the threat of abandonment), they may briefly lose reality testing and function on a psychotic level. Patients within cluster C (dependent, avoidant, passive-aggressive, obsessive-compulsive) typically can function at the neurotic or borderline level; it is only rarely with extreme stress that they function at a psychotic level (refer to Table 8.4).

PATIENT DEFENSES

Defenses are unconscious psychological processes used by the patient to help resolve internal conflicts, manage anxiety, or alleviate depression. They may also help mediate external dangers and facilitate adaptations to reality. Different personality disorders use specific constellations of defenses. By understanding the constellation of defenses used with each personality disorder, and when possible, the specific defense mechanisms used, the physician may be able to modify the pathologic functioning of the defenses interfering with good patient-physician interaction. Patients functioning at the neurotic level use higher-level defenses centered on repression. Patients functioning at the borderline level use splitting defenses, whereas patients functioning on the psychotic level may use primitive defenses and severe forms of splitting (Kernberg, 1975, 1984).

High-Level (Neurotic) Defenses

High-level (neurotic) defenses are centered on repression. To repress is to exclude from awareness (or consciousness) any threatening impulses, feelings, memories, ideas, or experiences. A patient who uses repression fails to see, hear, or attend to threatening impulses, wishes, desires, or fears. Some high-level defenses associated with repression are repression, displacement, and reaction formation (see Table 8.3).

Table 8.3 Defense Mechanisms

Neurotic Personality Defenses: Higher Level (Repression Center)

Repression: involuntary forgetting of a painful memory, feeling, or experience

Controlling: manipulation or control of events or people to avoid unconscious anxiety or inner conflicts

Displacement: transferring one's feeling from one person to another

Reaction formation: unacceptable impulses that are expressed as attitudes and behaviors which are the direct opposite of those impulses

Intellectualization: the unconscious replacing of feelings with facts or details

Suppression: a conscious choice to put a disturbing experience out of one's mind

Ambivalence: the coexistence of opposite feelings

Distortion: reorganization of external reality to fit internal needs and wishes

Phobia: attaching fear to an object or situation that is not objectively a source of danger

Inhibition: restricting thoughts, feelings, or behaviors for fear that unacceptable impulses will erupt and create anxiety or other damage

Rationalization: creating socially acceptable explanations for thoughts, motions, or behaviors

Isolation: unconscious process by which thoughts and memories are stored without emotion

Sexualization: transformation of functions or objects into sexual symbols to avoid unconscious anxieties

Passive-aggressive: superficial compliance and passivity disguising stubbornness and anger

Defenses of Borderline Personality Organization (Splitting Centered)

Splitting: dividing the view of self and others into all good or all bad (views are often highly fantastic and distorted); defenses based on the use of splitting mechanisms include:

Table 8.3 *(continued)*

Idealization: seeing self or others as powerful, ideal, or God-like
Omnipotence: seeing self or others as all-powerful
Devaluation: depreciating or exaggerating the badness of self or others

Projection: unconscious rejection of unacceptable impulses, which are attributed to others

Projective identification: a projection of a part of oneself onto the other person, who one then fears and attempts to control (control of the other person psychically controls the impulse in oneself)

Denial: refusal to acknowledge painful realities

Regression: unconsciously reverting to childlike thoughts, feelings, or behaviors

Hypochondriasis: irrational fears of having a physical illness (with a decreased threshold for pain and increased awareness of internal physiologic sensory perceptions) so as to avoid other unconsciously painful experiences

Defenses of a Psychotic Level of Functioning: Lower Level (Primitive Defenses and Severe Splitting)

Splitting defenses as listed above become more extreme

Acting out: expressing in action or behaviors things that cannot be expressed in words or emotions

Incorporation: the process of psychically taking something into oneself

Somatization: physical or medical symptoms caused by mental processes without known physical disease

Schizoid fantasy: retreat to idiosyncratic fantasy when faced with painful experiences

Splitting Defenses

The splitting defenses and related mechanisms observed with borderline personality functioning cause these patients to see themselves and others as all good or all bad. In other words, there is no emotional experience of self and others as consisting of a realistic mixture of good and bad qualities. Hence the patients see the world as black or white, good or bad, and things as totally right or totally wrong. They alternate between these two different feeling states at different times (refer to Table 8.3).

Primitive Defenses and Severe Splitting

Primitive defenses can encompass projection, projective identification, denial, somatization, and severe forms of splitting. These defenses help patients organize their psychotic processes into a mode that allows them some adaptive functioning. Challenging these primitive defenses, in the form of confronting the patients' reality distortions with other reality views of the same problem, may reveal the underlying psychotic processes they help defend against. These defenses are defined in Table 8.3.

PSYCHOTHERAPEUTIC MANAGEMENT AND INTERVENTIONS

After several office visits with a patient, the physician may have a general idea of the patient's personality diagnosis, an understanding of the physician's likely reactions to that patient, a sense of the patient's typical fears, the level of personality functioning, the patient's main defenses, and some anticipation of problematic interactions that may arise during the process of delivering medical care (see Table 8.4). With this information, the physician may be able to help the patient develop an alliance that allows good medical care. A physician cannot change the patient's personality disorder but may be able to help the patient function at a more adaptive level.

A review of the clinical management of a patient with a personality disorder involves establishing an alliance with empathy for the patient's fears, developing a therapeutic contract, agreeing upon a focal problem to resolve, and promoting more adaptive functioning by using the psychotherapeutic techniques of confrontation, clarification, and interpretation.

Establish an Alliance

To establish a good patient-physician alliance, a physician should begin every patient encounter with a friendly, open, available attitude that conveys a willingness to listen and help. When beginning the interview, the patient should be allowed to express any negative feelings about the physician or the patient's medical care to date. The physician should listen to the patient's complaints without reacting defensively. The physician may sometimes feel hurt, but it is important to realize that patients' complaints are often subjective feelings and do not necessarily represent any wrongdoing by the physician or a need for change. Listening with understanding to the patient's primary fears, and with empathy for the patient's worldview, then using commonly understood and simplified medical language, can facilitate a good patient-physician interaction and working alliance.

Therapeutic Contract

During a regular office visit, the physician should alert the personality disordered patient that a problem exists which is interfering with the patient's medical care. The physician may first ask for the patient's view of the present medical care. If the patient expresses the problem, the physician can join in the discussion. If time prohibits a discussion, a follow-up office visit can be scheduled. If the patient cannot identify the problem, or the physician believes there is a different problem, the latter may say, "I believe that there is a (different) problem in my ability to help you get the best medical care possible. I need to think about why this has happened, and I would like you to also think about this difficulty. I would like to see you next time for a longer office visit, when we can discuss your case in detail and find a better way to help you." With the patient's agreement, a time and future setting for a longer session can be established. Prior to the next visit, a focus should be chosen for that meeting.

Choose a Focus for the Interview

Patients with severe personality disorders often experience common problems in terms of cooperating with their medical care. There may be a problem in the doctor-patient relationship or in the patient's understanding or acceptance of the medical diagnosis or treatment, which may include requests by the patient for help with a psychological, interpersonal, familial, or social problem. The physician must identify the focus of the session at the beginning of the interview. Resolving problems in the patient-physician relationship may need to take priority over other problem areas. When possible, it is best to focus on one problem area before working on others.

Psychotherapeutic Techniques

After a brief period of immersion in the patient's complaints, the physician should respond with empathic and reassuring responses addressed to the patient's fears. Initially, the response may take the form of educational or informational instruction. If this response is insufficient, as it usually is for personality disordered patients, it may be necessary to respond with an empathic confrontation, clarification, or interpretations about the current problematic situation.

A *confrontation* is not a battle. It is an observation by the physician that is offered to a patient for his or her examination. It is usually a comment that draws attention to discrepancies or contradictions in the patient's perceptions or behaviors that are interfering with medical care. The physician may use confrontations in a nonjudgmental way and listen carefully for the patient's expanding self-awareness. Example: "I know that you want your medical condition to improve, yet your refusal to permit further diagnostic testing makes medical improvement unlikely."

A *clarification* is the doctor's request of the patient to add new information or perspective, or to clarify misunderstandings, miscommunications, or information that may seem vague or confusing. The need for repeated clarifications occur regularly with patients who have severe personality disorders. It is important to use clarifications before suggesting a new plan to correct the problem.

Interpretations integrate comments that link confrontations and clarifications with a patient's current problem regarding the goal of complete medical care. Interpretations in the medical setting generally should be made about the immediate situation. They may address the patient's defenses, a difficulty in the doctor-patient interaction, or the external reality of the disease process, medical work-up, medical treatment, or the patient's life circumstances. For example, an interpretation to a borderline patient with chronic pain might be: "I think you want relief from your pain. Yet your refusal to follow my recommendations makes relief from your pain unlikely" (confrontation). "You then get angry with me because your pain is not relieved, and so you do not keep your scheduled appointments" (clarification). "You do not use my help, but then blame me and feel frustrated. Your anger with me helps you avoid the frustration you feel with your husband, who has become less than sympathetic toward your pain" (interpretation). Such interpretations take practice but can powerfully restore a realistic, helpful doctor-patient relationship.

GENERAL INTERVENTION

By establishing that a patient's personality organization is functioning at the neurotic, borderline, or psychotic level, it may be possible to intervene at that level to improve the patient's ability to function. Management strategies for patients functioning at the neurotic level involve correction of subtle distortions in reality perceptions and the use of psychotherapeutic interventions to deal with the specific high-level defense mechanisms that are interfering with the patient's efforts to obtain optimal medical care. Patients functioning at the borderline level frequently suffer from short-lived disturbances in reality testing. These disturbances may manifest as transient simple hallucinations, dramatic distortions of what has been said, transient misperceptions of reality events, misunderstanding of the physician's or patient's role, feelings of unreality, or depersonalization. Such reality distortions are not severe and can be helped by the use of confrontation, clarification, and interpretation.

The general strategy for managing the splitting defenses involves intervening through the use of confrontations, clarifications, and interpretations; specifically, by making patients aware that half of their emotional feelings have been split off or dissociated. This exercise involves reminding a patient who is currently loving and idealizing that last week he or she considered the physican much less competent and not helpful. Alternatively, the patient who hates the physician and says that the physician is all bad can be reminded of other good experiences he or she has had with the physician in the recent past. Other, more specialized techniques of dealing with the related splitting defenses are mentioned under specific personality disorders (see below).

Patients functioning at the psychotic level require primary interventions geared toward improving reality testing. Such intervention is necessary to preserve basic trust in the doctor-patient relationship. Explaining the current medical condition and correcting the patient's distortions of medical realities can be extremely helpful. A patient suffering from hallucinations, delusions, or inappropriate or bizarre affect or behavior may require the use of medications, intervention with family members, or hospitalization. Occasionally, confrontations, clarifications, and interpretations may also be used to improve the patient's psychological functioning.

SPECIFIC INTERVENTIONS

A schema useful when working with personality disordered patients includes choosing the correct *DSM-IV* diagnosis, recognizing common physician reactions to each kind of personality disorder, understanding the patient's specific fears and reactions to those fears, and assessing the patient's level of personality functioning and main defenses. This conceptual framework may make it possible to formulate some helpful interventions for the specific personality disorder.

Paranoid Personality Disorder

When interacting with a paranoid patient, the physician commonly reacts with fear and mistrust and has a sense of danger. The physician may also feel blamed or accused. Such patients may have a similar fear of being hurt, exploited, or invaded. They often react to suggestions for medical care with mistrust, excessive fault finding, sensitivity to criticism, and hypervigilance; and they collect small insults that are used as proof of the world's injustices. When invasive procedures are performed, a male patient may react with full-blown panic and anxiety. This reaction may occur because many paranoid male patients unconsciously perceive body invasions as a homosexual assault.

Paranoid patients typically function at the level of a psychotic personality organization, as evidenced by severe and unwarranted suspiciousness of others. They rely most heavily on projection as their main defense. Using projection, they accuse the physician of a hurt that reflects their own aggressive style of hurting others.

A physician must empathize with the patient's mistrust and hypersensitivity and should avoid arguing or attempting to reason the patient away from his or her paranoid worldview. It is important to use confrontations and clarifications to help correct patient's distorted perceptions about his or her medical care. However, direct confrontation of a delusion or hallucination (the most troubling deficits in reality testing) often has the paradoxical effect of making the patients more suspicious of the physician. Acknowledging that the patient's suspicion has an emotional reality can be helpful. Rather than confront mistrust or suspicions directly, it is helpful to acknowledge responsibility for any actions the patient may have perceived as mistakes. For example, "I did not understand how it might have scared you when I took a throat culture." It may also help for the physician to openly express understanding and concern for the patient's rights. If there is a medical need for special testing of which the patient is suspicious, the physician should acknowledge his or her fears and describe openly and honestly the details of the procedures, the potential for pain, and the likely risks and benefits. If the patient still refuses to comply, the physician should not use direct persuasion. Rather, the physician should ask the patient, "Is it all right with you if we have different opinions?"

With the patient's consent to hearing a different opinion, the physician can then openly discuss the medical necessity of the testing without trying to resolve the problem (Kernberg, 1984). At future office visits, the physician can attempt new and ongoing discussions of the patient's fears of complying with requests for specialized testing. It may take months for the paranoid patient to trust the physician enough to consent to the appropriate treatment.

Counterprojective statements by the physician can diffuse the projections and distortions directed at the physician. The doctor can use counterprojective remarks to help the patient access his or her feelings while focusing angry or suspicious feelings away from the physician toward others who are not present. For example, a physician harassed by an angry, suspicious, or blaming patient could use a counterprojective statement, such as: "You felt angry and hurt when the lab technician drew your blood. You must have been hurt, and perhaps you are also fearful of the results of these tests."

Schizoid and Schizotypal Personality

When working with schizoid and schizotypal patients, physicians commonly feel uninvolved or detached, or they have a desire to break through the aloofness. Schizoid patients may give the physician the impression of the patient as a "loner." A common physician reaction to schizotypal patients is a feeling that the patient is both alone and "weird" or "strange." Patients with either diagnosis superficially fear personal contact and emotional involvement, and they fear that their privacy will be invaded. At the deepest levels, they long for emotional contact that is not overwhelming. In either situation, they may react to suggestions for medical care with avoidance, withdrawal, apparent emotional detachment, or denial of the medical problem.

Schizotypal patients function at a psychotic level with impaired reality testing manifested by magical, odd, or psychotic modes of thinking. Schizotypal patients use regression to schizoid fantasy and to a lesser extent denial as their main defenses. They appear increasingly idiosyncratic and withdrawn when stressed.

Schizoid patients do not appear psychotic, but rather, more detached and alone. They often can function at a borderline level of personality organization. When stressed by a medical problem, schizoid patients use psychotic denial of their illness and withdrawal as their main defense.

Efforts to reach these patients are often perceived as intrusions into their privacy and actually may drive them away from their physician. They are relieved when the physician is not present and prefer fewer medical appointments and contacts. It may be helpful to accept their unsociability at a level that does not demand involvement or permit total withdrawal. Medical information that is presented in a neutral or unemotional manner is most likely to be heard and utilized.

Antisocial Personality Disorders

Common physician reactions to a patient with antisocial personality disorder are feelings of being used, exploited, or deceived. These feelings lead to physician anger and a wish to be free of the patient, to uncover lies, and to punish or imprison the patient.

When ill, these patients fear that they will become vulnerable, lose respect or admiration from others, and become easy prey to manipulation. They expect to be exploited, demeaned, or humiliated. Like the narcissistic patient, they often have low self-esteem, excessive self-love, compensatory feelings of superiority, grandiosity, recklessness, emotional shallowness, and a lack of concern for others. They often react to medical care with entitled demands for special treatment. When caught in dishonesty, they may angrily attack or devalue the physician. They may resort to other psychopathic manipulations, such as deception, lying, cheating, or stealing.

Antisocial personality disordered patients typically function at the borderline level of personality organization, and their reality testing appears intact. In fact, their friendly, facile, slick, superficial charm and intelligent appearance are often beguiling for the physician. When stressed by the potential of getting caught in their deceptive practices, they may lose reality testing, manifested by impulsive actions that can reveal severely impaired or even psychotic judgments. When they are receiving medical care for a bona fide illness, they typically function at the same level as those with a narcissistic personality disorder (Kernberg,1992) and often can be managed similarly (see below).

To intervene with an antisocial patient, a physician needs to be alert and anticipate the possibility that the patient may be requesting unnecessary medical care. The patient may be seeking the secondary gain of illegal benefits or money, or seeking to avoid work or legal problems. It is important not to inadvertently collude with the patient's plans for secondary gain. For example, if the physician thinks a patient's request for disability is fraudulent or unwarranted, the patient should not be referred for additional evaluations. If deception is suspected, the physician can ask for verification of symptoms from other reliable sources. Often there is dishonesty in a patient's communication, in the form of partial truths or outright lying, cheating, or stealing. If dishonest communication occurs, the physician must avoid the common reaction of moralizing. Instead, the patient is granted the reality that if the patient chooses, he or she can fool all physicians. The patient can be told that the results of deception or giving false or inaccurate information is that the physician may make poorly informed medical decisions, which can ultimately result in the patient's receiving inadequate or poor medical care. The physician can wonder with the patient why the patient needs to act in a self-destructive manner. The patient may need to be reminded that the physician's role is to help the patient with medical problems, not to pass judgment.

Histrionic Personality Disorder

Patients with histrionic personality disorder have an emotionally expressive style, seek excessive attention, and are often dramatic. Physicians may feel flattered, captivated, seduced, or sexually aroused by these patients. Alternatively, a physician may feel overwhelmed by a patient's exaggerated or excessive emotions, embarrassed by his or her sexual overtures, or depleted. Such patients recruit others, through use of their sexuality, to satisfy their needs to be romantically pursued and dependently taken care of and satisfied. They fear that they are not desired and will lose the care of others.

There are two levels of functioning of patients with this personality disorder (Kernberg, 1984, 1992). Kernberg describes a neurotically functioning hysteric who has intact reality testing, defenses centered on repression, and stable and mature relations with others. The female hysteric has a flirtatious clinging, childlike dependence in intimate relationships but can function at mature levels in social and work situations (Kernberg, 1992). Male hysterics have similar psychological conflicts but may appear either as macho or effeminate (Kernberg, 1992). The hysteric of either sex often reacts to medical care with regression to a childlike, sexualized, dependent, clinging position. These individuals seek to gratify their wishes for dependent care by seducing or flattering others. Outside the physician's office, they typically function well.

In contrast, the histrionic patient who functions with a borderline personality organization (Kernberg, 1984, 1992) can display transient losses of reality testing, defenses centered on splitting, and chaotic sexualized relations with others. This patient is more self-centered and self-indulgent, with a pervasive childlike dependence that extends from intimate relationships into all aspects of social and occupational functioning. Female histrionics typically act flirtatious and may become indignant when a man shows sexual interest. Male histrionics also show the self-centered and dependent pattern but may additionally be severely hypochondriacal, or have antisocial features (Kernberg, 1992). The histrionic of either sex may react to medical care with regression but, unlike the hysteric, uses defenses centered on splitting. These individuals may see the physician as all good or all bad and can be devaluing. They may appear severely self-centered, attention seeking, diffusely sexual, frequently hypochondriacal, somatic, and exploitative, with an exhausting dependency on their physicians.

When working with both hysterics and histrionics, a physician must be friendly, neither overly warm or reserved. Hysterics often benefit from some gratification of their dependent wishes and a free discussion of their fears and emotions. They can often be reassured by an educational, informational approach to their medical illness and are capable of expressing gratitude to the physician. The intense dependence of histrionics is often made worse when their needs are gratified. Offering excessive emotional care may make them greedy or demanding of need satisfaction. Histrionics benefit from firm, kind limit setting (especially to their sexual overtures), with neutral acknowledgment and gratification of their *reasonable* needs. Additionally, they may be helped by focusing on their distortions in reality perceptions and interpretations of the splitting mechanisms.

Borderline Personality Disorders

Borderline patients frequently become dependent on their physicians in a demanding, clinging, helpless, or self-destructive manner (Gunderson, 1984; Kernberg, 1975, 1984). Physicians typically feel manipulated, angry, depleted, exhausted, or self-doubting, with wishes to either get rid of or rescue the patient.

These patients fear separation or abandonment and may react to potential losses with panic, emotional instability, anger, or impulsive (suicidal) actions. They often react to medical care by aggressively and dependently clinging to their physicians and other caretakers. When frustrated, they may angrily devalue others and make entitled demands for special treatment. They tend to relate to others as all good or all bad, which generally accounts for their poor life functioning.

Such individuals function on the borderline level of personality organization, where reality testing typically is intact (Gunderson, 1984; Kernberg,

1975, 1984, 1992). However, under stress, they may temporarily lose reality testing and manifest severe distortions in perception or sense of reality. They may misperceive the physician's intentions or instructions. They may also experience episodes of derealization, depersonalization, or brief psychotic episodes. Borderline patients have identity diffusion (extreme fluctuations from a grandiose perception of themselves to an excessively harsh underestimate of their abilities). They also suffer from stormy and chaotic relationships with others. They rely heavily on splitting, projective identification, projection, and devaluing.

Office management of these patients involves an empathic understanding of their feelings that their security is most threatened by fears of separation or abandonment and, secondarily, by rebuff or humiliation. They require firm limit setting (e.g., what the physician can realistically offer). When the physician attempts to satisfy these patients' intense needs, it often results in an exhausted or angry physician. This situation can be avoided by setting realistic limits while offering a patient several different ideas or options for more adaptive behaviors. Initial interventions should attempt to establish reality testing or to correct distortions. If reality testing is intact, the most helpful interventions can be aimed at decreasing the pathological splitting defenses by using confrontation, clarification, and interpretations of the problematic situation.

Narcissistic Personality Disorders

Physician reactions to narcissistic patients are often difficult to manage. The superior, entitled, self-loving, arrogant attitude of these patients can be intimidating. They may elicit in the physician feelings of being devalued and inferior, or fears of the patients' anger or criticism. Alternatively, the lack of empathy and interpersonal exploitation of these patients can readily provoke the physician to anger, a wish to retaliate with harsh criticism, or a wish to get rid of a patient.

The core fear of these patients is due to fragile self-esteem and their need for constant approval and praise from others. They fear loss of admiration, potency, power, and being exploited when vulnerable. Any perceived insult to their "grandiose self" (Kernberg, 1984, 1992) makes them feel rejected, deflated, and criticized, and frequently results in feelings of rage, shame, or humiliation.

The narcissistic patients who are most difficult to manage function at the level of borderline personality organization. Their reality testing is typically intact yet can undergo severe distortions when they perceive slights or rejection. Those narcissistic patients who have paranoid and antisocial features (Kernberg, 1992) have a worse prognosis. They have a fragile identity that frequently swings from the grandiose to the worthless.

These patients rely heavily on splitting mechanisms to regulate their self-esteem. They portray themselves as grandiose and superior, which helps defend against split-off feelings of inadequacy and vulnerability. When they act self-importantly, they can devalue, viciously attack, or degrade those around them. Alternatively, as splitting operates, they may idealize and envy others who for the moment are seen as more powerful or successful. In this position, their self-esteem plummets, as evidenced by their sense of worthlessness and their reports of deprecating and degrading self-attacks.

Office management of the narcissistic patient requires that the physician not mistake the patient's superior and entitled manner for genuine confidence. When being assaulted by a devaluing attack, it may help the physician to see the attacking patient as a wounded child having a disruptive outburst. This recognition may prevent a retaliation from the physician, which would only escalate a worsening situation. Intervention in the face of a devaluing attack involves acknowledging that the patient feels hurt and has a right to his or her opinions. If this patient can discuss the hurt feelings with a nonjudgmental, empathic physician, the problems generally resolve, and a good doctor-patient alliance is restored. If this type of discussion is not possible, the patient should be offered without malice, defensiveness, or apology the right to seek another expert for consultation. Such an offer may help the patient to calm down and reconsider his or her position. In a long-term relationship with a narcissistic patient, the current splitting can be interpreted, by reminding the patient that in the recent past he or she has praised the skill and abilities of the physician. The patient can be asked why he or she is now so critical and angry. When this technique is effective, it allows patients to discuss their perceptions of insults to their self-esteem.

Self-Defeating (Masochistic)

Self-defeating patients are often suffering, depressed, and self-sacrificing (Spitzer & Williams, 1987). They repeatedly make bad choices that lead to failure or pain. A common physician reaction to these patients is a wish to rescue them from their own self-destructiveness. Trying too vigorously to help these patients frequently results in worsening of the patients' complaints and symptoms, leaving the physician frustrated, angry, defeated, self-doubting, self-blaming, or hopeless. Alternatively, these patients can arouse sadistic fantasies in the physician, such as a wish that the patient would suffer or die.

Patients in this group are excessively dependent on love, support, and acceptance from others. They cannot directly express their anger and may be harshly self-judgmental. They fear recovery, which to them means losing love and care. Improvement of their medical condition can lead to the development of multiple new complaints that have no somatic basis.

Within this group, patients may function on either the neurotic or the borderline level of personality organization. Neurotically functioning masochistic patients can make the physician feel mildly guilty that they are causing pain or suffering or are not adequately helping. The patient and physician both suffer. However, these patients ultimately can be helped and can express genuine gratitude toward the physician. Borderline functioning masochistic patients are passive-aggressive "help seeking rejecters" (Groves, 1978) who make their physicians feel both helpless and responsible for their severe suffering or self-destructiveness.

Physicians can manage these patients by empathizing with a patient's realistic medical suffering, symptoms, or complaints due to the illness. It should not be suggested that the patient's symptoms are psychological or that the patient will improve or be cured quickly. Such misstatements paradoxically may increase the patient's symptoms, complaints, telephone calls, and office visits. Potential recovery can be presented as a likely, but distant reality. If the patient cannot permit or admit relief of the symptoms or suffering, he or she can be asked to speak less about symptoms for the benefit of other family members.

Schema for Personality Disorders

The schema for office-based management of personality disorders that was presented in this chapter is summarized in Table 8.4, which outlines the *DSM-IV* classification of personality disorders, physician reactions to these patients, patient fears, psychopathological level of personality functioning, patient's main defenses, and some interventions.

Table 8.4 Personality Disorders Schema

DSM-IV	Common Physician Reactions	Patient Fear and Psychological Reaction	Neurotic Borderline Psychotic	Patient Defenses	Interventions
CLUSTER A Paranoid	Fearful, sense of danger, mistrust; feels accused or blamed.	Fears being hurt, exploited, invaded; reacts with mistrust and anger; homosexual panic with invasive procedures.	PPO[a] or BPO[b]	Primitive defenses: projection, projective-identification, denial, splitting defenses.	(1) Empathize with patient's fear of being hurt and acknowledge complaints without arguing or ignoring. (2) Openly and honestly explain medical illness, nature of tests, etc. (3) Correct reality distortions and do not confront delusions. If patient refuses care out of mistrust, ask if it is OK if you can disagree about the need for the test; don't insist. (4) Interpret defenses, use counterprojection.
Schizoid	Detached or removed; wish to involve patient with others or to break through the isolation.	"Loner"; Fears intrusion or violation of privacy, then withdraws more from personal contact.	BPO[b] or PPO[a]	Primitive defenses: denial regression splitting defenses.	(1) Empathize with patient's need for both privacy and contact. (2) Accept the patient's unsociability. (3) Neutrally impart medical information. (4) Do not demand involvement and do not permit total withdrawal. (5) Test reality. (6) Interpret specific defenses.
Schizotypal	Detached, removed, "weird and alone" feelings; wish to involve or to break through the isolation.	Fears intrusion or violation of privacy; may withdraw from personal contact.	PPO[a] or BPO[b]	Primitive defenses: schizoid fantasy, regression, denial, splitting defenses.	As above

DSM-IV	Common Physician Reactions	Patient Fear and Psychological Reaction	Neurotic Borderline Psychotic	Patient Defenses	Interventions
CLUSTER B Antisocial	Used/exploited, deceived, causing anger and wish to uncover lies, punish, or imprison.	Fears exploitation or sudden vulnerability; may lie, manipulate, cheat, exploit, steal, seek secondary gain.	BPO[b] with stress PPO[a]	Acting out, somatization for secondary gain, splitting defenses.	(1) Empathize with the patient's fear of exploitation and low self-esteem. (2) Are you being used for a secondary gain? (3) If you suspect dishonesty, verify symptoms and illness progression with others. (4) Do not moralize; explain that deceiving results would mean you are giving the patient poor care. (5) Test reality. (6) Interpret defenses.
Histrionic	Flattered or captivated, seduced, or sexually aroused; flooded by emotions; embarrassed; depleted.	Loss of the caretaker; loss of desirability, attractiveness, or sexuality; seduces, flatters, or angrily devalues.	BPO[b] or NPO[c] with stress PPO[a]	Splitting defenses: sexualization, acting out, dissociation/ regression, somatization defenses.	(1) Empathize with patient's fear of losing love or care. (2) Interact in a friendly way, not too reserved or too warm. (3) Discuss patient's fears; reassure when possible. (4) Limit set if patient regresses. (5) Correct reality distortions. (6) Interpret specific defenses.
Borderline	Feels manipulated; fearful of anger; angry; impotent; depleted; self-doubting; wish to rescue or get rid of the patient; guilty.	Fears separation, loss, abandonment; may panic, be angry, impulsive, lose reality, reject help, devalue, manipulate; may make suicidal gestures.	BPO[b] with stress PPO[a]	Splitting defenses: projection, projective-identification, idealize/devalue, omnipotence, acting out, mini-psychotic breaks.	(1) Empathize with patient's fear of abandonment and separation. Plan for absences. (2) Express wish to help and satisfy reasonable needs. (3) Set firm limits and do not punish. (4) Test reality. (5) Interpret splitting and other defenses. (6) If suicidal, the patient must go to the emergency room. If the patient refuses, inform the patient of your wish to keep him or her alive, but that after the patient is safe, you will terminate the relationship.

(continued)

Table 8.4 *(continued)*

DSM-IV	Common Physician Reactions	Patient Fear and Psychological Reaction	Neurotic Borderline Psychotic	Patient Defenses	Interventions
Narcissistic	Devalued/inferior; fearful of patient criticism or anger; wish to retaliate with anger, devalue, or get rid of patient.	Fears loss of self-esteem or potency; acts entitled or viciously devalues, counterattacks, or idealizes physician.	BPO[b] or NPO[c] with stress PPO[a]	Splitting defenses: idealize/devalue, omnipotence, projection, projective-identification, acting out, denial, regression.	(1) Empathize with the patient's vulnerability and low self-esteem. (2) Do not mistake patient's superior attitude for real confidence and don't confront entitlement. (3) When you are devalued or attacked, acknowledge the patient's hurt, your mistakes, and express your continued wish to help. (4) If devaluing continues, offer a referral as an option, not as punishment. (5) Correct reality distortions. (6) Interpret splitting and other defenses.
Self-Defeating (DSM III-R Appendix A)	Wish to rescue; sadistic fantasies that patient will suffer or die; defeated, self-blaming, self-doubting, or hopeless.	Loss of love/care; fears recovery; when improved may intensify complaint, depression, dependence; guilty, judg-mental, harsh, self-destructive.	BPO[b] or NPO[c] Rarely PPO[a]	Splitting defenses: denial, projection, projective-identification, idealize/devalue, repression, reaction formation.	(1) Empathize with patient's suffering and acknowledge and appreciate the difficulty of the illness or treatments. (2) Emphasize that recovery may be a slow, steady process. (3)The need for recovery can be presented as necessary to benefit others. (4) Inquire about obviously self-destructive or self-defeating behaviors. (5) Do not abandon. (6) Interpret specific defenses.

[a]PPO = Psychotic Personality Disorder Organization
[b]BPO = Borderline Personality Organization
[c]NPO = Neurotic Personality Organization

REFERENCES

American Psychiatric Association. (1987). *Diagnostic and statistical manual of mental disorders* (3rd ed., revised). Washington, DC: Author.

———. (1994). *Diagnostic and statistical manual of mental disorders* (4th ed.). Washington, DC: Author.

Goldstein, W. N. (1988). Kernberg on the borderline: A simplified version. In J. M. Ross, (Ed.), *Concepts in psychoanalytic psychotherapy.* (pp. 169–186) Washington, DC: American Psychiatric Press.

Groves, J. E. (1978). Taking care of the hateful patient. *New England Journal of Medicine, 298*, 883–887.

Gunderson, J. G. (1984). *Borderline personality disorder.* Washington, DC: American Psychiatric Press.

Kahana, R. J., & Bibring, G. L. (1969). *Lectures in medical psychology: An introduction to the care of patients.* New York: International University Press.

Kernberg, O. (1975). *Severe personality disorders: Borderline conditions and pathological narcissism.* New York: Jason Aronson.

———. (1984). *Severe personality disorders: Psychotherapeutic strategies.* New Haven, CT: Yale University Press.

———. (1992). *Aggression in personality disorders and perversions.* New Haven, CT: Yale University Press.

Siever, L. J., & Davis, K. J. (1991). A psychobiological perspective on the personality disorders. *American Journal of Psychiatry, 148*, 1647–1658.

CHAPTER ***9***

Schizophrenia and Other Psychotic Disorders

Lewis A. Opler

Schizophrenia is a psychotic disorder characterized by a worsening in social functioning accompanied by characteristic active or positive symptoms (e.g., loose associations, delusions, and hallucinations) and deficit or negative symptoms (e.g., emotional flattening or lack of motivation). Schizophrenia affects 1% of the population worldwide. In the United States, it accounts for 10% of all disability payments (Rupp & Keith, 1993).

The introduction of antipsychotic medication and more effective psychosocial interventions has improved the treatment of schizophrenia over the past 50 years. The stigma associated with the disease in the past has been replaced by an enlightened understanding of schizophrenia as a medical disorder requiring treatment and not a sign of personal weakness or of a bad upbringing. It is important to underscore that schizophrenia is a treatable medical disorder. It is a chronic illness that has exacerbations and remissions and a more promising prognosis given the availability of new and improved treatments.

This chapter provides basic tools for treating schizophrenia and other psychotic disorders in a primary care setting. The chapter reviews diagnostic criteria, course of schizophrenia, and etiology; discusses the key role of antipsychotic medication and pharmacological management; reviews specific interpersonal, or "psychosocial," interventions, which, when used in combination with antipsychotic medication, significantly improve the course and outcome of schizophrenia; and offers a brief glimpse into a future in which preventive measures may decrease the prevalence of schizophrenia.

DIAGNOSIS OF SCHIZOPHRENIA

The first step in making a diagnosis of psychosis is to rule out a medical condition that could cause the psychosis, such as seizures, brain lesions to the posterior nondominant cerebral hemisphere, and other conditions affecting the central nervous system. Chapter 5, Psychiatric Symptoms Due to Medical Illness, reviews these conditions and suggests appropriate medical evaluations. The second diagnostic step is to rule out substance-induced psychosis such as that caused by drugs of abuse (e.g., cocaine, amphetamines, and phencyclidine), over-the-counter medications (e.g., antihistamines), and physician-prescribed medications (e.g., steroids). See chapter 4, Substance Abuse, and chapter 5 for a review of drugs that can cause psychosis. The third step is to rule out other mental disorders that can present with psychosis, such as bipolar and depressive disorders.

The diagnostic criteria for schizophrenia as specified in the *DSM-IV* (1994) are a decrease in social or occupational functioning manifested by poor work performance, interpersonal difficulties, or a decrease in ability to care for oneself, accompanied by at least two or more of the following characteristic symptoms: (1) delusions, (2) hallucinations, (3) disorganized speech, (4) grossly disorganized or catatonic behavior, and (5) negative symptoms (e.g., emotional restriction or lack of motivation). Only one of these characteristic symptoms is required to be present during a 1 month period (or for less than 1-month if successfully treated) for a diagnosis of schizophrenia if a patient's delusions are bizarre or if hallucinations consist of a voice that keeps up a running commentary on the patient's behavior or thoughts, or if two or more voices converse with each other. Otherwise, two or more of these symptoms must be present during this time period to make the diagnosis of schizophrenia. Finally, a *DSM-IV* diagnosis of schizophrenia is made only if persistent signs of disturbance have been present for 6 months or more. If less time has elapsed, a diagnosis of schizophreniform disorder is made.

DIFFERENTIAL DIAGNOSIS OF PSYCHOTIC DISORDERS

Other psychotic disorders that are similar to but distinguishable from schizophrenia are schizophreniform disorder, brief psychotic disorder, schizoaffective disorder, delusional disorder, shared psychotic disorder (*folie à deux*), and psychotic disorder not otherwise specified.

Schizophreniform disorder is identical to schizophrenia with two exceptions: The total duration of this illness is more than 1 month but less than 6 months, and impaired social or occupational functioning is not required for a diagnosis. A diagnosis of schizophreniform disorder is often used provisionally, since some patients will fully recover with no future illness, while others will continue to have symptoms for more than 6 months, at which point the diagnosis is changed to schizophrenia.

In brief psychotic disorder, the patient typically experiences positive psychotic symptoms for at least a day but less than a month and subsequently returns to normal functioning. A brief psychotic episode is often precipitated by events that anyone would experience as markedly stressful, such as the sudden loss of a spouse, a reaction to combat, or a reaction to a natural disaster such as an earthquake, or flood. This disorder can also manifest without any obvious stressor or as part of the postpartum period (see chapter 14, Women's Health Through the Reproductive Cycle).

In schizoaffective disorder, the patient experiences a mood disorder in conjunction with symptoms of schizophrenia, as described above. To qualify for this diagnosis, the patient must meet criteria for major depressive, manic, or mixed episode disorder at least once while schizophrenic symptoms are present (see chapter 3, Depression). The patient must also have had a period of 2 weeks or more in which delusions or hallucinations were present in the absence of prominent mood symptoms.

In delusional disorder, the patient suffers with a nonbizarre delusion that does not meet criteria for schizophrenia. For example, a patient may feel that he or she is being persecuted by others, be certain that he or she has an illness or is loved by a famous person, or be jealous and suspicious that his or her spouse is unfaithful despite objective evidence to the contrary. The patient's delusions are not otherwise fantastic, absurd, or unusual but simply not true. The patient generally does not exhibit impaired social or occupational functioning nor other bizarre behavior (in contrast to schizophrenia) except in relation to the specific delusion. The prognosis is quite variable, and delusions may totally remit, subsequently relapse, wax and wane in intensity, or follow a chronic course. There is some evidence that the jealous form of delusional disorder may have a better prognosis than the persecutory form.

In shared psychotic disorder, delusional thinking develops in a patient in the context of a close relationship with a person who is already delusional (e.g., a delusional mother raises her daughter to believe in the delusion). Typically, the primary sufferer influences the development of delusion in his or her partner (*folie à deux*). This disorder may be more common in women than men, but little is known about its true prevalence and course.

Psychotic disorder not otherwise specified is the diagnosis used when a patient presents with a psychosis that does not meet criteria for any of the other psychoses described here.

COURSE OF SCHIZOPHRENIA

Schizophrenia usually presents in the late teens or early 20s, either after a period of normal social or occupational functioning or after a period of deteriorating or poor premorbid social functioning. Schizophrenia frequently afflicts young people at a time when they are preparing for or launching careers. In earlier times, being diagnosed with schizophrenia usually meant the end of youthful dreams and aspirations and the beginning of a marginal existence marred by frightening and disruptive symptoms with frequent and, in some cases, lifelong hospitalizations. Before the introduction of antipsychotic medication in the 1950s, at any one time in the United States alone, roughly 100,000 individuals with schizophrenia resided in state or county hospitals. Today, the vast majority of patients with schizophrenia receive treatment in ambulatory care settings. Partial control of symptoms is now the norm, allowing patients to participate in rehabilitation programs. Many patients graduate from rehabilitation programs and can resume studies or work. However, those patients who are able to return to work often will function at a level below what they were able to achieve before becoming ill (e.g., someone who had been a medical student may, after rehabilitation, be able to work 5 to 10 hours a week sorting mail in the hospital where he or she had once hoped to practice medicine).

A small but growing minority of persons with schizophrenia achieve remission; that is, characteristic symptoms resolve. A smaller number even achieve recovery and become their "old selves" again, with both symptom remission and social skills returning. It is exciting that we are seeing recovery in a disorder once considered untreatable. However, those who do recover do so after an extended period of time, sometimes decades, making it impossible to pick up relationships, studies, or careers at the point at which the patient stopped functioning years earlier. Although recovery occurs in only a minority of cases, the possibility of recovery can offer hope to patients and family members experiencing the anguish of a diagnosis of schizophrenia. Knowing that there is at least a chance that a loved one may recover at some time in the future can be a comfort to everyone involved, including family, friends, physicians, and mental health care providers.

ETIOLOGY OF SCHIZOPHRENIA

Genetic factors, not "schizophrenogenic" mothers (i.e., mother who supposedly caused schizophrenia), appear to create a vulnerability to schizophrenia. A person's risk of developing schizophrenia is 10% if a first-degree relative has the disease. The risk of developing schizophrenia if an identical twin is afflicted is 50% (Torrey, 1995).

The 50% chance of developing schizophrenia in identical twins, called a concordance rate, as compared to a 10% concordance rate in nontwin siblings (as well as in nonidentical twins), clearly suggests that genetic factors play a role. Although a genetic vulnerability to schizophrenia has yet to be definitively demonstrated, it is difficult to explain increased concordance rates in identical twins who were raised apart in any other way. The concordance rates argue equally that genetic factors are not the whole story. Otherwise, the concordance rate for identical twins would be 100%.

While genetics probably supply the underlying vulnerability to schizophrenia, most patients also require a "second hit," an environmental factor or factors that can lead to the expression of vulnerability in susceptible individuals. In identical twins, careful review of records demonstrates that the afflicted twin is more likely to have had environmental insults, such as exposure to certain viruses, head trauma, high fevers, poor in utero nutrition to the pregnant mother, or even brief periods of anoxia during the perinatal period (Torrey, 1995). In most cases, it is the combination of genetic vulnerability and environmental triggers, not bad parenting, that leads to schizophrenia.

PHARMACOLOGICAL TREATMENT OF SCHIZOPHRENIA AND OTHER PSYCHOTIC DISORDERS

Prior to the 1950s, psychopharmacological agents, or psychotropics, were used in a nonspecific manner as sedatives in managing dangerous behavior. In 1952, Dr. Henri Laborit, a French surgeon, reported good results using a new antihistamine as a preanesthetic sedative (Laborit, Huguenard, & Alluaume, 1952). Later that year, two French psychiatrists, Delay and Deniker, administered this new sedating antihistamine to an agitated psychotic patient (Deniker, 1983, pp. 155–164). To their amazement, this new drug—chlorpromazine—led to a decrease in hallucinations and delusions. Delay and Deniker subsequently used chlorpromazine to treat hallucinations and delusions in other patients. They noted that at the same time chlorpromazine treated psychosis, it often induced the stiffness, rigidity, difficulty initiating voluntary movement, slow small-stepped ("festinating") gait, stooped posture, and hand tremor characteristic of Parkinson's disease. Impressed by chlorpromazine's broad range of effects on the nervous system—in particular causing sedation, improving psychotic symptoms, and inducing parkinsonism—Delay and Deniker decided to call chlorpromazine a neuroleptic, meaning literally an agent that seizes the nerves. To this day, the terms *antipsychotic* and *neuroleptic* are often used interchangeably.

This chapter uses the term *neuroleptic* as originally conceptualized by Delay and Deniker, that is, to refer to those antipsychotics that treat psychotic symptoms at doses that simultaneously produce clinically significant early extrapyramidal symptoms (EPS). Because we have since learned that the antipsychotic clozapine can effectively treat psychosis without causing parkinsonism or other EPS, clozapine will be referred to as a "nonneuroleptic," or "atypical" antipsychotic. The new antipsychotics risperidone (Risperdal, introduced in 1994), olanzapine (Zyprexa, introduced in 1996), and quetiapine (Seroquel, introduced in 1997) have not yet been shown to possess other atypical features (e.g., an ability to treat neuroleptic-refractory schizophrenia or schizophrenia that has failed to respond to reasonable trials with several standard neuroleptics). As a group, they will be referred to as "novel antipsychotics," because they cause fewer EPS than the older neuroleptics.

Antipsychotics

Indications for Uses

Antipsychotic medications are used to treat not only schizophrenia but also a broad spectrum of psychotic disorders. These include schizophrenia, schizophreniform disorder, brief psychotic disorder, bipolar disorder (manic-depressive illness), depressive disorders with psychosis, schizoaffective disorder, delusional disorder, shared delusional disorder, paranoid symptoms, dementia or delirium with psychosis, psychotic disorders due to a general medical condition (e.g., postictal psychosis and systemic lupus cerebritis), and substance-related psychosis (e.g., cocaine psychosis and alcoholic hallucinosis).

Traditional neuroleptics are most helpful in treating the positive symptoms of psychosis, such as hallucinations, delusions, thought disorder, disorganized speech, and catatonic behavior. Only 70% of schizophrenics (mostly those with positive symptoms) will respond to neuroleptics with symptom reduction (Kane, 1997). Fortunately, the negative symptoms of schizophrenia (restrictions in emotional expression such as emotional flattening, decreased speech output, and decreased motivation) are responsive to clozapine and the novel antipsychotic medications.

Neuroleptic antipsychotics share the following additional limitations:

1. Neuroleptics cause both early and late motor side effects. Specifically, neuroleptics can cause dystonias, akathisia, and drug-induced parkinsonism, as well as the late and at times irreversible movement disorder tardive dyskinesia (TD).
2. Neuroleptics cause hyperprolactinemia, leading to neuroendocrine side effects.
3. By definition, neuroleptics are ineffective in the approximately 30% of patients who suffer from neuroleptic-refractory schizophrenia.

Neuroleptic-induced Side Effects

Neuroleptic antipsychotics can produce EPS, which include acute dystonia, drug-induced parkinsonism, akathisia, tardive dyskinesia, and they can also cause neuroleptic malignant syndrome (NMS).

Acute dystonia (asymmetrical contraction of muscle groups), drug-induced parkinsonism, and akathisia (restlessness) usually respond to adjunctive anticholinergics such as benztropine (Cogentin) 1 to 6 mg/day and trihexyphenidyl (Artane), 1 to 10 mg/day, as well as to the indirect dopamine agonist amantadine (Symmetrel), 100 to 300 mg/day.

Akathisia, a motor restlessness syndrome easily confused with agitation or exacerbation of psychosis, sometimes does not respond adequately to either the anticholinergics or dopamine agonists. If this is the case, lorazepam (Ativan), 2 to 8 mg/day, or propranolol (Inderal), 20 to 120 mg/day, should be administered as alternative treatments of akathisia.

Tardive dyskinesia is a late-onset movement disorder caused by neuroleptics. TD is characterized by choreo-athetoid movements affecting primarily the tongue and lips, but often also involving the extremities and occasionally the diaphragmatic musculature (Opler, Katz, Kobayashi, & Ruiz, 1980). There is some evidence that giving vitamin E (1,200 IU/day) provides some protection against TD (Lohr et al., 1988).

NMS is a rare but potentially life-threatening condition characterized by severe muscle rigidity, high fever, rapid heartbeat, rapid breathing, excessive perspiration, abnormal blood pressure, and kidney failure. To successfully manage NMS, it is critical to discontine neuroleptics while beginning supportive measures (e.g., providing a cooling blanket to reduce hyperthermia and pushing fluids to prevent dehydration). To reverse NMS, anecdotal evidence additionally supports the use of dopamine agonists such as bromocriptine (Parlodel), 7.5 to 30 mg/day, and dantrolene (Dantrium), 240 to 600 mg/day, which is used in treating malignant hyperthermia.

All neuroleptics cause an increase in serum prolactin (also called hyperprolactinemia), which leads to such neuroendocrine side effects as increased weight, breast tenderness and/or swelling, decreased libido in men and women, and lactation and amenorrhea in women. Often the physician learns about these side effects only upon direct questioning. This is because many patients have difficulty discussing such highly personal and often confusing matters as changes in breast size, changes in sexual desire, the beginning of lactation, or the cessation of menstruation in women of childbearing age, even with a clinician. It is important to inform patients about the possibility that these side effects may occur during treatment with neuroleptics, as well as to inquire about the presence of these symptoms. Patients experiencing these side effects are relieved to know that they are common and due to their medication, and that symptoms can be treated by adding the indirect dopamine agonist amantadine (Correa, Opler, Kay, & Birmaher, 1987).

The neuroleptic antipsychotics fall into six major chemical classes: phenothiazines, butyrophenones, thioxanthenes, dihydroindolones, dibenzoxazepines, and diphenylbutylpiperidines. The clinical uses of neuroleptic antipsychotics, including chemical class, dosing, desirable effects, and common side effects, are summarized in Table 9.1. The doses suggested apply to medically healthy adults. Lower doses should be used for children, the elderly, or persons with certain concurrent medical conditions.

Clozapine: The Prototypical Atypical Antipsychotic

Like chlorpromazine, the development and subsequent discovery of clozapine's special properties was serendipitous. Clozapine was initially synthesized as a drug similar in structure to the antidepressant imipramine (Tofranil) as part of an attempt to synthesize new antidepressants. Only subsequently was clozapine found to be an antipsychotic, but, unlike the neuroleptic antipsychotics, one that caused neither EPS nor TD. Additionally, clozapine was shown to cause only transient hyperprolactinemia, with prolactin levels returning to normal within days.

Clozapine was released in Europe in the early 1970s. In 1975 clozapine was found to be associated with agranulocytosis, a potentially life-threatening condition, as without an adequate number of granulocytes, patients are unable to combat opportunistic infections (Idänpään-Heikkilä, Alhava, Olkinuora, & Palva, 1977). Because of reports of clozapine-induced agranulocytosis, in the United States between 1975 and 1982, only patients who had been started on clozapine before 1975 who were showing significant benefit, and who agreed to comply with weekly white blood cell (WBC) monitoring were allowed to remain on the drug through a compassionate use protocol.

By 1982 clozapine had been successfully introduced in other countries to patients who agreed to close monitoring so that those developing agranulocytosis could be withdrawn from clozapine and, if necessary, treated for infection. Not only was it reported to treat psychosis without causing EPS or TD, but additionally it was found to be effective, and, in some cases, dramatically effective in patients with schizophrenia refractory to standard neuroleptics. Furthermore, clozapine treated negative as well as positive symptoms. Given these reported advantages, the U.S. Food and Drug Administration (FDA) and Sandoz Pharmaceuticals, the manufacturer of the drug, agreed on a research design in which clozapine was compared to chlorpromazine plus benztropine in the treatment of patients with schizophrenia who had by history failed to respond to adequate trials with three or more standard neuroleptic medications (Kane, Honigfeld, Singer, Meltzer, & the Clozaril Collaborative Study Group, 1988). In this 6-week phase III study, 30% of patients with neuroleptic-refractory schizophrenia receiving clozapine achieved significant clinical improvement, as compared with only 4% in the control group receiving chlorpromazine and benztropine. In longer trials, even higher percentages of neuroleptic-refractory schizophrenics have been shown to benefit from clozapine treatment.

In 1990 clozapine was released as a second-line drug for patients with schizophrenia who had failed to respond to standard neuroleptics. At the time of its release, the calculated risk of developing agranulocytosis, based on data collected from the open label humanitarian protocol, was 1.6%, so that patients using clozapine were required to obtain weekly WBC counts as a condition of treatment with the drug.

This author considers clozapine the only true, atypical antipsychotic because it is the only antipsychotic that has at this time been demonstrated to possess all of the following properties: (1) treats negative as well as positive symptoms, (2) causes little or no EPS, (3) does not cause TD, (4) does not cause prolonged hyperprolactinemia, and (5) treats neuroleptic-refractory schizophrenia.

Despite being the "gold standard" (Kane, 1997) for maximal efficacy with neuroleptic-refractory schizophrenia, clozapine is underutilized as a second-line antipsychotic because of the risk of agranulocytosis. For several reasons the use of clozapine is likely to increase. First, in the United States, the risk of developing clozapine-induced agranulocytosis has dropped from 1.6% in 1990 to 0.4% in 1996. This is presumably because obtaining a complete blood count (CBC) with differential allows detection of granulocytopenia and if necessary, discontinuation of clozapine before agranulocytosis occurs. Second, accumulated data make it clear that the risk of developing clozapine-induced agranulocytosis decreases dramatically after the first 6 months. Third, it has been reported that subcutaneous administration of granulocyte colony stimulating factor (GCSF) rapidly restores both WBC and granulocyte counts, whereas previously, the mean time before WBC and granulocyte counts normalized was 16 days after discontinuing clozapine (Lamberti, Bellnier, Schwarzkopf, & Schneider, 1995). With clozapine-induced agranulocytosis rapidly reversible, the risk that a patient will develop a life-threatening infection is greatly diminished. Standard practice for treating clozapine-induced agranulocytosis should now include administering 300 μg/day of GCSF along with instituting reverse isolation procedures and beginning prophylactic antibiotics.

Clozapine is usually begun at a low dose (e.g., 25 mg at bedtime), then slowly titrated upwards to allow patients to develop tolerance to the

Table 9.1 Neuroleptic Drugs

Subclass	Dose	Desirable Effects	Side Effects
Aliphatic: chlorpromazine (Thorazine)	30–400 mg/day with bid dosing Increase 20–50 mg/day Max: 2,000 mg/day	Treats positive symptoms (hallucinations, delusions, thought disorder).	Anticholinergic (+3) Orthostatic hypotension (+4) Sedation (+4) EPS (+2) Seizure risk, Arrhythmia/EKG effects Photosensitivity/dermatitis
Piperidine: thioridazine (Mellaril)	150–300 mg/day with bid dosing Max: 800 mg/day	Treats positive symptoms.	Anticholinergic (+4) Orthostatic hypotension (+3) Sedation (+3) EPS (+1) Arrhythmia/EKG effects, retinitis pigmentosa, sexual dysfunction
mesoridazine (Serentil)	100–400 mg/day with bid dosing Max: 400 mg/day	Treats positive symptoms.	Anticholinergic (+4) Orthostatic hypotension (+3) Sedation (+3), EPS (+1) EKG effects
Piperazines: trifluoperazine (Stelazine)	15–40 mg hs Max: 80 mg	Treats positive symptoms.	Anticholinergic (+1) Orthostatic hypotension (+1) Sedation (+1) EPS (+3)
fluphenazine (Prolixin)	5 mg/day Max: 60 mg/day 12.5–50mg Decanoate q 2–4 weeks	Treats positive symptoms. Less seizure risk. Decanoate for adherence. Use nondepot test dose of IM, then decanoate for adherence.	Anticholinergic (+1) Orthostatic hypotension (+1) Sedation (+1) EPS (+4)

Subclass	Dose	Desirable Effects	Side Effects
Piperazines: perphenazine (Trilafon)	8–24 mg/day Max: 64 mg/day	Treats positive symptoms.	Anticholinergic (+2) Orthostatic hypotension (+2) Sedation (+2) EPS (+3)
Butyrophenone: haloperidol (Haldol)	1–15 mg/day Max: 100 mg/day Decanoate 25–100 mg q 4 weeks	Treats positive symptoms. Geriatric psychosis. Use nondepot test dose IM, then decanoate for adherence.	Anticholinergic (+1) Orthostatic hypotension (+1) Sedation (+1) EPS (+4)
droperidol (Inapsine)	2.5–15 mg/day Max 50 mg/day	Use for extreme agitation.	Anticholinergic (+1) Orthostatic hypotension (+1) Sedation (+4) EPS (+4)
Thioxanthene: thiothixene (Navane)	6–15 mg/day Max: 60 mg/day	Treats positive symptoms.	Anticholinergic (+1) Orthostatic hypotension (+1) Sedation (+1) EPS (+4)
Dihydroindolones: molindone (Moban)	50–100 mg/day Max: 225 mg/day	Treats positive symptoms. Less seizure risk. Less or no weight gain. Geriatric psychosis.	Anticholinergic (+2) Orthostatic hypotension (+1) Sedation (+2) EPS (+3)
Dibenzazepine: loxapine (Loxitane)	60–100 mg/day Max: 250 mg/day	Treats positive symptoms. Less or no weight gain.	Anticholinergic (+1) Orthostatic hypotension (+1) Sedation (+1) EPS (+4)
Diphenylbutyl-piperidine: pimozide (Orap)	1–2 mg/day Max: 20 mg/day	Treats nonbizarre delusions (e.g., pathological jealousy monosymptomatic hypochondriacal psychosis). Used for Tourette's syndrome.	Anticholinergic (+3) Orthostatic hypotension (+2) Sedation (+3) EPS (+4) Arrhythmia/EKG effects

+4 = Most 0 = Least All raise prolactin levels and all cause +1 weight gain.

sedation and orthostatic hypotension that frequently occur when clozapine is first taken. In patients being switched from another antipsychotic, a slow cross-over works better in most cases than an abrupt cessation of the previous antipsychotic, since upward titration of clozapine can take several weeks. A standard dose is 300 to 450 mg per day, although higher doses may be required. Because clozapine lowers seizure threshold in a dose-related manner, doses above 900 mg/day are not recommended. Clozapine is usually administered twice a day, with the larger dose administered at night. Other side effects associated with clozapine include weight gain, constipation, and excessive salivation.

The demonstration that the nonneuroleptic antipsychotic clozapine (i.e., a drug that treats psychosis without causing motor side effects) is superior to standard neuroleptics in a number of ways has changed the way pharmaceutical companies look for new and better antipsychotics. This has led to the development in recent years of several new antipsychotics, with others still in development.

The Novel Antipsychotics: Risperidone, Olanzapine, and Quetiapine

Table 9.2 summarizes the clinical use of clozapine and novel antipsychotics, including dosing, desirable effects, and common side effects. Following is a brief review of these novel medications.

The marketing of risperidone began in 1994, olanzapine in 1996, and quetiapine in 1997. All three drugs have been shown to have some of clozapine's advantages, but none of them are associated with a high risk of agranulocytosis. All have been referred to in the literature by various terms, including *atypical neuroleptic* and *atypical antipsychotic*. As previously noted, these three antipsychotics are referred to in this chapter as novel antipsychotics, because, at least at the present time, none has been demonstrated to have all of clozapine's unique advantages.

Because clozapine blocks the S2-serotonin receptor more potently than the D2-dopamine receptor, scientists at the Janssen Research Foundation synthesized a series of combined serotonin-dopamine antagonists (SDAs) and subsequently launched clinical trials with one of these, risperidone (Risperdal), including an 8-week, phase III, randomized, double-blind trial comparing risperidone to placebo and to haloperidol. The Positive and Negative Syndrome Scale, or PANSS (Kay, Opler, & Fiszbein, 1992), was used in the trial as the primary outcome measure in order to examine effects on negative as well as on positive symptoms. The group receiving

6 mg/day of risperidone showed the best overall clinical effects. Additionally, the risperidone group demonstrated significantly greater improvement in both negative and positive symptoms and was statistically indistinguishable from placebo on measures of EPS. These findings, and subsequent clinical experience, demonstrate that risperidone is useful for patients with schizophrenia who respond to neuroleptics but still suffer from negative symptoms and/or EPS. Risperidone, however, does increase serum prolactin and has been reported to cause TD. Risperidone's role in treating neuroleptic-refractory schizophrenia has not been established.

Risperidone is a novel antipsychotic with a low EPS profile and an ability to treat negative as well as positive symptoms. It should be started at a low dose of 1 mg twice a day, then titrated upward to a target dose of 6 mg/day. Dosing needs to be individualized, with the optimal dose appearing to be 1 to 2 mg below that at which clinically significant EPS emerges; therefore, EPS should suggest a lowering of the dose rather than the need to use antiparkinsonian agents concurrently. It is not advisable to exceed 16 mg/day. Many patients respond to daily doses below 6 mg; however, maximal effects usually occur at doses of 4 to 6 mg/day.

Olanzapine (Zyprexa), in addition to blocking the S2-serotonin receptor and the D2-dopamine receptor, possesses other biochemical features that suggest that it is clozapine-like: (1) A member of the thienobenzodiazapine class, olanzapine is structurally similar to clozapine. (2) Like clozapine, olanzapine exhibits high to moderate affinity for receptors of serotonin, dopamine, acetylcholine, and histamine. (3) Olanzapine substitutes for clozapine in animals trained to discriminate clozapine from a test vehicle.

A series of phase II and phase III clinical studies have shown that olanzapine treats both positive and negative symptoms at doses at which it induces only minimal EPS as well as only moderate prolactin elevation (Kane, 1997). Olanzapine was FDA-approved, and marketed in 1996. It has since emerged as a well-tolerated and easily administered novel antipsychotic.

Olanzapine is generally started at 10 mg at bedtime and often needs to be tapered upward to 20 mg/day or more. It can cause a transient rise in serum hepatic enzyme levels, which has not been shown to be significant clinically but which still suggests avoiding use of this drug in patients with preexisting liver disease. Because olanzapine is sedating, the entire dose is usually administered at bedtime. Olanzapine can also cause significant weight gain. A special role for olanzapine in the treatment of neuroleptic-refractory schizophrenia has not been established.

Table 9.2 Clozapine and Novel Antipsychotics

Name	Dose	Desirable Effects	Side Effects
Clozapine (Clozaril)	25 mg/hs initial Slowly increase to 300–600 mg /day Max: 900 mg/day	Treats positive and negative symptoms. Only medication shown to treat neuroleptic refractory schizophrenia. Little or no EPS. Does not cause tardive dyskinesia (TD). No prolonged hyperprolactinemia.	Anticholinergic (+4) Orthostatic hypotension (+4) Sedation (+4) EPS (0/+1) Agranulocytosis (0.4%) in monitored populations 5% seizure risk >600 mg/day 70% gain weight (+4) 32% excessive salivation Arrhythmia/EKG effects (0) Approx. cost: $6/100-mg tablet Average daily cost: $30/day
Risperidone (Risperdal)	1 mg bid initial Effective dose: 6 mg/day Max: 16 mg/day	Good for positive and negative symptoms. As good as traditional neuroleptic; better for negative symptoms. Has not been shown to treat neuroleptic refractory. schizophrenia (like clozapine).	Anticholinergic (+1) Orthostatic hypotension (+2) Sedation (+1) EPS (0/+1) TD/NMS? Weight gain (+2) Transient hepatic enzyme elevations (+1) Increase prolactin level (0/+3) Arrhythmia/EKG effects (0/+1)

Name	Dose	Desirable Effects	Side Effects
Olanzapine (Zyprexa)	10 mg hs initial Effective dose: 10–30 for negative symptom relief Max: 40 mg/day	Treats positive and negative symptoms. Has not been shown to treat neuroleptic refractory schizophrenia.	Anticholinergic (+2) Orthostatic hypotension (+1) Sedation (+2) EPS (0/+1) TD/MNS? Weight gain(+2) Transient hepatic enzyme elevations (0/+1) Increased prolactin level is moderate and possibly transient. Arrhythmia/EKG effects (0)
Quetiapine (Seroquel)	25 mg bid initial Effective dose: 150 mg bid Max: 750 mg/day	Treats positive and negative symptoms. Has not been shown to treat neuroleptic refractory schizophrenia.	Anticholinergic (+1) Orthostatic hypotension (+2) Sedation (+2/+3) EPS (0) TD/NMS? Weight gain (+2) No increased prolactin level Arrhythmia/EKG effects (+1)

+4 = Most 0 = Least ? = Insufficient data

Quetiapine (Seroquel), a dibenzothiazepine derivative, combines serotonin with dopamine antagonism. In placebo-controlled clinical trials, quetiapine has been found to be an effective and well-tolerated antipsychotic that treats both negative and positive symptoms at doses at which EPS ratings and prolactin levels were no greater than in patients receiving placebo. Quetiapine's role in neuroleptic-refractory schizophrenia has not yet been demonstrated, and it is too early to draw conclusions regarding whether or not it causes TD.

Quetiapine is usually started at 25 mg twice a day, then titrated upwards to a target dose of 300 mg/day in divided dose. Some patients may require higher doses, but 750 mg/day is the recommended upper limit. Side effects may include orthostatic hypotension, somnolence, and weight gain.

Medical Evaluation for Antipsychotic Drug Treatment

The expert consensus guidelines for medical evaluation prior to the use of antipsychotic medications (Frances, Docherty, & Kahn 1996) recommend that the initial medical screen include medical history, routine physical, and first-line laboratory testing, which includes screening for drugs of abuse, a complete blood count (CBC), general chemistry screens, and urinalysis. Second-line laboratory testing that should be considered on a case-by-case basis includes pregnancy test; EKG, MRI, or CT of the brain; EEG; neuropsychological testing; and general psychological testing.

Neuroleptics vs. Novel Antipsychotics vs. Clozapine: How Do You Choose?

The choice of an antipsychotic medication for a first psychotic episode is based on the symptomatic presentation. Patients presenting with positive symptoms can be treated first line with a high-potency conventional neuroleptic, with risperidone, or with one of the other novel antipsychotic medications. Second-line drug treatment would be low-potency conventional neuroleptics. Patients presenting with predominantly negative symptoms generally are treated with risperidone or other novel antipsychotic medications first line and conventional neuroleptics second line. For patients who fail to respond to either neuroleptics or novel antipsychotics, clozapine is the treatment of choice.

For patients who are on maintenance medications and doing well, there is no compelling reason to switch to one of the newer agents. However, if negative symptoms or EPS symptoms remain problematic, the novel antipsychotics should be considered. Clozapine remains one of our most effective medications and should always be considered for use in patients who are refractory to other medications, including patients with persistent negative symptoms and /or intolerable EPS.

Tables 9.1 and 9.2 summarize the clinical use of neuroleptics, novel antipsychotics, and clozapine, including dosing, desirable effects, and common side effects.

PSYCHOSOCIAL TREATMENT OF SCHIZOPHRENIA

Forming a Therapeutic Alliance

Persons with schizophrenia suffer from extreme isolation. Former friends and relatives who do not understand or cannot cope with schizophrenia drift away; paranoid delusions make it at times impossible for the schizophrenic patient to trust anyone, even those still trying to help. Breaking through this isolation and distrust is often the first challenge. Many patients in the acute phase of illness lack insight into the nature of their condition and may refuse to take antipsychotic medication. At times, if the patient is dangerous to himself or herself or others, lacks insight into his or her condition, and is unable or unwilling to go along with a less restrictive form of treatment, the only choice is to commit the patient involuntarily to a hospital that has mechanisms for administering medication over objection (see chapter 7, Violence and Suicide). However, coercive hospitalization and medication over objection should be avoided if at all possible. The patient often experiences this as traumatic and demeaning, and later work between the patient and those involved in the commitment process may become difficult or even impossible.

How, then, can one form a working alliance with a delusional, often paranoid, patient? In past decades, before we relied so heavily, and perhaps at times too exclusively, on pharmacotherapy, techniques were articulated for working with delusional thinking, including paranoia. One way to work with a paranoid patient is to form an alliance based on affect as opposed to content. Consider the example of a man brought to the clinician's office who believes everyone is trying to poison him and who is therefore refusing to eat. You can tell the patient that you think there is another explanation for his fear of being poisoned. Inform the patient that you believe a treatable biochemical change in the brain function is causing these false beliefs.

It is not helpful to argue with patients, and challenging their sense of reality seldom leads a patient to give up his or her delusions. If anything, confronting delusions can lead the patient in this example to believe that you are in cahoots with the "others" who are trying to poison him, making it more difficult to form a working relationship. Rather, empathic statements like "It must be difficult to believe that your friends and family wish to poison you" are most helpful. By speaking to the patient's emotions (while not agreeing or disagreeing with the delusions), you can somewhat allay the pain and isolation the person must be experiencing simply by acknowledging what he or she is feeling. This emotional alliance can form the basis of an ongoing discussion and, over time, may lead to the development of trust and adherence with treatment.

If the patient remains reluctant to take antipsychotic medication and is not dangerous to self or others, the primary care physician can consider using another medication. For example, many patients with schizophrenia can benefit from low doses of lorazepam to help with anxiety or sleep. This choice of medication may be a good first step and may set the groundwork for both psychotherapeutic work and future pharmacotherapy with an antipsychotic medication.

Psychotherapy

Once a therapeutic alliance has been established, ongoing psychotherapy may be helpful in addition to pharmacotherapy. There is a general misunderstanding that psychotherapy always means psychoanalytically oriented therapy. This is not the case. Although persons with schizophrenia may benefit from understanding how early childhood experiences have an impact on maladaptive behavior patterns in adulthood, there is no evidence that schizophrenics as a group benefit from insight-oriented psychotherapy. Supportive psychotherapy—providing a safe setting in which the person can express concerns and fears and receive advice regarding specific strategies for solving problems—is helpful and can be provided at the same time that one is evaluating the patient's response to antipsychotic medication (see chapter 16, Consulting and Counseling in Primary Care).

Additionally, social skills training for patients, educational work with families, and social support for both patients and their families can improve the course of schizophrenia when combined with pharmacotherapy and supportive psychotherapy.

Social Skills Training

Social skills training involves helping persons with schizophrenia to learn and practice concrete tasks required to carry out day-to-day functions. This training can be conducted individually, but it is more often carried out in a classroom or group setting by mental health practitioners. Topics are spelled out clearly and include managing money, carrying on a conversation, exhibiting a fuller range of emotions, and shopping and cooking.

Social skills training is geared toward helping patients develop the cognitive, verbal, and nonverbal behaviors necessary to interact better with those around them. Ideally, social skills training helps patients learn both to interpret correctly the social messages given to them by others and to get across to others the message that they themselves mean to give. These skills are taught in elementary steps. For example, to help persons with schizophrenia learn how to carry on a conversation, they are first taught to maintain eye contact and to maintain an appropriate level of volume when speaking (Bellack & Mueser, 1993).

Other skills addressed may include attention-focusing, social problem-solving, and vocational and recreational skills (Liberman et al., 1986). Attention-focusing training consists of brief training sessions in which the patient practices conversational skills with a partner. The partner provides conversation "openers" as well as instructions, prompts, and reinforcement. If the patient's attention falters, the partner is there to provide a prompt. The training session is ended after three prompts. Social problem-solving addresses many social situations that may come up, including medication management, friendship and dating, shopping, and money management. These scenarios may be explored through hypothetical questioning, role-playing, and self-assessment. Vocational skills training encompasses job-seeking skills, interview presentation, and the coping skills needed to deal with on-the-job problems. Recreational skills training teaches the patient how to construct a recreational plan. Studies have shown that patients who are engaged in structured leisure activities show a lower incidence of bizarre behavior than those with unstructured leisure time.

For schizophrenic patients who suffer from worsened social functioning, this breakdown of social skills to more elementary tasks may make successful social interaction less frightening and more feasible. Although social skills training can be an important tool in learning how to interact with others, it is best used in combination with other psychosocial and psychopharmacological treatments.

Educational Work With Families

Educational work with families, also called psychoeducational family therapy, has been shown to improve the course of schizophrenia (see chapter 18, Family Counseling). First, families are taught, often in a class-room setting, about the neurobiological models of schizophrenia. They are presented with the evidence that genetic factors, not "schizophrenogenic" mothers, create the vulnerability to schizophrenia and that the environmental insults that cause this vulnerability to be expressed appear to be biological. In other words, it appears that what triggers schizophrenia in genetically vulnerable individuals is not growing up in a dysfunctional family, but rather being exposed to infectious agents such as influenza. Families are taught that schizophrenia is present in 1% of the general population and that the risk of developing schizophrenia is probably genetically controlled. Families are also educated that the genetic vulnerability to schizophrenia is often brought out not by a bad emotional environment but by biological factors, such as infection with high fever early in life, and that it may occur in children with a lower birth weight or who have suffered a period of anoxia at birth. Learning about the neurobiological model of schizophrenia is a great relief for most families. It relieves family members who previously have been burdened with guilt and self-recriminating thoughts that they caused schizophrenia by poor communication, mixed messages, or by not allowing separation-individuation. Families need to know that they did not cause schizophrenia in their loved one and that they deserve assistance, not blame.

Once families understand that schizophrenia is a neurobiological disorder, the fog and guilt lift. Many families are then able to explore new ways to improve the coping and functioning of their family member with schizophrenia. It is very useful to talk with families about pacing themselves. It helps to tell families that what they are undertaking is more like a cross-country run than a 100-yard dash. Families should be encouraged to get help and to make sure they don't burn out so that they can be there for the long haul. They need the realistic hope that, for reasons we do not understand, roughly one third of schizophrenics get better in late midlife just as mysteriously as they became ill in young adulthood.

After explaining the cause of schizophrenia and lessening the guilt, the family can progress to look at new ways to help the patient. Members can be taught that they can have a positive impact on the course of schizophrenia by monitoring and decreasing critical or judgmental remarks. Just as families have been unjustly accused of causing schizophrenia, the person with schizophrenia often receives similar unfair criticism. It is common for a patient with schizophrenia to be told that he or she is lazy, is not trying hard enough, and just has to pull himself or herself out of it. Schizophrenics have no more ability to will their symptoms away than diabetics have to will their blood sugar levels into the normal range. Often it is the negative symptoms of schizophrenia that family members have the most trouble seeing as part of their loved one's neurobiological brain disease. Negative symptoms are deficits in normal functioning such as blunted affect and emotional withdrawal that appear to be caused, at least in part, by dysfunction of the prefrontal (anterior) cortex (Opler, Ramirez, Rosenkilde, & Fiszbein, 1991).

Families can be taught either in individual family sessions or in multifamily groups to recognize and decrease their critical inputs or judgments. The technical term for these negative inputs or criticism is expressed emotionality (EE). Families should learn to lower their EE, because low levels of EE reduce the numbers of relapses and hospitalizations in the schizophrenic patient and improve the overall course of schizophrenia.

In summary, successful educational work with families conveys the following: (1) Families are not bad people whose pathological ideas or behaviors caused schizophrenia in a family member. (2) Families can have a positive impact on the course of the disease by not blaming their loved one who is ill and by reducing critical comments and judgment regarding the patient's difficulties with daily functioning. For families wishing additional information about schizophrenia, as well as about other psychiatric disorders and their treatment, *Surviving Schizophrenia: For Families, Consumers, and Providers,* 3rd ed. (Torrey, 1995) and *Prozac and Other Psychiatric Drugs* (Opler & Bialkowski, 1996) provide easy-to-read practical information.

Social Support

Social support for persons with schizophrenia as well as for their families is extremely important. For families, the development of the advocacy movement has provided a social support network that in previous eras was lacking. Mental health advocacy groups also give families a place to put their energies (e.g., educating others and lobbying for more funding for treatment and research). Additionally, support from others who are going through a similar process allows families to feel that they are not alone and provides them with an opportunity to hear from others and to learn what has helped and what has not.

Recently, patients have banded together both to advocate for themselves and to receive social support from peers. Patients often prefer to refer to themselves as consumers or recipients rather than patients in order to distance themselves from the stigma that has been inappropriately associated with being a "mental patient." They are increasingly speaking for the need for more self-help, peer advocacy, and recipient empowerment.

The National Alliance for the Mentally Ill (NAMI) is a national umbrella organization of over 1,000 groups that is a resource for both patients, friends, and families interested in support and/or advocacy groups. The quickest way to learn about local support and advocacy groups is by calling the NAMI Helpline (800-950-NAMI). Also helpful are the National Depressive and Manic-Depressive Association (800-82-NDMDA) and the National Mental Health Association (703-684-7722).

Psychiatric Consultation or Referral

Primary care physicians and other clinicians should have a low threshold for consulting for schizophrenic patients and should refer such patients to a psychiatrist, particularly if treating psychotic disorders is a new aspect in the physician's practice, if the physician feels uncomfortable with a particular case, or when the patient's clinical picture is worsening. Psychiatrists can consult on differential diagnosis of psychosis and medications and can make recommendations about the broad range of psychosocial treatments that can be utilized. The primary care physician should seek occasional routine consultation with a board-certified psychiatrist to ensure that nothing is being missed and that state-of-the-art treatment is being applied to every patient. Referral to a psychiatrist for primary management is indicated if the patient becomes acutely dangerous to self or others, is floridly psychotic, is in need of sophisticated psychopharmacology, or requires hospitalization for either persistent and troubling positive or negative symptoms.

FUTURE DIRECTIONS

Schizophrenia remains a devastating disorder. Once we learn more about its pathogenesis and treatment, future goals that may be realized include making recovery from schizophrenia the norm rather than the exception and preventing schizophrenia. Prevention may include the following: (1) learning how to identify those at risk before the emergence of schizophrenia (e.g., finding a marker in the blood or urine); (2) developing early intervention programs for those showing prodromal signs, as well as learning what preventive measures need to be implemented to ensure that those at risk never develop symptoms; and (3) identifying those whose family history suggests they are at some genetic risk, then intervening to prevent the "second hit"—an environmental factor or factors that can precipitate the expression of vulnerability in susceptible individuals. This may mean preventing exposure to certain viruses, head trauma, high fevers, and poor nutrition to the pregnant mothers, or preventing brief periods of anoxia during the perinatal period. Someday, through preventive interventions, we will be able to reduce, perhaps even eradicate, schizophrenia.

As the multifactorial etiology of schizophrenia is elucidated, it will become important to use medications to treat active symptoms and as part of strategies aimed at preventing the development or worsening of schizophrenia in vulnerable individuals. Prophylactic approaches in schizophrenia are suggested by work indicating that antioxidants may have a role in preventing the development of symptoms such as depression and apathy (Lohr et al., 1988); that anticonvulsants may prevent increased dopamine sensitivity in the brain (Csernansky, Murphy, & Faustman, 1991), and that central nervous system infections and/or autoimmune reactions may trigger schizophrenia in vulnerable individuals (Kirch, 1993).

Someday, the identification of individuals at risk for schizophrenia will allow for interventions that will prevent the eruption of this devastating disorder. When that day comes, the extremely important and effective treatment interventions discussed in this chapter will be of historical rather than pragmatic interest. Until that day, however, it is extremely important and gratifying to know that during the latter half of the 20th century, highly effective treatments for schizophrenia were introduced, allowing reintegration, rehabilitation, and, for some, even recovery from what was once an untreatable condition.

REFERENCES

American Psychiatric Association. (1994). *Diagnostic and statistical manual of mental disorders* (4th ed.). Washington, DC: Author.

Bellack, A. S., & Mueser, K. T. (1993). Psychosocial treatment for schizophrenia. *Schizophrenia Bulletin, 19*, 317–336.

Correa, N., Opler, L. A., Kay, S. R., & Birmaher, B. (1987). Amantadine in the treatment of neuroendocrine side effects of neuroleptics. *Journal of Clinical Psychopharmacology, 7*, 507–518.

Csernansky, J. G., Murphy, G. M., & Faustman, W. O. (1991). Limbic/mesolimbic connections and the pathogenesis of schizophrenia. *Biological Psychiatry, 30*, 383–400.

Deniker, P. (1983). Introduction of neuroleptic chemotherapy into psychiatry. In M. J. Parnham & J. Bruinvel. (Eds.), *Discoveries in pharmacology: Psycho and neuropharmacology* (Vol. 1, pp. 155–164). New York: Elsevier Science Publishers.

Frances, A., Docherty, J. P., & Kahn, D. A. (1996). The expert consensus guideline series. Treatment of schizophrenia. *Journal of Clinical Psychiatry, 57*(Suppl. 12B), 15–27.

Idänpään-Heikkilä, J., Alhava, E., Olkinuora, M., & Palva, I. P. (1977). Agranulocytosis during treatment with clozapine. *European Journal of Clinical Pharmacology, 11*, 193–x198.

Kane, J. M. (1997). The new antipsychotics. *Journal of Practical Psychiatry and Behavioral Health, 3*, 343–354.

Kane, J., Honigfeld, G., Singer, J., Meltzer, H., & the Clozaril Collaborative Study Group. (1988). Clozapine for the treatment-resistant schizophrenic: A double-blind comparison versus chlorpromazine. *Archives of General Psychiatry, 45*, 789–796.

Kay, S. R., Opler, L. A., & Fiszbein, A. (1992). *Positive and Negative Syndrome Scale* (PANSS) manual. Toronto: Multi-Health Systems.

Kirch, D. G. (1993). Infection and autoimmunity as etiologic factors in schizophrenia: A review and reappraisal. *Schizophrenia Bulletin, 19*, 355–370.

Laborit, H., Huguenard, P., & Alluaume, R. (1952). Un nouveau stabilisateur vegetatif (b 4560 R.P.). *Press Médecine, 60*, 206–208.

Lamberti, J. S., Bellnier, T. J., Schwarzkopf, S. B., & Schneider, E. (1995). Filgrastim treatment of three patients with clozapine-induced agranulocytosis.*Journal of Clinical Psychiatry, 56*, 256–259.

Liberman, R. P., Mueser, K. T., Wallace, C. J., Jacobs, H. E., Eckman, T., & Massel, H. K. (1986). Training skills in the psychiatrically disabled: Learning coping and competence. *Schizophrenia Bulletin, 12*, 631–647.

Lohr, J. B., Cadet, J. L., Lohr, M. A., Larson, L., Wasli, E., Wade, L., Hylton, R., Vidoni, C., Jeste, D. V., & Wyatt, R. J. (1988). Vitamin E in the treatment of tardive dyskinesia: The possible involvement of free radical mechanisms. *Schizophrenia Bulletin, 14*, 291–296.

Opler, L. A., & Feinberg, S. S. (1991). The role of pimozide in clinical psychiatry: A review. *Journal of Clinical Psychiatry, 52*, 221–233.

Opler, L. A., & Bialkowski, C. (1996). *Prozac and other psychiatric drugs.* New York: Simon & Schuster.

Opler, L. A., Katz, I., Kobayashi, J., & Ruiz, P. (1980). Tardive dyskinesia and institutional practice: Current issues and guidelines. *Hospital and Community Psychiatry, 31*, 239–245.

Opler, L. A., Ramirez, P. M., Rosenkilde, C. E., & Fiszbein, A. (1991). Neurocognitive features of chronic schizophrenic inpatients. *Journal of Nervous and Mental Disease, 179*, 638–640.

Rupp, A., & Keith, S. J. (1993). The cost of schizophrenia: Assessing the burden. *The Psychiatric Clinics of North America, 16*, 413–423.

Torrey, E. F. (1995). *Surviving schizophrenia: For families, consumers, and providers* (3rd ed.). New York: Harper & Row.

CHAPTER 10

Sexual Disorders and Sexual Trauma

Anne A. Brewer

Human sexuality occurs over the entire continuum of life. Sexuality plays a major role in well-being, but it can also be the source of much suffering. Because of the effect sexuality has on health, it is a proper concern for primary care physicians. However, many primary care physicians do not address issues of sexuality in their practices. Time constraints and other pressing medical problems that need to be addressed often crowd out discussions of sexuality and sexual health. Many physicians receive little or no training in sexuality and feel ill-prepared to discuss it with their patients. Moreover, some physicians, because of upbringing or personality, feel uncomfortable discussing such a sensitive area of life with their patients. The shame and guilt about sexuality that many clinicians and patients share contribute to the secrecy that often shrouds sexuality in our culture. Unfortunately, silence about sexual issues leaves people alone in their confusion or distress, and this can have adverse effects on health.

American society presents a paradox: The media are sex-saturated, and sexual issues are discussed openly on television talk shows. Yet misinformation, shame, and discomfort in discussing sexuality abound. Primary

Special thanks to Linda Palermo, M. A., M.F.T., who read this chapter and made many helpful suggestions.

care physicians, who often are a patient's first contact with the medical care system, have a unique opportunity to dispel misinformation and assist people in dealing with this important, often painful, area of their lives.

SEXUAL DEVELOPMENT

Sexual development begins before birth, when hormonal influences control the development of reproductive organs and genitalia. Occasional anomalies such as intersex or hormonal pseudohermaphroditic conditions point up the complexity of prenatal development. Gender role assignment often begins at birth or even before, with the advent of ultrasound and amniocentesis for prenatal sex determination. All societies have expectations for male and female traits and behaviors, although some of these vary from society to society. A person's gender identity is based on internalization of these expectations. However, the degree to which these role expectations are incorporated into personality varies among individuals, which may influence the security of their gender identity (Tiefer & King, 1995). Strong discordance between role expectations and individual traits and personality may cause difficulties in gender identity or societal rejection.

Sexual feelings and behavior begin in infancy, with the oral gratification the infant receives from feeding and with early self-exploration of eyes, ears, mouth, and genitalia. In early childhood, self-exploration continues; children may also engage in sex play with peers and siblings. These behaviors may continue into later childhood as well. Adolescence brings physical, hormonal, and emotional changes and an upsurge in sexual feelings and sometimes in sexual activity. Increased adolescent sexual activity may have such adverse consequences as pregnancy, sexually transmitted disease, and emotional harm. In the adult years, establishing sexual identity and partnerships and sometimes undertaking parenthood are major life tasks. As adults age, some experience a diminution of sexual potency as a result of aging, concomitant disease, or medication side effects. However, sexual feelings and activity often continue throughout the later years of the life cycle. Therefore, at every stage of life, primary care physicians, with their concern for health promotion, can play an important role in assisting people with sexual health issues or concerns about their sexuality.

TAKING A SEXUAL HISTORY

Sexuality is as much a part of a patient's medical history as are past medical problems and use of medications. Many of the published forms for sexual history taking are extensive and thus impractical for a primary care office practice. However, by incorporating sexual history into the medical history, the physician conveys the message that sexuality is as much the doctor's concern as are immunizations. Taking a sexual history in a matter-of-fact, nonjudgmental way gives the patient permission to raise this often-difficult subject. It is most appropriate to ask about sexual issues during either the review of systems or the social history. A general question, such as "Are you having any sexual concerns or problems?" is a good opener. This can be followed by questions about sexual orientation (e.g., "Are you sexually active with men, with women, or both?"). Then, issues of contraception, protection against sexually transmitted diseases, and high-risk behaviors can be addressed. With adolescents, questions about dating can be a helpful opening to this discussion. If concerns or problems are raised, further history can be elicited. For more extensive history taking, published outlines are available that can provide a guide (Risen, 1995).

Taking a sexual history also provides the opportunity for anticipatory guidance, which is a major part of health promotion. When working with parents of infants and young children, physicians can educate them about the normalcy of sexual exploration, both with self and with peers. Such education may help parents respond to normal sexual behavior in a low-key way instead of becoming upset. Some parents may need discussions about the difference between healthy parental physical contact with their children and sexually abusive behavior. Well-child visits can also be occasions to discuss "good touch" and "bad touch" with children and parents and to offer guidance about appropriate responses.

With adolescents, separate interviews with parents and the adolescent provide the opportunity to discuss normal development, including the physical and emotional changes of puberty. Questions of sexual identity often arise during adolescence, and the primary care physician can give guidance and appropriate referral. If adolescents are not having sexual intercourse, anticipatory guidance about contraception and safe sex can be given, as well as the message that the physician is a resource for the adolescent if these concerns should arise. The clinician can also support an adolescent's decision to abstain from sexual intercourse, despite peer pressure or pressure from the partner. If an adolescent is engaging in sexual intercourse, the physician can address needs for contraception and for testing for and protection from sexually transmitted diseases (STDs).

Adolescents often deny the risks associated with unprotected sexual intercourse. They may require education and counseling over time to overcome their resistance to using contraception and protection against STDs. Peer education and groups in which teens learn assertiveness about safe sex and refusal skills are sometimes effective. Legally, physicians can evaluate and treat minors for sexually transmitted diseases and prescribe contraception without parental permission. For many adolescents, the physician can encourage discussion with parents. However, in certain situations, disclosure of sexual activity may lead to severe repercussions for the adolescent. Unless the adolescent's life or health is endangered, confidentiality is appropriate, even if the parents are also patients.

Many of the issues facing adolescents are also relevant to adult anticipatory guidance. Premarital and prenatal visits, as well as physical exams, provide an opportunity to discuss sexual issues and concerns. Sexual concerns often surface at times of transition (e.g., marriage, parenthood, divorce, and bereavement), and the primary care physician can respond to these concerns and make referrals as appropriate. Illness and surgery, particularly myocardial infarction, hysterectomy, mastectomy, and prostatectomy, often raise sexual concerns because of fears of death, loss of physical attractiveness, or loss of sexual functioning. In these situations, brief counseling by a clinician can alleviate anxiety and assist in maintaining sexual function. For example, most people who recover from myocardial infarction have questions and fears about resumption of sexual activity. A brief explanation that intercourse puts no more strain on the heart than climbing a flight of stairs and that cardiac death associated with intercourse is very rare may prevent much sexual dysfunction for couples.

Office visits with geriatric patients also offer an opportunity for sexual discussions and guidance. One of the myths of American society is that the elderly are asexual. Many elderly people maintain a high level of sexual interest and activity, which for some is determined by the availability of a partner. Physical changes, such as those resulting from estrogen deficiency, reduced erectile capacity, arthritis, and heart disease, may affect sexual function. Many of these problems can be ameliorated by relatively simple interventions, such as advising a patient to take nitroglycerine before sexual intercourse or recommending changes in coital positions, such as the female-superior or side-to-side positions, which may put less stress on arthritic joints or lessen exertion. Estrogen deficiency can be treated with oral or topical estrogens, and lubricants can be used to relieve vaginal dryness. Manual stimulation can be prolonged to improve erections to facilitate intercourse. Noncoital activities can also foster closeness.

SEXUAL DYSFUNCTION

The prevalence of sexual dysfunction is high. In a survey of 100 well-educated, self-described happily married couples, 75% noted sexual unhappiness at least some of the time (Frank, Anderson, & Rubenstein, 1978). In order to evaluate and classify sexual dysfunction, it is first necessary to rule out sexual dysfunction due to a general medical condition or substance-induced sexual dysfunction. If there is no clear organic basis, the sexual dysfunction can be further classified as lifelong (primary) or acquired (arising secondarily after a period of satisfactory sexual function). Sexual dysfunction can also be generalized (occurring in all situations) or situational (occurring with a particular partner or in a particular setting). For an overview of the *DSM-IV* (1994) classification of sexual dysfunction, see Table 10.1.

The three major components of the sexual cycle are desire, arousal, and orgasm (Kaplan, 1979). Desire is a combination of the biologic urge to be sexual, a wish to be sexual, and the willingness to be sexual. Arousal is the state of physical excitement that is characterized by increased blood flow into the genital area, causing penile erection and vaginal engorgement and lubrication. Orgasm is the rhythmic contractions of penis and vagina. During orgasm in the male, semen is ejaculated. This cycle is governed by complex hormonal and neuronal influences. Sexual disorders that occur in the desire phase include hypoactive sexual desire disorder (decrease or absence of desire) and sexual aversion disorder. Not listed in the *DSM-IV* but clinically relevant is hyperactive sexual desire (exaggerated sexual desire or sexual addiction). Of these dysfunctions, absence of desire and sexual aversion are likely to be lifelong and related to events in childhood, such as child sexual abuse and sexual identity confusion. Hypo- and hyperactive desire can be lifelong or acquired. Hypoactive sexual desire is the most prevalent of the desire phase dysfunctions, occurring in 15% to 20% of the general population (Rosen & Leiblum, 1995). It is also the most common sexual dysfunction in patients presenting to sex therapy clinics.

Table 10.1 Sexual Dysfunctions

Sexual Dysfunction
Due to a General Medical Condition

Substance-induced Sexual Dysfunctions

Desire Phase Dysfunctions
- Hypoactive sexual desire disorder (decrease or absence of desire)
- Sexual aversion disorder
- Hyperactive sexual desire disorder *(Not in DSM–IV)* (exaggerated desire or sexual addiction)

Arousal Phase Dysfunctions
- Male erectile disorder
- Female sexual arousal disorder (impaired or lack of arousal)
- Dyspareunia
- Vaginismus

Orgasmic Phase Dysfunctions
- Female orgasmic disorder
- Male orgasmic disorder
- Premature ejaculation

Specify for Each Disorder:
- Lifelong vs. acquired
- Generalized vs. situational
- Due to psychological factors
- Due to combined factors

Reprinted and adapted with permission from the *Diagnostic and Statistical Manual of Mental Disorders*, Fourth Edition. Copyright 1994 American Psychiatric Association.

Desire Phase Sexual Dysfunction

The cause of hypoactive sexual desire disorder is multifactorial. Hypogonadal women and men experience lowered sexual desire, which is reversible with hormone replacement therapy (androgens in men and androgens or estrogens in women). Hypoactive sexual desire disorder also commonly occurs in persons with depression and in survivors of sexual abuse or trauma. Relationship difficulties are a major factor in hypoactive sexual desire, particularly infidelity, unresolved marital conflicts, problems in sexual communication, and lack of physical attraction. Pharmacological and psychotherapeutic approaches have met with varied success, partly dependent on the etiology of the disorder. For example, hypoactive sexual desire due to hypogonadism may be treated with hormonal replacement, whereas hypoactive sexual desire due to depression can be treated with antidepressants, and a marital problem can be treated in couples/sex therapy.

Arousal Phase Dysfunction

Disorders of arousal occur in both men and women. In men, male erectile disorder is most common. In women, female sexual arousal disorder includes impaired arousal with stimulation (absence of lubrication), vaginismus (the involuntary contraction of vaginal musculature), and other forms of dyspareunia (pain with intercourse).

Erectile dysfunction occurs in an estimated 10 million to 20 million men in the United States. In the Massachusetts Male Aging Study (Feldman, Goldstein, & Hazichriston, 1994), 52% of men between the ages of 40 and 70 years reported some erectile dysfunction. The frequency increases with age and with an increasing number of concomitant medical disorders. In the past, erectile dysfunction (a term preferred over impotence) was thought to be largely psychological in nature. More recent investigation has shown that a high proportion of erectile dysfunction is organic. Risk factors for erectile dysfunction include diabetes mellitus, heart disease, hypertension, hypercholesterolemia, cigarette smoking, ulcers, prostate conditions, and arthritis. Psychological factors often interact with biological factors to cause or perpetuate erectile dysfunction.

Many medications also cause erectile dysfunction. These include antihypertensives, especially diuretics, beta blockers, and central sympatholytics; antidepressants, especially the tricyclics; antipsychotics; lithium; cimetidine; and digoxin (Schiavi & Segraves, 1995). Chronic heavy use of recreational drugs such as alcohol, marijuana, cocaine, and narcotics also causes erectile dysfunction. In contrast, moderate use of these drugs may enhance sexual performance by lessening sexual inhibitions.

Evaluation and treatment of erectile dysfunction have become more sophisticated as the number of treatment options has expanded. A high proportion of medical conditions can cause erectile dysfunction, and psychological factors often interact with the medical conditions and can impede treatment if they are not addressed. A small percentage of cases of erectile dysfunction is largely psychogenic in origin.

Evaluation of erectile dysfunction by the primary care physician includes a thorough history of the problem, assessment of medications or substance abuse that might be responsible, and a physical exam with attention to the vascular and genital systems. If these do not reveal the cause of the dysfunction, or if medication adjustment or reduction in substance use does not bring improvement, referral to a specialized clinic that can perform more extensive evaluation is appropriate. At such a clinic, psychological assessment of the man and his partner, urological examination, and hormonal testing are performed. Evaluation of penile neurologic and vascular function may be done, as well as nocturnal penile tumescence testing.

Treatment options include psychotherapy and/or sex therapy (individual or couples), oral medication (yohimbine), hormone replacement, self-injection of vasoactive compounds, vacuum devices, penile prostheses, vascular surgery, and no treatment. Recent advances in the treatment of erectile dysfunction include intra-urethral alprostadil and oral sildenafil (Viagra).

The first published reports on oral sildenafil suggest substantial improvements in sexual function among men with erectile dysfunction, both organic and psychogenic (Goldstein, Lue, Padma-Nathan, Rosen, Steers & Wicker, 1998). Men in Goldstein's study had erectile dysfunction from organic and psychogenic causes, as well as mixed causes. The initial dose of sildenafil is 25 mg., approximately one hour before intercourse. The dose can be increased up to 100 mg., depending upon the response. In the initial studies, there was a dose-response effect, with the highest response to the maximum dose. Sildenafil was generally well-tolerated. Side effects included headache, flushing, dyspepsia, and rhinitis; but these side effects were transient, and few men withdrew from the study because of them. In the initial studies, the contraindications to use of sildenafil were poorly controlled diabetes, recent myocardial infarction or stroke, active peptic ulcer disease, substance abuse, major psychiatric disease that was poorly controlled, major hepatic, renal, or hematologic disease, and therapy with nitrates.

Sildenafil attracted great media attention when it was first released. More experience with this medication will establish its place among the therapeutic options. In deciding among these options, patients can be guided by the primary care physician as well as specialists. A large minority of patients (28% in one study) improve spontaneously without treatment (Althof & Seftel, 1995).

Less research has been devoted to the female disorders of arousal, which include impaired arousal with stimulation, vaginismus, and dyspareunia. Impaired arousal may be caused by hypoestrogenic states; depression; sexual trauma; marital discord; and medications, notably antidepressants, antipsychotics, digoxin, and cimetidine. Sexual trauma or abuse, painful gynecologic procedures or exams, and anxiety may cause vaginismus, the involuntary contraction of vaginal muscles. Dyspareunia, or painful intercourse, may be caused by vaginal atrophy after menopause, vaginitis, chronic interstitial cystitis, reduced lubrication resulting from childbirth or lactation, or inadequate foreplay.

The primary care physician can often diagnose these problems by thorough history and physical examination, with attention to the gynecological exam. This needs to be done with care and gentleness, particularly in women who have experienced sexual trauma or are troubled by vaginismus. It is helpful to explain each step of the examination, to raise the head of the exam table so that the patient and examiner can see one another, to use a warmed speculum, and to avoid sudden movements. The presence of vaginismus can be detected by digital exam before insertion of the speculum. The presence of vaginal discharge or atrophy should be noted. Many of these disorders are treatable by the primary care physician with medication and education (e.g., use of vaginal lubricants or changes in coital position or technique). Some cases of vaginismus respond to education and home programs of self-digital dilatation. Women who are severely depressed or anxious and those who have experienced sexual trauma should be referred to a mental health specialist.

Orgasmic Dysfunction

Disorders of this phase include female orgasmic disorder (formerly known as inhibited female orgasm, difficulty achieving orgasm, or anorgasmia), male orgasmic disorder (formerly known as inhibited male orgasm or retarded ejaculation), and premature ejaculation.

Masters and Johnson (1970) pioneered behavioral treatment for many of these disorders, which had previously been considered the province of psychotherapy. They reported good results with short-term intensive sex therapy, which persisted in long-term follow-up.

Premature ejaculation, in which a man ejaculates too quickly following minimal stimulation, is the most common disorder of the orgasmic phase in men, with a prevalence of 30% to 40% according to some self-report studies (Althof, 1995). It is a common occurrence in men following a period of sexual abstinence or with a new partner. Performance anxiety can convert this common occurrence into an acquired pattern. Treatment includes exercises that help a man regain control of ejaculation (stop-start and squeeze techniques) and sensate focus exercises, in which the emphasis is shifted from intercourse to other ways of exchanging pleasure. Selective serotonin reuptake inhibitor antidepressants offer potential benefits in delaying orgasm in men who do not respond to these exercises.

Anorgasmia in women can be primary or secondary. If a woman has never had an orgasm (lifelong anorgasmia), the most effective treatment is a program of self-exploration and self-stimulation. Once she experiences orgasm in this way, she can involve her partner. Acquired anorgasmia is usually caused by difficulties in the relationship such as conflict with the partner, inability to communicate about sexual matters, and sexual technique. These difficulties may interfere with a woman's ability to experience orgasm. Couples therapy is the treatment of choice.

COMPULSIVE SEXUAL BEHAVIORS

Compulsive sexual behaviors (either paraphilic or nonparaphilic) are sexual activities that are potentially harmful to oneself or others. Paraphilias, which formerly were called perversions, are recurrent, intense, sexually arousing fantasies, sexual urges, or behaviors generally involving nonhuman objects, the suffering or humiliation or oneself or one's partner, or children or other nonconsenting persons. These behaviors occur over a period of at least 6 months (*DSM-IV*). Paraphilias include exhibitionism, fetishism, frotteurism, pedophilia, sexual masochism, sexual sadism, transvestic fetishism, voyeurism, and paraphilia not otherwise specified. Most paraphilias involve nonconsenting partners and are against the law (e.g., exhibitionism, voyeurism, frotteurism, and pedophilia). Other paraphilias are potentially dangerous (e.g., sadism and masochism). Treatment of these disorders requires specialty referral and can involve medication, psychotherapy, use of cognitive-behavioral techniques, and hospitalization if the behavior is dangerous to oneself or others.

Compulsive sexual behavior of the nonparaphilic type is likely to be encountered in primary care practice. Common behaviors include compulsive masturbation, compulsive sexual activity within a relationship, multiple sexual partners, and frequent contact with prostitutes. Patients may present with anxiety, depression, marital discord, or sexually transmitted diseases.

The difference between compulsive and noncompulsive sexual behavior depends on the underlying motivation and the consequences of the behavior for the individual and the partner.

One model of this type of compulsive sexual behavior is the addiction model proposed by Carnes (1983). In this model, sexual activity is analogous to alcohol for the alcoholic. Sexual addicts generally feel a deep sense of shame and unworthiness about themselves. They believe that no one could ever love them and that their needs will never be met. Sex becomes a way of self-medicating against painful feelings and hence becomes the focus of their lives. Treatment of compulsive sexual behavior may involve psychotherapy (individual and couples), medication (particularly antidepressants), and self-help groups modeled on Alcoholics Anonymous.

HOMOSEXUALITY

Homosexuality, in which the primary sexual attraction and orientation is to members of the same sex, is controversial in our society. Most primary care physicians have homosexual patients in their practices, although such patients may not identify themselves as homosexual. Widespread debate surrounds the etiology of homosexuality, although recent research suggests that much homosexuality is inborn. Many homosexuals describe same-sex attraction as their earliest experience of sexual feelings. Homosexuality is no longer listed as a psychopathology in the *DSM-IV*. Because of widespread family and societal condemnation, many homosexual persons experience shame and guilt about their sexual orientation. Shame and guilt, however, can drive people to engage in compulsive or unsafe sexual behaviors. Primary care clinicians who can be nonjudgmental are in a unique position to provide a safe forum in which patients can discuss issues of sexual orientation, sexual concerns, and specific health needs.

SEXUAL ABUSE AND SEXUAL TRAUMA

Primary care physicians are likely to encounter survivors of sexual abuse and sexual trauma in their practices. These forms of violence occur more frequently than was previously suspected and often go unreported, making accurate estimates of incidence difficult. A 1986 study (Feldman et al., 1994) reported the incidence of child sexual abuse to be 15% among girls and 7% among boys. Statistics have shown a steady increase in the number of rapes reported, but many rapes are not reported (Abel & Rouleau, 1995).

Contrary to popular myths of stranger molestation, most perpetrators of child sexual abuse are known to the victim and usually are trusted adults or adolescents. Child molestation can involve fondling, oral-genital sex, and vaginal or anal penetration. Perpetrators known to the child rarely need to use force because of the child's lack of knowledge and inability to resist adult authority.

Child molesters generally fall into four major categories (Abel & Rouleau, 1995). The first are adolescents who have ready access to younger children and may use them as they learn about sex. Such molestation is different from sex play between age mates, which is generally benign, because the age of the adolescent and the power difference render the younger child unable to consent. The second group of child molesters are adults who involve themselves with their children, stepchildren, and friends of their children. The third group comprises older adults (over age 55 years) who may have nervous system disease or cognitive impairment or turn to children in the wake of bereavement. The fourth group comprises pedophiles, who experience arousal to children throughout their lives and frequently molest large numbers of children.

Children who have experienced sexual abuse may present to the primary care physician in a number of ways. Because the clinician may be a trusted adult, the child may first disclose the abuse to the clinician. Physicians are obligated by law to report suspected child abuse, including sexual abuse, to the child protective services of their state. This may be difficult for the physician, particularly if the perpetrator is also a patient and the physician experiences conflicting loyalties. However, the potential for harm to the child is so severe that these considerations should not deter the physician from making the appropriate referral. Evaluation of the child, especially obtaining evidence that may be used in legal action, is best done by an expert in the field.

Physicians who provide primary care to children should also suspect child sexual abuse in a number of clinical settings. These include the presence of a sexually transmitted disease in a child (which usually is definitive evidence of molestation), children with perineal or anal injuries, those with recurrent pelvic or urinary tract infections, sexual acting out by a child, unexplained depression, and school failure. Evaluation of these children may require gentle but nonleading questioning by the clinician. If the clinician has a strong suspicion of sexual abuse, referral to a child protective services agency for further evaluation is warranted. The mandated involvement of child protective services may cause conflict with the parents or within the family. At the present time, child protective services are often overloaded with these highly charged situations. However, the clinician's first responsibility is the child's safety. If possible, the clinician should maintain contact with the family during the process to provide ongoing support.

Physicians also may care for children whose abuse has been reported. In these situations, family disruption and stress are common. The clinician can provide education about normal behavior, reassurance to the family and child that reporting the abuse was the right decision despite the turmoil, and ongoing stability and medical care.

Prevention of child sexual abuse is also a proper role for physicians caring for children. This may include assessing families for abuse potential and referring stressed families to supportive services. Education of parents and children about "good touch" and "bad touch" and about boundaries and appropriate sex education for children may also be helpful.

Adult survivors of sexual abuse are present in all primary care practices. Some survivors are aware of the abuse and have taken steps to deal with it. Others remember the abuse but have tried to lock it away. Still others do not remember abuse or later retrieve memories. Patients for whom the index of suspicion for sexual abuse is high include those with chronic pain, especially pelvic, back, and headache; functional gastrointestinal disease; sexual problems, particularly hypoactive sexual desire; severe depression; dissociative identity disorder (formerly known as multiple personality disorder); posttraumatic stress disorder; and eating disorders.

Working with survivors of sexual abuse can be challenging for the primary care physician. Survivors are often distrustful of authority because their trust was betrayed. They have high needs for control and yet have high dependency needs. Neglect of self or self-destructive behaviors are common results of sexual abuse, and survivors may have unaddressed medical (especially gynecological) and dental needs. A stepwise approach is often helpful, as well as allowing the survivor control over some aspects of medical care. However, if serious health problems arise, the physician may need to work with the patient to overcome resistance to treatment. This may involve mobilizing the patient's support network. Pelvic exams, genital and rectal exams, dental work, and anesthesia are particularly difficult for many survivors. When performing pelvic exams on female survivors, the physician can make it easier for the patient by raising the head of the exam table, doing everything possible to ensure the patient's comfort, and allowing the patient to call a halt to the exam if she feels overwhelmed. A chaperone is mandatory for male physicians giving any pelvic exam, not just those performed on survivors. Sexual abuse survivors may benefit from having a support person present during the exam. If the physician suspects that the patient has severe anxiety or a dissociative identity disorder, psychiatric consultation is warranted.

Most survivors of sexual abuse find psychotherapy helpful in addressing the sexual abuse. Pharmacotherapy may be considered if a patient's depression or anxiety is severe. It is important for survivors to work with therapists who are experienced in dealing with sexual abuse or trauma. Other resources that survivors may find helpful are support groups and alternative therapies such as yoga, tai chi, massage therapy, and meditation. Unless alternative therapies are supplanting conventional medical treatment for serious problems, physicians should refrain from criticizing them. Physicians who work with survivors of sexual abuse may find first-hand accounts of recovery helpful.

Recently, there has been controversy about recovered memories, particularly with the use of hypnosis. A number of highly publicized court cases and the formation of the False Memory Foundation have called into question the entire concept of recovered memories. On the opposing side, many survivors and therapists strongly support the concept of recovered memories. Studies by Terr (1994) and others support the existence of memories of trauma that can be dissociated for many years and then surface, either spontaneously or with hypnosis. However, these studies also demonstrate that memories can be altered or planted in children by adults in positions of authority. Thus caution is advised in undertaking confrontation or legal action based on recovered memories.

RAPE

Rape, which is nonconsensual sexual relations with an adult, produces effects similar to those experienced by survivors of child sexual abuse. Rape can occur between strangers, often in the course of an assault or robbery, or between acquaintances, as in date or acquaintance rape. Rape can also occur within a marriage or other relationship. It is primarily a crime of power rather than sex.

Evaluation of a rape victim should be performed as soon after the rape as possible and in a hospital emergency room where forensic evidence can be collected. Rape crisis centers and hotlines offer support and counseling to rape survivors. The primary care physician's approach to rape survivors is similar to the approach to survivors of child sexual abuse.

Symptoms resulting from sexual trauma, both child sexual abuse and rape, are similar to those resulting from other types of trauma. Post-traumatic stress disorder, which was officially recognized in 1980 in the *DSM-III*, has been described since ancient times as a reaction to battle. This disorder is marked by recurrent distressing recollections of the event, flashbacks, and severe anxiety and arousal. If PTSD is untreated, it frequently results in substance abuse, psychiatric illness, or distorted relationships with others (Bursztajn, Joshi, Sutherland, & Tomb, 1995). Treatment involves psychotherapy, medication, relaxation therapy, or a combination of these approaches.

PROFESSIONAL SEXUAL MISCONDUCT

Since ancient times, medical ethics has condemned doctor-patient sexual relations. The Hippocratic oath states, "I will come for the benefit of the sick, remaining free of all intentional injustice, of all mischief, and in particular of sexual relations with both male and female persons." Despite this blanket condemnation, sexual contact with patients does occur. Surveys of health care professionals report that up to 10% of professionals have been sexually involved with patients (Lazarus, 1995). This behavior is damaging to patients and risky for professionals. Effects on patients can include depression and risk of suicide, inability to trust, identity disturbances, and cognitive dysfunction. Risks for professionals include malpractice suits, professional censure, and loss of license. Sexual misconduct of medical professionals is now reported to the National Practitioners Data Bank.

Risk factors for professional sexual misconduct include substance abuse, marital or professional conflict, depression, isolation, and bereavement. If a clinician experiences recurrent sexual arousal with a patient or is experiencing any of these stressors, seeking treatment is mandatory. Prevention of professional sexual misconduct requires awareness of risk factors, education about appropriate professional boundaries, and keeping a balance in life and work to avoid loss of perspective and burnout. It is often difficult for physicians, who are accustomed to the role of healer, to ask for help in these areas. However, because the damage to both patients and physicians can be so great as a result of professional sexual misconduct, seeking help is essential.

Primary care physicians are in a unique position to assist patients in dealing with sexual issues, concerns, and disorders. Despite the constraints of time in busy primary care practices, physicians can have a profound impact on their patients by engaging in relatively brief discussions of sexuality as a part of the patient's life.

REFERENCES

Abel, G., & Rouleau, J. (1995). Sexual abuses. *Psychiatric Clinics of North America, 18*, 139–153.

Althof, S. (1995). Pharmacologic treatment of rapid ejaculation. *Psychiatric Clinics of North America, 18*, 85–94.

Althof, S., & Seftel, A. (1995). The evaluation and management of erectile dysfunction. *Psychiatric Clinics of North America, 18*, 171–193.

American Psychiatric Association (1994). *Diagnostic and statistical manual of mental disorders* (4th ed.). Washington, DC: Author.

American Psychiatric Association. (1980). Diagnostic and statistical manual of mental disorder (3rd ed.). Washington, DC: Author.

Bursztajn, H. J., Joshi, P. T. Sutherland, S. M., & Tomb, D. A. (1995, March 30). Recognizing post-traumatic stress. *Patient Care*, pp. 40–61.

Carnes, P. (1983). *Out of the shadows: Understanding sexual addiction* (2nd ed.). Minneapolis: Compcare Publications.

Feldman, H. A., Goldstein, I., & Hazichriston, D. G. (1994). Impotence and its medical and psychosocial correlates: Results of the Massachusetts male aging study. *Journal of Urology, 151*, 54–61.

Frank, E., Anderson C., & Rubenstein, D. (1978). Frequency of sexual dysfunction in "normal" couples. *New England Journal of Medicine, 299*(3), 111–115.

Goldstein, I., Lue, T. F., Padma-Nathan, H., Rosen, R. C., Steers, W. D., & Wicker, P. A. (1998). Oral Sildenafil in the treatment of errectile dysfunction. *New England Journal of Medicine, 338*(20), 1397–1404.

Kaplan, H. S. (1979). *Disorders of human sexual desire*. New York: Brunner Mazel.

Lazarus, J. (1995). Ethical issues in doctor-patient sexual relationships. *Psychiatric Clinics of North America, 18*(1), 55–70.

Masters, W., & Johnson, V. (1970). *Human sexual inadequacy*. Boston: Little, Brown.

Peters, S. D., Wyatt, G. E., & Finkelhor, D. (1986). Prevalence. In D. Finkelhor (Ed.), *A source book on child sexual abuse* (p. 15). Beverly Hills, CA: Sage Publications.

Risen, C. (1995). A guide to taking a sexual history. *Psychiatric Clinics of North America, 18*, 39–53.

Rosen, R., & Leiblum, S. (1995). Hypoactive sexual desire. *Psychiatric Clinics of North America, 18*(1), pp. 107–122. Philadelphia: W. B. Saunders.

Schiavi, R., & Segraves, R. (1995). The biology of sexual function. *Psychiatric Clinics of North America, 18*, 107–122.

Terr, L. (1994). *Unchained memories*. New York: Basic Books.

Tiefer, L., & King, B. (1995). Gender and the organization of sexual behavior. *Psychiatric Clinics of North America, 18*, 25–37.

CHAPTER 11

Psychological Disorders and Problems of Childhood and Adolescence

Marion Hart and Stanley Kaye

Family physicians, pediatricians, and other primary care clinicians are usually the first to encounter mental conditions in children and are often the first to uncover the serious psychosocial problems of childhood and adolescence. National estimates reveal that several million youths in the United States suffer psychological impairment and are in need of mental health services, and many of these children are not receiving adequate treatment. Approximately 13% of children visiting pediatricians have a mental health or behavioral problem, which is often expressed or is disguised by somatic complaints, such as headaches, stomach aches, and sore throats (Achenbach & Howell, 1993).

PSYCHIATRIC CONDITIONS IN CHILDREN AND ADOLESCENTS

Attention Deficit/Hyperactivity Disorder

Attention deficit/hyperactivity disorder (ADHD) is a disorder of the ability to stop, look, and listen. Although its cause is not yet clear, there is much evidence pointing to a complex interaction of genetic, biologic, and psychosocial factors. Prevalence estimates for this disorder vary from 2.2% to 12.6% within the general child population (McCracken, 1992). A child may have symptoms that include carelessness, forgetfulness, problems with sustaining attention when passively listening, or difficulty sustaining a mental focus when actively engaged in tasks. At school, children with ADHD do not raise their hands, cannot wait their turn, and may spend half the school day chasing their pencils into the aisle or constantly falling off their seats. Children with ADHD are often hyperactive, impulsive, and unfocused and are unable to utilize social cues to predict social outcomes and consequences. Not surprisingly, the child with this disorder is often socially isolated, develops a reputation in school as a trouble maker, and may have limited capability for school, work, or play. Table 11.1 presents the diagnostic criteria for ADHD as established in the *DSM-IV* (1994).

> Both the mother and school describe 8-year-old Paul as uncontrollable. His history reveals dramatic levels of activity since infancy. His mother portrays Paul as having vaulted out of his crib, hitting the ground running, and not stopping until he dropped from exhaustion. He has been running ever since. Incredibly, even although he is prone to carelessness and has dreadful organizational skills and poor study habits, his reading and arithmetic skills are at grade level.

Etiology

The etiology of ADHD is still controversial despite extensive studies. Parental uncertainties easily parallel professional controversies in the search for primary causal factors. The diagnostic predecessor to ADHD, minimal brain dysfunction (MBD), carried the implication of perinatal brain damage. Although most children with ADHD do not show this history, some major studies have noted the presence of significant health problems in infancy.

Temperamental factors are likely contributors to the development of ADHD and continue to exert effects throughout adulthood. Neurobiologic hypotheses are focusing on dopamine receptor interactions, a major area of study. The most consistent and convincing genetic data indicate that a single major gene is probably responsible for many cases of ADHD. A complicating factor is the high level of comorbidity between ADHD and other psychiatric disorders including mood, anxiety, and conduct disorders. The major implication of these combined data is that ADHD is most likely a heterogeneous group of conditions with a multifactorial etiology and with psychosocial factors encouraging different outcomes.

Table 11.1 DSM-IV Criteria, Attention Deficit/Hyperactivity Disorder*

Inattention
- Poor attention to detail or careless mistakes
- Poor attention in tasks or play
- Poor listening when spoken to directly
- Poor follow-through on instructions, school, chores, or duties
- Difficulties organizing tasks and activities
- Avoids tasks requiring sustained mental effort
- Loses things
- Easily distracted
- Often forgetful

Hyperactivity/Impulsivity
- Fidgets or squirms
- Leaves seat
- Runs or climbs when not appropriate
- Poor at quiet play and leisure
- On the go as though driven by a motor
- Talks excessively

Impulsivity
- Blurts out answers
- Has problem awaiting turn
- Interrupts and intrudes on others

*6 or more of these symptoms for 6 months

Reprinted with permission from *Diagnostic and Statistical Manual of Mental Disorders*, Fourth Edition. Copyright 1994 American Psychiatric Association.

ADHD is not only a condition of childhood. For many patients, ADHD persists throughout adulthood, continuing to create concentration, social, emotional, and impulse problems. There are some ADHD children who grow to normal adulthood with only residuals effects. For others, the ADHD symptoms in adulthood are complicated by persistent symptoms of other psychiatric disorders, such as depression and antisocial behavior.

Diagnosis and Clinical Management

The primary care physician is often the first clinician to make the diagnosis of ADHD. There are now some excellent questionnaires to facilitate differential diagnosis. The Attention Deficit Disorders Evaluation Scales (ADDES/Conners scales, Hawthorne Educational Services, 1995) were developed specifically to meet *DSM-IV* criteria for ADHD and to reflect an awareness of that condition as observable from early childhood into adulthood. There are specific scales for the preschooler, the school-age child, and the adolescent, as well as the Conners Parents Questionnaire and Conners Teachers Questionnaire (Hawthorne Educational Services, 1995). The Conners Parents Questionnaire explores five behavior clusters or factors, which include conduct problems, learning problems, psychosomatic problems, impulsivity-hyperactivity, and anxiety. There is also a parent guide for appropriate interventions in response to "What do you do when . . ." questions. For example, the parent is guided in helping an impulsive child settle down or preparing a child in advance for changes in routines. The ADDES can be an invaluable addition to the clinician's office.

To make the diagnosis of ADHD, the clinician must establish the presence of symptoms that appeared prior to age 7 years. The parent may describe an infant who seemed completely disinterested in exploring his or her crib environment. Subsequent behavioral patterns may not demonstrate hyperactivity but, instead, a more focal problem with focused attention. Core clinical signs or symptoms may be observable as early as age 3 and include excessive gross motor activity, disorganization of behavior, easy distractibility, low frustration tolerance, and inability to sustain attention or remain focused on a task. In some instances, the first indication of emerging ADHD is excessive motor activity in a toddler who is developing locomotion skills. In many more instances, problems with early elementary school adjustment are the first signs. By late childhood, excessive motor activity and inability to sit and attend may have largely given way to more subtle evidence of excessive motor activity, such as fidgeting, restlessness, an inability to wait one's turn, or a distaste for reading and other quieter activities. The child may be thought of as "not with it" because he or she cannot stay focused on social conversations any more than on social studies at school.

Primary care physicians should not rely on reported symptoms alone for diagnosis. Instead, they need the full clinical picture, which minimally includes direct observation, teacher and parent reports, the completion of Conners or other scales by teacher and parent, and psychological or neuropsychological testing. The psychological testing is particularly helpful in establishing the need and nature of special educational services that might facilitate school adjustment. For example, a child with impaired concentration might require additional time for exams, or an impatient/impulsive child might require teaching in smaller, more digestible doses.

Parents have numerous questions about ADHD: What can we expect for the future? Will this run its course by the time he gets through adolescence? We hate the idea of medication. After all, it is a kind of amphetamine, isn't it? Won't medication set him up to become drug dependent? Will his growth be stunted? The families of these children are often under enormous stress and are also likely to benefit from psychological counseling or family therapy. Children are frequently in need of psychological counseling that will help them to understand their problem and to develop methods of behavioral control and coping.

Pharmacotherapy

Psychostimulant medication with methylphenidate (Ritalin) has become the ubiquitous treatment modality for ADHD. It accounts for over 90% of the use of stimulants in the United States (Bernstein, 1995) with well-documented effectiveness. Following the administration of psychostimulants, teachers' global reports support improvements in motor restlessness, on-task behavior, compliance, and success with classroom tests. There is also clear evidence of reduced aggressivity and improved arithmetic productivity and efficiency. However, social problem-solving deficits do not appear to be affected by the medications.

Psychostimulants are rapidly absorbed from the gut. Food enhances absorption, and they act quickly at relatively low concentrations. Methylphenidate (MPH) 5 mg bid is a common initial dose, which may prove sufficient. A standard MPH tablet acts quickly, within 30 minutes of ingestion, peaks in plasma in 2 to 2.5 hours, and falls to half the peak in 3 hours. The short half-life of MPH prevents steady-state plasma concentration, so that a standard tablet must be given several times a day for sustained benefit. Medications are best administered before school and just after breakfast (8 A.M.), just after lunch (noon), and just before homework (about 3:30 P.M.). Obviously, administration of the noon pill requires assistance from school personnel. There are sustained-release forms of MPH (Ritalin-SR) available in 20-mg tablets. This preparation makes it possible to give the psychostimulant just once, in the morning. There is some controversy as to whether the sustained-release form is as effective as the standard form.

Pemoline (Cylert) and dextroamphetamine have longer half-lives than MPH and consequently can be administered once a day. The efficacy of the three psychostimulants is reported to be roughly equal, but the safety record and extensive studies using MPH make it the first choice for most patients. Before beginning MPH, a baseline white blood count (WBC) is indicated, with a follow-up within 3 to 6 months. This is because MPH can lower the WBC. Dextroamphetamine may have greater adverse effects, particularly in the area of weight and height suppression. Pemoline has a delayed onset of action. If pemoline is used, baseline liver function studies should be made, with repeated monitoring every 3 to 6 months to avoid potential hepatotoxic effects.

Dextroamphetamine can be started with 2.5 mg as the first dose. Pemoline's lowest dose unit is 18.75 mg. Doses can be increased at 1-week intervals, although more rapid advances using 3-day intervals can reduce the delayed response and appear to produce no additional side effects. Some children experience "behavioral rebound" at the end of the day, a consequence of psychostimulant withdrawal. Irritability, overtalkativeness, motor hyperactivity, and insomnia may occur. If rebound occurs, the primary care physician can add a small afternoon MPH dose. Concerns that the psychostimulants might stunt growth have been reduced by recent research findings (Greenhill, 1992). If growth suppression does occur, it is transitory, and the child eventually attains normal height. Pemoline is the least likely to suppress growth in height or weight. However, it frequently cause insomnia and has been linked with choreoathetoid movements.

There is, as yet, no evidence that the positive effects of stimulants are sustained over an extended period of time. Most research has focused on short-term use, and it appears that stimulant medications fail to maintain improvement in either academic skills or social problem-solving skills beyond a 6-month period. Stimulants for ADHD may cause problems in children who have comorbid disorders. For example, stimulant use exacerbates Tourette's syndrome, autism, conduct disorders, and learning disorders. This has led to the exploration of other drugs in controlling ADHD (Bernstein, 1995), especially antidepressants such as imipramine, bupropion, and fluoxetine. These alternative medications may be appropriate in some situations, but there has been little research about their relative dangers and efficacy in children.

Prescriptions for methylphenidate, dextroamphetamine, and pemoline have tripled between 1990 and 1994. That fact has engendered substantial professional disagreement as to whether ADHD is being increasingly diagnosed with greater accuracy, is indeed becoming more prevalent, or is being overdiagnosed. Some physicians report as many as 20% of the children they see as having ADHD (McGee, 1991), whereas other clinicians report rarely encountering it.

Anxiety Disorders in Children

Anxieties, fears, and worries are common in a large number of children who go through phases of fearing strangers, animals, or the dark. An early epidemiological survey showed that more than 40% of mothers reported that their children were having many fears and worries, including separation concerns (Bell-Dolan, Last, & Strauss, 1990). In this study, phobias and overanxious disorders were noted in 10% of the children, with one third of the children showing excessive concerns about competence and extensive needs for reassurance. More obvious anxiety disorders, such as separation anxiety in association with school phobias, appear in some 3.5% to 5.5% of the general population of children (Messer & Bidel, 1994).

Anxieties appear to be specific to ages and to gender. Younger children tend to fear sudden, intense, and novel stimuli and separation from caretakers. Older children's fears involve school, peers, and health-related issues. Overanxious disorders seem to affect older children, and separation anxiety, younger children. Girls tend to report more fears than boys and are more likely to fear animals, illness, and injury. Girls are also more likely to experience separation anxiety in the form of fear of harm befalling the caretaker or fear of calamitous events befalling the child.

Separation Anxiety Disorder

The *DSM-IV* diagnosis of separation anxiety disorder requires developmentally inappropriate and excessive anxiety concerning separation from home or from those to whom the individual is attached, as evidenced by three or more symptoms that persist for more than 4 weeks. A summary of *DSM-IV* symptoms includes (1) excessive distress when separation from home or a parental figure is anticipated; (2) worry about losing, or possible harm to, caretakers; (3) worry about separation from parental figures; (4) persistent refusal to go to school or elsewhere; (5) excessive fear of being alone; (6) persistent refusal to go to sleep without a parental figure nearby; (7) nightmares with the theme of separation; and (8) repeated complaints of physical symptoms, such as headaches and stomachaches, in anticipating separation from attachment figures. Primary care physicians and other clinicians may be helped by understanding that these anxieties are anchored to the child's sense of his or her own dependency and vulnerability. Therefore, it is important to consider that somatic complaints such as headaches, stomachaches, and nausea may be physical manifestations of separation anxiety.

Separation anxiety disorder may not be recognized until there is clear functional impairment (e.g., a camper with separation anxiety becomes miserable, inconsolable, and preoccupied with a determination to return home as soon as possible). It may also present in more subtle ways.

> Harold's separation anxiety was demonstrated in several ways. He refused to go on errands to local stores or to do other chores in the neighborhood. On several occasions, he refused to leave his father in the parked car and dash into a store. His parents characterized him as selfish, and when he persisted, as stubborn and defiant. He adamantly refused to go to his room to do homework, was constantly underfoot, and insisted on doing his homework at the kitchen table.
>
> In this case, it was possible to help the mother to see that her son's intense attachment served to keep a continual eye on her. He was underfoot to fend off massive overwhelming separation anxieties and difficulty in being alone.

Separation anxiety appears commonly in children and adolescents. A child may speak of fears of what will happen to him or her at school or on the way to school and may occasionally protest about to going to school. School phobia is a more severe crystallized form of school aversion in which the child suffers overwhelming anticipatory fear and phobic avoidance of school. School phobia can present with persistent tantrums and total refusal to go to school. It often signals more global separation fears.

A child with underlying separation anxiety may also present with a sleep disturbance. The child may insist on a parent staying with him or her until he or she falls asleep or demand that space be granted in the parental bed. Children manifesting anxiety around sleep often show other problems with separation. The onset of puberty, with accompanying fears of growing up, can commonly arouse separation anxieties and sleep disturbances. For example, a high school senior may experience a dramatic drop in grades, seriously jeopardizing his college acceptance. His separation anxiety causes him to unconsciously sabotage his moving out and leaving home. In many cases, the varied manifestations of anxiety will require evaluation by a child or adolescent mental health practitioner who can help uncover social determinants such as stresses within the family or even dysfunctional family interactions that may be fueling the child's anxieties.

Clinical Management/Intervention

The primary care physician or clinician can assume a supportive, educational, and counseling role in the treatment of anxiety in children. When the disorder manifests in sleep problems, the clinician can help the parent to understand the child's sense of dependence and fragility. The clinician should inquire about stresses, separations, loss, and changes in the child's life. If the child actively seeks a place in the parental bed in order to soothe his or her anxieties and sleep, the clinician can counsel the parents that acceding to this wish will be counterproductive, because it will reinforce the child's anxiety. The clinician can help the parents to deal with the guilt of saying no and suggest to the parents that returning the child to his or her own room with parental support is the best long-term solution. The clinician may uncover subtle and unwitting collusion by the parents in the child's separation anxieties. For example, if the parents are having marital or sexual difficulties, the child may be invited into the marital bed to be a buffer against spousal conflicts or sexual demands.

The separation anxiety that manifests in school phobia usually calls for the physician to be empathetic to parental guilt. A frightened, possibly sobbing child whose stomachache appears at exactly the same time as the school bus arrives can stir parental guilt and fear. The clinician's reassurance can do much to relieve the parents' guilt and thus relieve the child's anxieties. The clinician can educate the parents about some applications of "tough love," (e.g., how to send the child back to school). The clinician can support both the parents and the child in what can feel like a daily crisis. The parents can be counseled that the longer the child is absent from school, the more difficult it will be for the child to return. The clinician may suggest that the child go off to school with someone other than the parents. The vast majority of school-phobic children will successfully return to school with the clinician guiding the parent-child interaction. The primary care clinician should refer the child to a mental health specialist if anxiety symptoms or school phobia persists. Involving the entire family may permit a greater exploration of psychosocial factors or family issues that are intensifying the child's insecurities.

In some situations, the parents' separation anxiety is as great as the child's. The clinician often becomes aware of the parents' conflicts and anxieties when they report failure of efforts to get the child back to school. The parent might complain, "He lay down, screaming, in the middle of the street. I couldn't drag him all the way to school, could I?" In situations in which the parents' separation anxiety undermines "tough love" treatment, mental health evaluation and treatment may be appropriate.

Psychopharmacology

When a child's anxiety is overwhelming, the child may require treatment with an antidepressant or antianxiety medications. There is no definitive evidence that tricyclic antidepressants (TCAs) in children are better than placebo. Despite this fact, the TCAs imipramine, desipramine, or nortriptyline are often prescribed. Children who receive a TCA need a baseline blood pressure and EKG, with a repeat blood pressure and EKG at target dose levels to check for delayed conduction, increased heart rate, and increased blood pressure. Plasma levels should not exceed 250 mg/ml of the combined imipramine and desipramine levels. Plasma levels, not mg/kg, should be used to guide therapeutic dosage. A child may begin at 1 mg/kg/day with a gradual titration upward toward a maximum of 3.5mg/kg/day (Maxmen & Ward, 1995). A treatment response may be expected within 1 to 6 weeks. Many children will be totally symptom-free after 3 to 4 months. Fluoxetine may be as effective as the TCAs and has recently been utilized in treating anxiety, particularly to treat the early symptoms of a developing school phobia. It is available in liquid form for children who have difficulty swallowing pills. It is important to start with a low dosage, 5 mg/day, and increase slowly to lessen the risk of agitation and heightened anxiety.

Benzodiazepines have shown some effectiveness in treating anxiety symptoms in children. Alprazolam in dosages ranging from 0.5 to 1.5 mg/day has proved helpful with overanxious or avoidant disorders in children. Clonazepam in the dosage range of 0.5 to 3.5 mg/day has been employed in the treatment of panic symptoms. With either, the clinician should begin with a low dose and gradually increase the dose until symptoms are relieved. These antianxiety medications are well tolerated on a short-term basis, but the risk of dependence dictates short-term usage. Discontinuance should be gradual to avoid withdrawal symptoms such as tremors or seizures. Prolonged treatment of anxiety might warrant the use of nonaddicting, sedating antihistamines such as hydroxyzine or diphenhydramine. Sedating antihistamines have proved particularly effective with sleep disturbances, including night terrors. However, their side effects, especially drowsiness, may preclude their use.

There has been relatively limited research concerning the use of buspirone, a nonbenzodiazepine anxiolytic agent, in the treatment of childhood anxiety disorders. Buspirone can be prescribed in a dose of 5 mg/day for children and 5 mg bid for adolescents. It takes 4 to 6 weeks to reach maximal efficacy. The side-effect profile of buspirone is favorable with a low risk of dependency and abuse and with a good margin of safety.

Mood Disorders

Epidemiological studies have documented that mood disorders are among the most common major psychiatric disorders affecting children and adolescents (McCracken, 1992). Incidence varies greatly with setting, age, gender, and other symptomatology. Dysthymia or major depression is frequently accompanied by anxiety, conduct, or attention-deficit hyperactivity disorders. In pediatric settings, children evaluated for headaches and for educational problems showed a 60% incidence of depression (McCracken, 1992). The rate of depression in late adolescence surpasses the highest rates noted at any other point along the life span.

DSM-IV criteria for major depression in children and adolescence require either a depressed mood or a loss of pleasure that is present continually for 2 weeks in association with five or more symptoms, including significant weight loss, insomnia or hypersomnia, psychomotor agitation or retardation, fatigue or loss of energy, feelings of worthlessness or excessive and inappropriate guilt, diminished concentration or indecisiveness, recurrent thoughts of death or suicide, or a suicide attempt. In general, children have depressive symptoms similar to those of adolescents and adults. Criteria for a major depression diagnosis in children are only slightly different from the core *DSM-IV* criteria for adults. In children, irritable mood can replace a sad mood as a major diagnostic criterion, and a failure to make expected weight gains can replace the adult criterion of a change of more than 5% of body weight in a month. According to the *DSM-IV* (pp. 3.1–3.8), "Somatic complaints and social withdrawal are common in children, whereas psychomotor retardation, hypersomnia, and delusions are less common in prepuberty than in adolescence or adulthood."

> Adam, who is now 15 years old, was 13 when his parents separated. He was a good student, socially active, and a fine athlete. Adam began to give up things. First, he gave up his baseball church league with the explanation that he had so many things to do. Then, he didn't bother to try out for soccer. His grades held up pretty well, but he seemed to be having less and less time for friends. He spent a lot of time alone, especially on weekends. His friends continued to call him for quite a while, but they gradually got the message that he wasn't interested. His mother sought professional guidance for what was now recognizable as a serious depression.

Diagnostic Considerations

Conditions that are frequently comorbid with depression in both children and adolescents include disruptive behavior disorders, attention deficit disorders, and anxiety disorders. These may present as psychosomatic reactions, refusal to attend school, antisocial behaviors, fire setting, and learning disabilities. There appears to be a strong relationship between depression and anxiety in young children, particularly the comorbidity of depression and separation anxiety and/or school refusal. This may explain why, in major studies, more than 80% of school-phobic children return to school after treatment with imipramine, an antidepressant.

Depression accompanied by symptoms of impaired cognition, attention, and concentration often resembles ADHD. One fourth of those children suffering with both anxiety and depressive disorders have been found to have attention deficit disorders as well. In adolescence, major depression is also frequently associated with substance-related disorders and eating disorders.

There has been some tendency to think of mood and anxiety disorders in children and adolescence as transient. However, an untreated episode can last for 6 or more months. Some depressive symptoms, although they may fall below the threshold for major depressive disorder, can last for years. Mood disorders can be both severe and enduring requiring diagnosis and appropriate treatment.

Clinical Management/Intervention

Antidepressant treatments for children and early adolescents do not show the same clear efficacy that they do with adults. However, combining psychotherapy and antidepressant treatments in children and adolescents does lead to recoveries that are of longer duration than those that result from medication alone (McCracken & Cantwell, 1992). Cognitive-behavioral therapy has proven to be a highly effective treatment, even in the absence of medication, for both social adjustment and vegetative symptoms. In cognitive-behavioral therapy, children are taught skills of self-rewarding, self-monitoring (for awareness of good things and good thoughts that occur), cognitive restructuring as "thought detectives" trained to reevaluate evidence supporting their negative beliefs (see chapter 20, Behavioral Counseling and Medical Adherence, for a discussion of cognitive behavioral therapy). Children may also be taught stress management, relaxation, and problem-solving skills.

Psychopharmacology

Research has shown that children and early adolescents do not have the same excellent response to antidepressants as adults. This may be explained partly by the fact that depression in the younger age groups is associated with many comorbid conditions. There also is concern that children and adolescents are being placed on powerful medications without evidence of efficacy and with insufficient understanding of the impact of these medications on physical development. Nevertheless, tricyclic antidepressants and the SSRIs remain the mainstay of psychopharmacological treatments of depressive disorders in children. Imipramine has been the best studied, along with amitriptyline, desipramine, and nortriptyline. Of these four medications, desipramine is the least sedating and anticholinergic and often the best tolerated by children. Imipramine, the best studied TCA in children, more frequently causes sedation and anticholinergic side effects. The anticholinergic symptoms of dry mouth can be a significant problem in children, because it can lead to a marked increase in dental cavities (Maxmen & Ward, 1995).

The maximum dose of imipramine is 3.5 mg/kg/day for children and 5 mg/kg/day for adolescents. A common dose of amitriptyline is 5 mg/kg/day for treatment of adolescent depression. Tricyclic antidepressants may provoke anger outbursts in children. For children complaining of low energy levels, depression, or excessive sleep, desipramine is best tolerated. However, desipramine has been implicated in some cases of arrhythmia, sudden collapse, and sudden death.

Because of the questionable efficacy and potentially toxic side effects of TCAs (conduction delay, seizures, and delirium in children with brain injuries, or dental caries with prolonged anticholinergic exposure), SSRIs may be the safest option in treating children with depression (Maxmen & Ward, 1995). These medications generally are used in lower doses than in adults. Table 11.2 reviews antidepressant dosing schedules. Although SSRIs alone appear to be less cardiotoxic than tricyclics, this may not be true when SSRIs are prescribed in combination with other drugs.

PROBLEMS IN CHILDHOOD AND ADOLESCENCE

Physical and Sexual Abuse

Abuse affects every aspect of the child's psyche and development. In 1992 approximately 3 million children were alleged victims of maltreatment. Of this total, 800,000 were reported to be victims of physical abuse and 500,000, of sexual abuse (McCurdy & Daro, 1993). The number of unreported cases probably exceeds that of reported cases, which makes child

Table 11.2 Antidepressant Dosing for Major Depression in Children and Adolescents*

Medication	Suggested Dosage	Plasma Level Response Range [ng/ml]
Imipramine	3–5 mg/kg/day	150–300
Desipramine	3–5 mg/kg/day	> 125
Nortriptyline	1–2 mg/kg/day	60–100
Amitriptyline	3–5 mg/kg/day	unknown
Fluoxetine	5–40 mg/day	unknown
Clomipramine	2–3 mg/kg/day	unknown
Phenelzine	30–90 mg/day	unknown
Tranylcypromine	10–40 mg/day	unknown

*Plasma level based on 12 hours after the last dose.

Source: McCracken, J. T., & Cantwell, D. P. (1992). Management of child and adolescent mood disorders. *Child and Adolescent Psychiatry Clinics of North America, 1*(1), 229–256.

abuse a national epidemic. Nationally, close to 1,000 children each year never get to their second year of life as a result of maltreatment. The incidence of severe physical injury in the abused school-age child appears to be small compared to its incidence in the abused infant. Signs of child abuse may be hidden by clothing or concealed behind "shaken baby syndrome." Some children are kept home from school until the evidence of abuse fades.

Adolescents are at twice the risk of abuse as are preschoolers (Kaplan, 1994). One-third to one-fourth of girls and one-fourth to one-sixth of boys will be sexually assaulted by the age of 18 (McCurdy & Daro, 1993).

The psychological residue of all forms of abuse may be severe. These may include cognitive damage, developmental delay, psychosocial impairments, and childhood depression and anxiety disorders. Childhood sexual or physical abuse has been identified as a primary or contributing factor to many cases of adult disorders such as dissociative identity disorder, borderline personality disorder, and PTSD.

Many factors related to the parent and child are known to increase the likelihood of abuse. Table 11.3 provides a comprehensive list of risk factors for child abuse, which can be observed in either the parent or the child. Prematurity, low birth weight, difficult infant temperament, a physical handicap, and failure to develop a secure mother-infant attachment are

Table 11.3 SUSPECT CHILD ABUSE

When the Child:

1. Shows evidence of unexplained dehydration and/or malnutrition or has been given unusaul medications, drinks, or food
2. Shows evidence of overall poor care
3. Seems unusually fearful
4. Shows evidence of sexual abuse
5. Observable evidence of repeated injury, particularly where the injury is not readily explainable, e.g. stocking or glove type burns
6. Has multiple healing abrasions
7. X rays show multiple fractures or long bone damage
8. Shows unusual changes in physical, emotional, or mental make up
9. Assumes the role of parentified child

When the Parents:

1. Describes the child as "different"
2. Appears psychologically disturbed or mentally limited
3. Is grossly unrealistic about the child's capacities
4. Appears to lack empathy for the child experiences or shows a lack of empathy for the child's injury
5. Refuses consent for medical work up or further diagnostic studies
6. Does not recognize the seriousness of the situation or seem intent on diverting the discussion to other matters
7. Acts or thinks impulsively, appears psychotic, or shows indifference to the child
8. Witholds information or provides a history which does not explain the injury
9. Appears to lack social support from others who might assist the parent who is angry or stressed with the child
10. Appears guarded during the interview
11. Repeatedly changes the child's physicians or health care institution
12. Abuses substances
13. Makes the physician feel uncomfortable about the parent's child care practices.

associated with child maltreatment. Psychopathology, immaturity, social isolation, and chronic illness are among the parent factors linked with abuse and maltreatment. A new parent with unrealistic expectations who is uninformed about child care and the nuances of a baby's crying might be at risk for harming that infant. See chapter 14, Women's Health Through the Reproductive Cycle, for additional discussion.

The presence of risk factors for child abuse should alert the primary care clinician to interview the parents, directly observe parent-child interaction, perform a complete physical examination of the child, and review medical records. The physician needs to interview the parents as to the cause of childhood fractures, healed fractures, burns, and bruises. Parents of failure-to-thrive children need careful interviewing to determine probable cause. Parental explanations of poor growth or injury should be evaluated for their plausibility. Glove-like or sock-like burns may be caused by hot water immersion and should not be dismissed by parental stories of boiling pots of water falling from stoves. The physical exam will also reveal signs and symptoms of physical trauma. The consequences of shaking injuries, for instance, can be detected through examination of the child's eyes.

Sometimes parent-child interactions will suggest abuse. Episodes of violent discipline in the office or a detached or excessively frightened child are suggestive of abuse. When there is suspicion of child abuse, the clinician should review the child's entire lifetime medical record, including records from other doctors.

Most abused children also show problems in management of aggression and modulation of affect. Abused children who become depressed often grow up to be depressed adults. As many as one third of abused children maintain abuse as a family tradition and grow up to be abusers themselves.

Clinical Management/Intervention

All providers who suspect child abuse or neglect have a legal responsibility to report even the suspicion of child abuse. Beyond the role in diagnosing, investigating, and reporting abuse, the primary care physician can be supportive and provide education to the entire family. Many parents who abuse children are highly receptive to learning. At least some abuse reflects parental misinformation and inexperience, and in such cases, parents may be open to educational interventions. The clinician can help parents to set realistic expectations for their child's developmental level. Some parents require education about effective discipline techniques that do not employ hitting or violence. It is important that the clinician maintain ongoing and regular contact with potentially abusive parents to provide regular guidance and education in their understanding of their child's needs throughout the many stages of development. A parent who cannot manage his or her own anger, a parent who is overwhelmed, or a parent with poor parenting skills will need a preventative referral to a social service agency and/or referral to mental health practitioners with special expertise in this area.

Suicide of Children and Adolescents

In the United States, adolescent suicide is the third-leading cause of death in teenagers, after accidents and homicide. In the 10- to 11-year-old age group, there are 14 attempts made for every successful suicide (Rotheram, Tiacentini, Miller, Graae, & Castro-Blance, 1994). Within the child population, the risk of suicidal behavior is linked to depression, preoccupation with death, aggression, and the presence of psychopathology, such as overanxious disorder, dysthymic disorder, or oppositional disorder. The presence of some acute distress seems important in understanding the precipitants of suicide in children, preadolescent, and adolescent populations.

> Alfred, age 6, began his day with an argument with his 4-year-old sister, which ended when he punched her and left her crying. His mother intervened and harshly reprimanded him. Alfred, upset, struggled to open the window so he could jump out. His mother became terrified and brought her son in for evaluation.

Psychological autopsies after completed suicide reveal that suicidal action in teenagers can be precipitated by an acute disciplinary crisis; by ridicule, rejection, humiliation, or failing at some event; or by a dispute with a girlfriend or boyfriend. In general, adolescents attempting suicide report higher levels of perceived distress than do nonsuicidal teenagers. Psychological autopsies have also revealed that feelings of hopelessness, suicidal ideation, negative self-evaluation, hostility, and a previous history of suicidal attempts may help assess risk and prevent suicide in adolescents. These traits can be measured by a suicide probability scale (Larzelere, Smith, Batenhorst, & Kelly, 1996). The Beck Depression Inventory can be used as a self-report measure to determine level of depression, because severe mood disorders should raise the question of increasing suicidal potential. Many children and adolescents who attempt or succeed at suicide have poor coping skills and/or suffer with depression or chronic anxiety.

Children suffering with suicidal ideation or behavior need to be seen and heard. If not heard, a child may well "up the ante," try harder, and eventually succeed at suicide. Children do take pills, run in front of cars, or put plastic bags over their heads. The cognitive limitations of young children make for greater difficulty in gauging serious suicidal intent. A 5-year-old may well have intended to die by ingesting two aspirins. On the other hand, a 9-year-old might mean to die, be seriously suicidal, but still believe that death is reversible.

Reliable information can more easily be obtained by formulating questions about the frequency of the child's symptoms in a more concrete fashion, such as "Do you think about killing yourself more than once or twice a day?" Several studies have indicated that parents are less likely to report suicide attempts or even suicidal ideation than the children themselves. Asking the parents broad questions about the child's global functioning may be more productive than direct questions, such as "Has your child been suicidal?"

Clinical Management /Intervention

A clinician should take seriously any suicidal gesture or suicidal ideation as well as a patient's expression of feelings of helplessness or hopelessness. Rather than labeling a child "mentally ill," it is more effective to speak to the child in a straightforward manner about suicidal feeling or actions and to frame the child's suicidal feelings as an attempt to resolve an acute problem or overwhelming stress. It is generally better to speak directly to the child in such terms as "your wish to kill yourself" rather than taking a less direct approach and asking, "Do you intend to do yourself harm?" One critical moment of emotional distress can precipitate suicide. Thus even knowing whether or not a youngster has a plan of action is not necessarily helpful in predicting whether that child will attempt suicide.

There are various options available to the clinician and the family when a child is suicidal. The clinician can refer a child or family to a crisis intervention service or an emergency room if psychiatric care is required. Crisis hotlines can offer help; however, these have more appeal to female than to male patients, and only a small percentage of crisis callers actually take the advice offered on the hotline. Patients referred to the emergency room will receive acute psychiatric treatment but rarely follow up on referrals for psychotherapy. Thus it is important that the primary care clinician maintain contact with the family and facilitate the referral process.

Some suicidal adolescents and children may be hospitalized for psychiatric care. It is not uncommon for these children to make a new suicide attempt after discharge. It is important for the primary care physician to continue to monitor the patient's mood disorder, because suicidal patients, even those on antidepressants, are at an ongoing risk for a new suicide attempt. Management, evaluation, and treatment approaches to the suicidal patient are detailed in chapter 7, Violence and Suicide. General treatment approaches are also reviewed in the last four chapters in this book.

The primary care physician should have a low threshold for consultation and referral in the treatment of suicidal children and adolescents. If a child appears suicidal, the clinician should establish and coordinate psychiatric treatment by a mental health professional (see chapter 7, Violence and Suicide).

Psychopharmacology

In some cases, the primary care physician may prescribe antidepressants while the child or adolescent is in psychiatric treatment with a psychologist or social worker. Most adolescents will be treated with the SSRIs. Refer to chapter 3, Depression, for medication guidelines.

Advising Parents on Dealing With a Child's Concerns About Death

It is not uncommon for parents to seek advice from their primary care physician on how to handle a child's questions about death. The death of a family member or classmate can precipitate a child's preoccupation and concern about death. Also, parents are often unsure as to whether or not to take a child to a funeral or to the cemetery.

> Charley is 6 years old. His 7-year-old brother recently died of a congenital disorder after prolonged suffering. The brothers were very close, and Charley seems shattered by his brother's death. His parents have misgivings about taking Charley to the cemetery. The parents are not aware that Charley believes that his normal rivalrous feelings led to his brother's death.

Clinical Management/Intervention

Children of 3 years of age and older can be allowed to attend funerals and visit cemeteries. Attending funeral rituals and witnessing burials are part of learning and preparation for other inevitable losses. Parents need to know that excluding a child from participation with the family at the time of tragedy can be harmful. A child who is excluded from death and dying rituals may feel overlooked, alone, and unable to perceive the parents' support.

The primary care physician can also help the family and child to better understand the meaning of death at various developmental levels of the child. As in the case above, the child believed that his rivalrous thoughts killed his brother. Children often believe in the magical powers of their thoughts and fantasies. In this case, the clinician can advise the parents to explain to the child that no thoughts or feelings are able to cause a death. This counsel can greatly allay the child's feelings of guilt and improve the parents' coping, which can prevent future problems.

Childhood questions about death can be handled as they occur. Learning about death should be part of the gradual experience of daily life, such as learning about a dead bird found lying in the street or the loss of a pet. It is through these experiences that children learn to cope with losses.

In helping parents talk to their child about death, the clinician should advise parents not to explain death with the euphemism that the deceased is "sleeping." This explanation may make the child fearful of nighttime sleeping or nap time. The child will best adapt to dealing with death by witnessing the rituals surrounding death and the parents' coping with it.

The loss of family members can be devastating for children. The sadness that young children demonstrate is likely to be of a relatively short duration, because they are not cognitively able to understand the permanency of loss. The trauma of the loss for a child relates more to the parents' unavailability if they become absorbed by their own experience of loss. A parent may withdraw from the child in self-absorbed despair because of pain related to the death. In these circumstances, the clinician might suggest that other family members be recruited to fill in the void of responding to the child. The child must not experience the devastation of abandonment. If parents become emotionally unavailable to the child or if there is no support system, the primary care physician should refer the entire family to a mental health practitioner.

Mourning about a childhood loss may not occur for many years, as the capacity to mourn begins to develop in adolescence. When mourning begins in adolescence, it is often a new loss that precipitates the mourning, as well as working through of the older childhood loss.

Divorce

When a child presents with such psychological symptoms as anxiety, depression, concentration impairment, behavioral problems, suicidal preoccupation, and changes in levels of academic proficiency, the clinician should inquire about the status of the parents' marriage and parental relationships. Divorce has the potential to affect every important aspect of the child's psyche, regardless of the child's age at the time of divorce. At least one major study found that the impact of divorce on children is both devastating and long-standing (Wallerstein & Blakeslee, 1990). However, one problem with this study was its failure to consider the predivorce condition of the children. For example, many of the children in the study who demonstrated long-standing depression subsequent to the divorce were found to have been depressed before the divorce.

Clinical Management/Intervention

Divorce is traumatic for both parents and children. Not uncommonly, conflicts between parents persist after divorce and continue to be perpetuated over the phone or in driveways at visitation pick-up times. Divorced parents often experience diminished ability to discipline their children and provide care, and many parents have difficulty staying sensitively focused on their children's needs. When the family structure breaks down, parental effectiveness declines and children commonly experience loss, insecurity, grief, and feelings of abandonment.

Divorce can be particularly traumatic for the adolescent. Newly created one-parent families may have difficulty setting limits for their adolescent children. Under these circumstances, the normal sexual and aggressive impulses of the adolescent may be difficult for the parent to manage.

Adolescent acting out, such as drunk driving, sexual experimentation, and difficulties with school or friends, may occur. For the adolescent experiencing his or her parents' divorce, acting out becomes a tension reducer in a climate of uncertainty.

The primary care clinician can be a compassionate constant when the parental support base is dysfunctional or when parents are entangled in partisan warfare. The clinician can serve as a guide for the rebuilding process by providing support for all parties and reminding parents of their children's needs for extra support. The physician should refer any family member who is struggling to deal with divorce to individual therapy. Sometimes, a family referral for either the parents or a subset of the family can markedly reduce the hostilities and improve the function of the entire system. Remaining an active and interested participant in the follow-up of this traumatic event is a critical role for the physician.

REFERENCES

Achenbach, T. M., & Howell, C. T. (1993). Are American children's problems getting worse? A 13-year comparison. *Journal of the American Academy of Child and Adolescent Psychiatry, 32*, 1145–1154.

American Psychiatric Association. (1994). *Diagnostic and statistical manual of mental disorders*. (4th ed.). Washington, DC: Author.

Bell-Dolan, D. J., Last, C. G., & Strauss, C. C. (1990). Symptoms of anxiety disorders in normal children. *Journal of the American Academy of Child and Adolescent Psychiatry, 29*, 759–766.

Bernstein, J. G. (1995). *Handbook of drug therapy in psychiatry* (3rd ed.). New York: Mosby.

Greenhill, L. L. (1992). Pharmacotherapy: Stimulants: In: Attention deficit hyperactivity disorder. *Child And Adolescent Psychiatric Clinics Of North America, 1*, 411–449.

Hawthorne Educational Services. (1995). *Attention Deficit Disorders Evaluation Scales (ADDES) for the preschooler, the adolescent and the adult as well as the school age child.* Columbia, MO: Author.

Kaplan S. (1994). Adolescent physical abuse. *Child and Adolescent Psychiatric Clinics of North America, 3*(4), 695–713.

Larzelere, R. E., Smith, G. L., Batenhorst, L. M., & Kelly, D. B. (1996). Predictive validity of suicide probability scale among adolescents in group home treatment. *Journal of the American Academy of Child and Adolescent Psychiatry, 35*, 166–175.

Maxmen, J. S., & Ward, N. G. (1995). Psychotropic drugs: Fast facts. (2nd ed.). New York: Norton.

McCracken, J. T. (1992). The epidemiology of child and adolescent mood disorders. *Child and Adolescent Psychiatry Clinics of North America, 1*(1), 88–111.

McCracken, J. T., & Cantwell, D. P. (1992). Management of child and adolescent mood disorders. *Child and Adolescent Psychiatry Clinics of North America, 1*(1), 229–256.

McCurdy, K., & Daro, D. (1993). *Current trends in child abuse reporting and fatalities: The results of the 1992 annual fifty state survey.* Chicago: National Committee for the Prevention of Child Abuse.

McGee, R., Partridge, F., Williams, S., & Silva, P. A. (1991). A twelve year follow up of preschool hyperactive children. *Journal of the American Academy of child and Adolescent Psychiatry, 30*, 224.

Messer, S. C., & Bidel, D. C. (1994). Psychosocial correlates of childhood anxiety disorders. *Journal of the American Academy of Child and Adolescent Psychiatry, 33*, 975–976.

Rotheram, M. J., Tiacentini, J., Miller, S., Graae, F., & Castro-Blance, D. (1994). Brief cognitive-behavioral treatment for adolescent suicide attempters and their families. *Journal of the American Academy of Child and Adolescent Psychiatry, 33*, 508–517.

Wallerstein, J. S., & Blakeslee, S. (1990). *Second chances: Men, women and children a decade after divorce.* New York: Ticknor & Fields.

PART 2

Behavioral Medicine in Primary Care

CHAPTER **12**

Cardiovascular and Psychosocial Risk Factors Reduction: Office-Based Interventions

Robert E. Feinstein, Laurel Carey, Peter M. Rabinowitz, Joyelle Gallicano, Anne A. Brewer, Abraham Bornstein, Joseph V. Connelly, Pamela F. LeDeaux, and Dewees H. Brown

In order to maximize cardiovascular health, a primary care physician must be able to assess and intervene with patients who have modifiable cardiovascular risk factors. Assessing the broad sweep of medical and psychosocial risk factors requires office-based assessments and intervention strategies. However, intervention is usually complicated by psychosocial factors that neither the patient nor the physician is aware of and that preclude success in reducing risk. This chapter will review the medical and psychosocial risk factors for cardiovascular disease; provide brief assessment strategies and intervention plans for nutrition/obesity/eating disorders, exercise, and smoking cessation; and discuss barriers to changing lifestyle.

MEDICAL AND PSYCHOSOCIAL RISK FACTORS FOR CARDIOVASCULAR DISEASE

Nonmodifiable Cardiovascular Risk Factors

There are three main nonmodifiable risk factors associated with cardiovascular disease.

Age: The risk for cardiovascular disease begins at age 45 in men and 55 in women and increases with age and the slow, progressive development of atherosclerosis. Atherosclerosis often leads to vascular compromise and vascular events, such as a stroke or myocardial infarction.

Gender: Women who are premenopausal or on hormone replacement therapy have greater protection from heart disease than men. Estrogen exerts its cardio-protective effect by decreasing low-density lipoprotein (LDL) and increasing high-density lipoprotein (HDL), and it may directly protect the arterial lining, by decreasing fat deposition in injured artery walls.

Family history of early coronary artery disease (CAD): Heart disease runs in families as an independent risk factor when adjusted for other CAD risk variables. A family history is positive if a first-degree relative, before age 55 in men and age 65 in women, has (1) clinical evidence of heart disease, such as angina or shortness of breath, or (2) laboratory evidence and/or positive diagnostic tests that reveal cardiovascular atherosclerosis, peripheral vascular disease, or cerebrovascular disease. This genetic risk of cardiovascular disease (CVD) is mediated through defects in lipoprotein, cholesterol production, homocysteine, or other metabolic pathways. The genetics of CVD can be used clinically to motivate patients to make necessary lifestyle changes. For example, a father's heart attack can greatly motivate his son to reduce his own CAD risk. Additional facts about these important nonmodifiable risk factors are summarized in Table 12.1.

Modifiable Cardiovascular Risk Factors

Modifiable cardiovascular risk factors include blood pressure, diabetes, smoking, nutritional habits, weight reduction, and sedentary lifestyle. Change of these risk factors typically requires changes in lifestyle and/or the use of medications. Modifiable risk factors are reviewed in Table 12.2.

Table 12.1 Nonmodifiable Cardiovascular Risk Factors

Age

Risk doubles every 10 years
Significant risk in men >45 years old and women >55 years old
Mean age of infarction: men, 55; women, 65

Gender

Women:
- Females have relative protection against CHD
- Estrogen decreases LDL and arterial wall damage
- Hormonal replacement therapy:
  - Decreases risk of CHD and osteoporosis
  - Slightly increases uterine cancer risk if estrogen is given alone
  - Questionable increase in breast cancer rates
- Women who suffer a myocardial infarction
  - Often present without chest pain
  - 37% present with shortness of breath
  - 9% present with epigastric pain
- Women on oral contraception increase CHD risks
- Women on contraception and smoking have 20x risk

Men:
- Men at 40 have 4x mortality risk of women
- Men at 70 have 2x mortality risk women
- At 80 the mortality risk is equal for men and women

Family History

Independent risk factor for CAD

+ Family Hx: if a first degree relative has angina, sudden death, or myocardial infarction, male <55 or female <65

Familial abnormal lipid profiles increase the risk

Existing CAD: if clinical or lab evidence of cardiac, peripheral vascular disease, or cerebrovascular diseases

50% of myocardial infarctions and 70% mortality occurs in patients with existing disease

Sources: Anderson, K. M., Castelli, W. P., & Levy, D. (1987). Cholesterol and mortality: 30 years of follow-up from the Framingham Study. *Journal of the American Medical Association, 257*, 2176–2180.

Castelli, W. P., Garrison, R. J., & Wilson, P. W. F. (1986). Framingham Heart Study: Incidence of coronary artery disease and lipoprotein cholesterol levels. *Journal of the American Medical Association, 256*, 2835–2838.

Centers for Disease Control. (1987). Protective effect of physical activity on coronary heart disease. *Morbidity and Mortality Weekly Report, 36*, 426–430.

Healthier People Version 4.0 [Computer software]. (1991). Atlanta: Carter Center of Emory University (Health Risk Appraisal Program 1988. Vol 4: Scientific Documentation, July).

Table 12.2 Modifiable Risk Factors

Blood Pressure

Clinical issues (JNC-V):

BP should be taken 2x each office visit. Patients should be sitting, with no emotional arousal

BP >140/90 requires lifestyle modification

Lifestyle changes for 3–6 months before medications are used:

1. reduce alcohol to 2 oz/day
2. regular exercise can lower blood pressure
3. restrict salt intake–may lower BP

Diabetes

Increase the risk of cardiovascular events 1.5x

In men: Increases the risk of CHD by 3x

In women: Increases risk by decreasing estrogen's protection

Type 1: Increases atherosclerosis, CAD, stroke, vascular disease

Type 2: Insulin resistance increases BP and coronary/cerebro-/peripheral vascular disease

Syndrome X: Insulin resistance with 4 features:
abdominal obesity, increased BP, diabetes, lipid abnormalities

Smoking

Associated with 20% of all deaths

400,000 deaths/yr, 53,000 from passive smoke

Links to smoking: 20% heart disease, 85% lung cancer, 30% other cancers; increases chronic lung diseases, GI ulcers, gastritis, reflux, the risk of abortion and low birth weight

In childhood: increases asthma, ear infections, and cancers

CAD: Risk proportional to number of packs/year history

Smoking cessation in post-MI patient decreases mortality by 50%

Comorbid conditions complicating smoking cessation:
alcohol/drug use, depression, schizophrenia

Nutrition/Weight

CAD correlates with: increased total cholesterol, LDL, TG, and total cholesterol/HDL ratio and decreased HDL

Obesity: BMI ≥ 30% or a BMI of ≥ 27, ≥ 2 or more risk factors or overweight by 25% for men, 35% for women

Obesity adds a small independent risk of CHD

Obesity of > 20% : can increase risk of diabetes, increases BP and LDL, and decreases HDL

Sedentary Lifestyle
Causes 250,000 deaths/year

Not exercising = same risk as high blood pressure, smoking, high-fat diet

Exercising reduces premature death, CHD, diabetes, blood pressure and obesity

Exercise improves lipid and Glucose profiles, O_2 consumption, heart and lung efficiency, muscle strength, reaction time, sleep, and longevity

Sources: Anderson, K. M., Castelli, W. P., & Levy, D. (1987). Cholesterol and mortality: 30 years of follow up from the Framingham Study. *Journal of the American Medical Association, 257*, 2176–2180.

Bartecchi, C. E., MacKenzie, T. D., & Schrier, R. W. (1994). The human costs of tobacco use (Part 1). *New England Journal of Medicine, 330*, 907–912.

Castelli, W. P., Garrison, R. J., & Wilson, P. W. F. (1986). Framingham Heart Study: Incidence of coronary artery disease and lipoprotein cholesterol levels. *Journal of the American Medical Association, 256*, 2835–2838.

Centers for Disease Control. (1987). Protective effect of physical activity on coronary heart disease. *Morbidity and Mortality Weekly Report, 36*, 426–430.

Healthier People Version 4.0 [Computer software]. (1991). Atlanta: Carter Center of Emory University (Health Risk Appraisal Program 1988. Vol 4: Scientific Documentation, July).

Hughes, J. R. (1996). Practice guidelines for treatment of patients with nicotine dependence. *American Journal of Psychiatry, 153*(October Suppl.), 263–265.

Lee, I., Hsieh, C., & Paffenbarger, R. S. (1995). Exercise intensity and longevity in men: The Harvard Alumni health study. *Journal of the American Medical Association, 273*, 1179–1184.

MacKenzie, T. D., Bartecchi, C. E., & Schrier, R. W. (1994). The human costs of tobacco use (Part 2). *New England Journal of Medicine, 330*, 975–980.

Paffenbarger, R. S., Kampert, J. B., Lee, I., Hyde, R. T., Leung, R. W., & Wing, A. L. (1994). Changes in physical activity and other lifeway patterns influencing longevity. *Medicine and Science in Sports and Exercise, 26*(7), 857–865.

Pate, R. R., Pratt, M., Blair S. N., Haskell, W. L., & Macera, C. A. (1995). Physical activity and public health: A recommendation from the Centers for Disease Control and Prevention and the American College of Sports Medicine. *Journal of the American Medical Association, 273*, 402–407.

Psychosocial Risk Factors for Cardiovascular Disease

Acute Stress, Situational Disturbances, Sudden Death, and CAD

In patients with existing CAD, acute stress, such as a disturbing, stressful life event, death of a spouse, or divorce, or events such as public speaking, getting stuck in a traffic jam, or the expression of severe emotions such as an angry outburst, can produce an arrhythmia and sometimes cause sudden cardiac death. This stress-arrhythmia/sudden death connection is present in approximately 20% of patients with CAD who are hospitalized for dangerous arrhythmias (Goldstein & Niaura, 1995). This lethal connection is created through stress-induced sympathetic arousal.

One model that explains this connection (Kamarck & Jennings, 1991) is that psychological stress elicits a fight-or-flight response through the autonomic nervous system. The vagus nerve controls heart rate variability, and the sympathetic nervous system brings on the fight-or-flight response. Repeated activation of the fight-or-flight response can cause damage to the blood vessel lining, which fosters atherosclerotic heart disease. This process occurs over a matter of years. Repeated activation of the fight-or-flight response can cause constriction of the coronary arteries, platelet aggregation, and thrombogenesis. The fight-or-flight response can also cause an arterial fat plaque eruption, which can cascade into coronary artery occlusion and myocardial infarction. This process can occur in a matter of minutes to seconds. The adrenaline surge and fight-or-flight response can create contraction band lesions, resulting in pathologically distinct heart damage over a long period of time, or produce a lethal abnormal heart rhythm and sudden cardiac death (Eliot, 1994). Although the stress-mind-heart connection is not an issue for every patient, it is important for patients suffering with chest pain, angina, or existing CAD.

Personality Types and the Development of CAD

Although the mind-heart connection is well established for sudden death, the connection between personality style and CAD connection is more controversial. Friedman and Rosenman (Friedman, 1992) were the first to describe a mind-heart connection with the classic description of Type A personality. This personality type is characterized by hostility, time urgency, impatience, aggressiveness, competitiveness, and hard-driving behavior with speech and motor characteristics such as rapid body movement, tense facial/body muscles, explosive speech, and hand or teeth clenching. Their famous Western Collaborative Group Study (Friedman, 1992) suggested that men with Type A personality had twice the likelihood of developing CAD as men who did not have this behavioral pattern. This meant that Type A behavior carried a risk for CAD similar to that of smoking. Later studies with more sophisticated design, such as the Multiple Risk Factor Intervention Trial (Shekelle et al., 1985), failed to find any increased risk of heart disease in Type A men. Trends in the area of personality and CAD (Barefoot, Dahlstrom, & Williams, 1983) have moved the focus to the link between high expressed hostility and CAD. Reinterpretation of Friedman's data (Ketterer, Lovallo, & Lumley, 1993) has moved to AIAI (aggravation, irritation, anger, and impatience) and the hostility syndrome (cynicism. anger, and agression) (Williams & Williams, 1994), as the behavioral expressions of hostility responsible for increasing the risks of CAD.

Eliot (Eliot, 1994; Eliot & Morales-Ballejo, 1994) described "hot reactors," with potential links to the development of cardiovascular disease. Hot reactors are patients who appear outwardly calm but inwardly show autonomic arousal. Eliot performed autopsies on healthy men who had died mysteriously and discovered a new kind of stress-induced myocardial injury called contraction band lesions. These myocardial lesions are caused by stress-related releases of high doses of epinephrine and norepinephrine. Acute stress can produce massive lesions and induce sudden death. Chronic stress produces micromyocardial lesions (Eliot, 1994), which gradually increase the risk of arrhythmias and sudden death. Thus there is consensus that hostility or high-intensity emotion or the hot reactor personality probably increases the risk of developing sudden cardiac death and may increases the long-term risk of CAD in predisposed individuals.

Stress, Hostility, and CAD

The literature on stress and heart disease suggests that much of the mind-heart connection occurs through the fight-or-fight response. This vast literature can be summarized as follows:

1. Repeated arousal is responsible for some cases of chronic hypertension (Eliot, 1994; Eliot & Morales-Ballejo, 1994).
2. In the hot reactor personality style, excessive autonomic hyperactivity activates surges in blood pressure, which cause arterial damage and accelerate atherosclerosis (Eliot, 1994; Eliot & Morales-Ballejo, 1994).
3. Mental stress, especially anger, has been shown to increase platelet aggregability, which can lead to thrombogenesis and coronary events (Malkoff, Muldoon, Zeigler, & Manuck, 1993).
4. Mental stress, such as that experienced during public speaking, makes healthy arteries constrict, increasing the risk of angina, myocardial infarction (MI), and sudden death (Lacy, Contrada, Robbins, Tannenbaum, & Moreya, 1994).
5. Recall of angry events in patients with existing CAD can make atherosclerotic-narrowed arteries constrict and become narrower.

Anger recall also reduces the heart's efficiency as a pump (Jiang et al., 1996).

6. In some patients who have CAD, an episode of intense anger can bring on an MI within 2 hours (Follick et al., 1990).
7. Anger can cause a plaque in a narrowed artery to rupture and occlude the artery, producing an MI (Muller, Abela, Nesto, & Tofler, 1994).

A combined model (Krantz & Durel, 1983) links stress, personality, and biological factors to produce CAD. This model suggests that stress interacts with the personality styles of high hostility or hot reactor and with genetic tendencies. These interactions are mediated through the processes of hypertension, atherosclerosis development, clotting abnormalities, and lipid deposition and abnormalities, to produce CAD.

Depression and CAD

Primary care physicians and cardiologists fail to diagnose depression in as many as 30% to 50% of the patients they treat. Depression is easy to miss in a patient with CAD because many of the symptoms of depression are similar to the symptoms of patients who have recently suffered a myocardial infarction. Post-MI patients often complain of sad mood, fatigue, sleep problems, and loss of appetite, which may be incorrectly ascribed to CAD. Patients who have had an MI understandably may have depressive symptoms, which should trigger the physician to perform a more detailed evaluation to rule out or identify depressed mood or clinical depression. Because depression may require immediate treatment, it is important to be alert to its signs. The cardiovascular significance of depression only recently has been acknowledged. Depression affects cardiovascular disease in four ways: (1) Depression can cause sudden death. (2) Mortality rates increase for those who have a history of recurrent depression and coronary artery disease. (3) Depression is an independent risk factor for developing CAD and an MI. (4) Heart disease increases the chance of becoming depressed by 20% to 30%. Following is a review of these four aspects of the heart-depression connection.

SUDDEN DEATH AND DEPRESSION. Two prospective studies (Frasure-Smith, Lesperance, & Talajic, 1993, 1994) have begun to elucidate how depression may actually cause sudden cardiac death. Through the vagus nerve, depressed patients emit a low-frequency CNS nerve pulse, which, when less than 10 cycles per minute, affects heart rate variability, increasing the risk of arrhythmias and sudden cardiac arrest. In addition, through changes in serotonin, depressed patients also show changes in platelet aggregability, which may lead to thrombogenesis (Frasure-Smith et al., 1993, 1994).

RECURRENT DEPRESSION AND MYOCARDIAL INFARCTION. Other research (Barefoot & Schroll, 1996; Pratt et al., 1996) reveals that a history of recurrent depression increases mortality rates from a myocardial infarction 4 to 5 five times. A prior history of depression is a greater risk than is an acute first episode of depression following an MI.

DEPRESSION AS AN INDEPENDENT RISK FACTOR FOR CHD. Two studies (Barefoot & Schroll et al., 1996; Barefoot & Helms et al., 1996) showed that there is a spectrum of depressive moods, from sad to major depression, which gradually increases the risk of developing CAD. Three recent studies (Barefoot, 1996; Pratt et al., 1996; Barefoot & Helms, et al., 1996) have confirmed that depression is an independent risk factor for MI and the development of CAD when other cardiovascular risk factors are controlled. Depression decreases the chance of survival of cardiovascular events by 20%.

HEART DISEASE CAUSES DEPRESSION. Not only does depression increase the risk for heart disease, but reciprocally, CAD can cause depression. If one has never been depressed but develops CAD, the risk of becoming depressed at some time in the future is 20% to 30% (Carney, Rich, & Freedland, 1988).

TREATMENT OF DEPRESSION WITH CHD. Concern was raised in two prospective studies (Frasure-Smith et al., 1993, 1994) that antidepressant medication used to treat depression may have been responsible for increased risk of cardiac mortality. A more recent prospective study (Pratt et al., 1996) showed that tricyclic antidepressants and benzodiazepines do not increase the risk of MI, but that lithium, meprobamate, phenothiazine, and barbiturates do. The data collected from this study was accumulated in the1980s and therefore did not include SSRIs. Despite the fact that SSRIs have not been shown to be risk free, the clinical impression is that they are cardio-safe. Currently, treatment of depression is probabbly indicated to decrease overall morbidity. Additional data are forthcoming to determine if treatment of depression in the MI or CAD patient leads to increased survival. See chapter 3, Depression, for a complete discussion of depression and its treatment.

Anxiety and CAD

One major association between cardiovascular disease and anxiety is that phobic anxiety increases the risk of arrhythmias and sudden cardiac death (Kawachi, Sparrow, Vokonas, & Weiss, 1994), and high worry increases the risk of CAD in older men (Kubzansky et al., 1997). However, there is scant evidence showing that anxiety disorders cause or predict the development of CAD. A recent study (Jonas, Franks, & Ingram, 1997) has suggested that anxiety and depression predict a future incidence of hypertension. If anxiety confers any increased risk of CAD, it is likely through the effects of other cardiovascular risk factors. Although anxiety is not a major risk factor for the development of CAD, many patients seeing a cardiologist suffer unnecessarily with anxiety disorders that are not diagnosed or treated. Those patients who are not referred for treatment of their anxiety may progress from panic to health worries, phobias, demoralization, and depression. This is unfortunate, because anxiety disorders are very treatable through medication and through behavioral and psychotherapeutic means (see chapter 2, Anxiety Disorders).

Social Support

The relationship between social support and health became a research focus when it was determined that good social support, measured as being married, having frequent contacts with extended family and friends, and/or having involvement in religion, reduces mortality rates from all causes. In one study, those who lacked social support died at twice the rate of those who were socially connected (Berkman & Syme, 1979). A second study (House, Landis, & Umberson, 1988) showed that lack of social support affects health as dramatically as does cigarette smoking or high cholesterol. Poor social support and a sense of isolation put one at risk for CAD and increase the death rate from all causes. A patient with CAD who is alone has a three-fold increase in mortality (Williams & Williams, 1994). A more recent study (Pratt et al., 1996) has shown that being divorced or separated is an independent risk factor for MI.

Marriage has been examined as a main form of social support. It has been shown that a good marriage substantially decreases death rates from all causes, whereas chronic marital discord seems to lead to suppressed immunity and poor health (Brecht, Drawp, Moser, & Riegel, 1994). Support groups benefit patients with CAD in a similar way (Ornish, 1990), as they have been shown to increase longevity in breast cancer patients (Speigel, 1993).

The exact mechanism that explains these finding has not yet been elucidated. It is likely that social support provides benefits by modifying other risk factors, such as decreasing hypertension, acute and chronic stress, depression, and anxiety, or by improving medical adherence and adjustment or coping with cardiac disease.

Occupations and CHD

A high-strain job is defined as a job that allows little decision making and has high psychological demands (Karasek & Theorell, 1990). High-strain jobs are considered by many to be a risk factor for CAD, although the validity and study designs for assessing this relationship have been questioned (Goldstein, 1995). Telephone operators, bus or factory workers, and air traffic controllers have classic high-strain jobs. They have to complete repetitive tasks in tight time frames and have no control over the volume of work. On the other hand, Wall Street executives, physicians, and lawyers have active, high-demand jobs that have a wide latitude for decision making. These kinds of jobs have fewer health risks. The healthiest jobs, such as nature scientists and elective home-based businesses, have low demands and maximum latitude for decision making. Women have been shown to have high job strain and increased risk for CAD when they have jobs with high demands and little social support. Rotating-shift work for 6 or more years seems to increase the chance of CAD in female nurses (Kawachi et al., 1995).

The effects of high-strain jobs on health seem to be mediated predominantly through the increased risk for developing hypertension. It is probably through hypertension that work stress contributes to CHD, CAD, MI, and sudden death.

Work environments that create the "FUD factor"—fear, uncertainty, doubt (Eliot, 1994)—also seem to increase the risk of developing hypertension. Work stress contributes to poor health in other ways, through factors such as little exercise, excessive smoking, overeating, or by the ability of stress to decrease immunity.

Socioeconomic Factors and CAD

The links between socioeconomic factors and CAD are not well studied. CAD has been shown to be the leading cause of death in African Americans, and the differences in mortality rates between Blacks and Whites are widening dramatically. CAD mortality rates are 3% to 70% higher among Blacks than Whites of the same age until age 74, and CAD develops 5 years earlier in Black men.

A recent study suggests that place of birth, signifying sociocultural and socioeconomic factors, may be more important than race in determining mortality from CAD (Fang, Mandhaven, & Alderman, 1996). This study showed that Southern-born Black men and women had the highest mortality from CHD, Northeastern-born Blacks had moderate mortality rates, and Caribbean-born Blacks had the lowest mortality rates. Studies that attempt to determine whether race is an independent risk factor for heart disease have not been reliably completed. Differences between Blacks, other minorities, and Whites are usually explained by the following:

1. Higher levels of risk factors occur more frequently in lower socioeconomic groups. For example, African Americans show an increase in multiple risk factors, such as cigarette smoking, hypertension, diabetes mellitus, obesity, left ventricular hypertrophy, and physical inactivity.
2. Ethnic customs and geography can affect lifestyles and can often increase or decrease cardiovascular morbidity and mortality. For example, high-fat ethnic diets worsen lipid profiles. Japanese living in Japan, where the typical diet is low in fat, have the lowest risk for CAD, compared to a moderate risk in Hawaiian Japanese and the highest risk in American Japanese.
3. Living conditions can also affect the risk of CAD. For example, crowded ghetto living conditions increase the risk of hypertension. Sometimes, dangerous neighborhoods cause sedentary lifestyles, which increase the risk of CAD.

In addition, there may be a few genetic reasons for differences in CAD between races. For example, African Americans may have a clustering of cardiovascular risk factors in the form of syndrome X dyslipidemic hypertension. Patients suffering with this syndrome have severe risk of cardiovascular disease and associated complications.

OFFICE-BASED ASSESSMENTS AND BRIEF INTERVENTIONS

Nutrition

Conclusive epidemiological information correlates the incidence of CAD with the amount of total cholesterol and saturated fats in diets. High-fat diets increase total cholesterol and LDL and the risk of CAD. Low LDL, low total blood cholesterol levels, and high levels of HDL definitely lower the risk of CAD. A growing number of physicians now recommend heart disease prevention, as summarized in Table 12.3.

To reduce dietary risk factors for cardiovascular disease, it is important to assess a patient's nutritional lifestyle and offer basic nutritional and weight counseling. This can be accomplished by eliciting a nutritional history, evaluating for obesity, and screening for eating disorders. The physician can then offer nutritional counseling, dietary monitoring, and weight counseling to reduce the risks of CAD. The physician should refer the patient to a nutritionist or weight loss specialist, as necessary.

Dietary history can be obtained using a dietary screening instrument, such as the Duke University questionnaire, *How Does Your Diet Measure Up?* (Duke Center for Living, 1995). This instrument is a checklist of items that rate a patient's diet as healthy if the score is 14 or less, as needing improvement for scores 14 to 20, or as needing major improvement for scores above 21. Alternatively, a physician may use a clinical approach and ask the following questions:

1. How many meals/snacks per day do you eat? (The average person eats two to four meals and two snacks per day.)
2. What kinds of food do you eat, and how much of each?
3. Do you take vitamins, minerals, herbs, or any other nutritional supplements?
4. What foods do you avoid and why?

Many physicians will ask their patients to construct a food diary for a single day to facilitate a quick nutritional overview. If additional, detailed information is needed, a physician can ask the patient to complete a weekly detailed food diary. Food diaries with the format of "what, when, where, with whom?" are easy to construct and use with patients. Patients with a history of multiple diets or weight loss attempts should consider a 3- to 6-week daily food diary before attempting any dietary changes.

Table 12.3 Heart Disease Prevention

Exercise 3–5 times/wk for 20–60 min/day or 200 kcal/day
No smoking
Alcohol <2 oz/day
Waist to hip ratio ≤ .8
BP < 140/90
Glucose ≤ 100
If no heart disease: LDL ≤ 130, TG ≤ 150 mg/dl, T. chol/HDL ratio ≤ 4
If existing disease: LDL ≤100, TG ≤ 100 mg/dl, T. chol/HDL ratio ≤ 3
Homocysteine ≤ 10 mm/liter
Apolipoprotein A ≤ 20 mg/dl
Enteric aspirin 80–325 mg/day if not contraindicated. Increase soluble fiber
Fish 2x/week
5 servings of green, leafy vegetables/day
Vitamins that may prevent or decrease risk of CAD: folate and B complex vitamins, vitamin C, d-isomer of vitamin E (d-alpha tocopherol)

Sources: Hoff, G. L. (1997, May 30). Cardiovascular risk reduction: What really works? *Patient Care*, 47–60.
Summit on Cholesterol & Coronary Disease. (1997). *Proceedings of the 2nd National Conference on Lipids in the Elimination and Prevention of Coronary Artery Disease.*

Nutritional Counseling

After obtaining a 1-day food diary, the physician can review a basic primary care nutritional guideline for cardiovascular health with the patient, instructing the patient to:

1. Reduce foods high in saturated fat, such as butter, suet, spreads, lard, cooking oils, fast foods, and fried foods, and avoid hydrogenated or tropical oils and margarine. Switch to canola or olive oil.

2. Reduce consumption of red meat (beef, pork, lamb, veal, dark turkey, or chicken) and increase intake of skinless chicken, white turkey, fish, and shellfish. Limit meat to 6 oz/day.
3. Reduce whole-fat milk, egg yolks, butter, cheese, ice cream, cottage cheese, and yogurt, and increase intake of skim milk, nonfat yogurt, and low-fat cheeses.
4. Increase intake of fruit and vegetables. Increasingly, health prevention experts are suggesting that we all move toward plant-based diets or vegetarianism. Patients may also want to avoid high-fat fruits and vegetables, such as avocado, olives, and nuts.
5. Increase intake of soluble fibers and complex carbohydrates from foods, such as pastas, potatoes, cereals, beans, rice, whole-grain breads, oats, and bran. Reduce consumption of convenience foods, crackers, potato chips, movie popcorn, cakes, and pies.
6. Use all sweets sparingly.
7. Use nutritional supplements. For the average patient, these may include iron-free multivitamins for men and nonmenstrual women, multivitamins with iron for menstrual women, and multimineral supplements for adults of any age. For adults who wish to pursue heart disease prevention, this may include daily intake of 100 to 500 mg of vitamin C, 400 IU of vitamin E (d-alpha tocopheryl), 1 mg of folic acid (reduces blood homocysteine levels), and 1,000 mg of a calcium supplement. Men 50 years or older should consider taking 81 mg of enteric-coated aspirin, and women should consider hormone replacement therapy.

In addition, the physician can teach a patient to read a food label, provide an estimate of optimal fat grams per day, and estimate caloric intake based on desired weight goal. Table 12.4 shows how to estimate percentage of fat in food, daily caloric needs, and daily fat grams.

Obesity

Obesity is defined by a body mass index (BMI) of 30 or higher, a BMI of 27 with two or more cardiac risk factors, or a body weight 35% above height for weight as defined by the Metropolitan Life Insurance tables. Alone, it adds a small independent risk of CHD, and obesity greater than 20% increases the risk of diabetes. Obesity conveys additional overall risk of CAD because it increases the likelihood of glucose intolerance, diabetes, hypertension, high LDL, and low HDL.

Table 12.4 Worksheet for Estimating Dietary Fat and Caloric Needs

Percent of Calories From Fat

Step 1: Number of fat grams × serving on the label ______ gm

Step 2: Multiply grams × 9 calories = ______ total fat calories

Step 3: Total calories/serving divided by step 2 = ______ % calories fat
Food ≤ 30% good or ≤ 25%/20% optimal

Caloric Needs Estimates

Step 1: Body weight (lb) × 10 ______

Step 2: To maintain/lose ≤ 10 lb, add 500 + step 1 ______

Step 3: To loose 10–25 lb, use step 1 alone ______

Step 4: If patient is ≤ 350 lb, subtract 1,000 from step 1 ______

Total caloric need is ______ calories/day

Fat Grams Estimates/Day

Step 1: Decide on 30%, 25%, or 20% of calories from fat

Step 2: Total caloric need × .30 or .25 or .20 = ______

Step 3: Divide step 2 by 9 (1 gm fat = 9 calories) = ______ fat grams/day

A Roland BMI, converted from kilograms to pounds, can be used to determine if a patient is overweight. A BMI below 20 or above 25 increases the risk of health problems. The BMI can be calculated using the following formula:

BMI = 705 × weight (lb)/height (in.)^2

Alternatively, the Metropolitan Life Insurance tables developed in 1960 can be used.

Obesity can be characterized as overweight or as mild, moderate, severe, or morbid obesity. Visceral obesity, sometimes called android, central, or apple-shaped obesity, is an additional risk for CHD and is also associated with glucose intolerance, hypertension, and lipid disorders. Obesity-induced hyperinsulinemia and insulin resistance probably explain part of these associations. Waist-to-hip circumferences measurement is used to assess a patient for visceral obesity. Healthy ratios are less than .9 in men and .8 in women. An additional measure of body fat percentage can be estimated using calipers for skinfold measurements or by densiometry (underwater weighing), the gold standard of fat distribution measurements.

When taking a history from an obese patient, it is important to obtain a history, which can include:

1. Description of the number/frequency of previous attempts at weight loss/gain.
2. An understanding of the methods used to change the weight. Did the patient decrease fat intake? Increase exercise? Skip meals or fast? Take medications?
3. Determination of weight loss pattern. How long after each attempt was the weight loss maintained? The shorter the time the weight loss was maintained, the worse the prognosis. Stable weight change for 3 to 5 years predicts a good outcome for a new attempt.

WEIGHT COUNSELING. When working with obese patients, it is important to recognize that they often blame themselves for weight loss failures. This self-recrimination is never helpful and is often unjustified, as genetic or metabolic influences account for 40% of individual differences in responses to eating and exercise and 25% to 30% of individual differences in body fat distribution (Meyer & Stunkard, 1993). When setting goals for weight reduction, it is important to emphasize lifestyle change rather than weight loss. Most patients need healthy eating and exercise rather than a weight loss program. Don't assume that obese patients automatically eat poorly or excessively. Physicians should maintain a psychologically neutral attitude toward the etiology of a patient's obesity, as bias against the obese is extremely high in our society and often influences appropriate treatment recommendations.

It is also important to remember that some patients are obese and healthy. Many patients have a genetic inclination to obesity, some have a comorbid binge-eating disorder, and others may have a primarily psychobehavioral etiology to their weight gain. In most cases, obesity is a multifactorial illness.

Advocacy for lifestyle change includes nutritional education and an exercise plan. During this phase, ask the patient to keep a food diary as a self-monitoring intervention. Food diaries focus the patient's attention on (1) attitudes and beliefs about food; (2) environmental cues that trigger poor eating, such as snacking, binge eating, and binge/purge cycles; (3) factors that allow controlled eating and those that derail controlled eating; (4) learning about emotional eating, such as how moods such as anxiety, depression, loneliness, and boredom are often linked to overeating; (5) developing an individualized exercise program with the physician's help.

In general, realistic weight goals can be estimated by ascertaining the lowest weight a patient has had in his or her adult life and adding 10 pounds to this weight. Realistically, this is the lowest achievable weight goal. For many moderately to severely obese patients, the weight loss goal should be modest, because the chance of success in maintaining a specific long-term weight goal is small. Weight loss of 2 to 5 lb/month is reasonable for most patients. In fact, repeated cycles of weight loss and gain have significant health risks. The Harvard Alumni Study (Lee, Hseih, Paffenbarger, & Kampert, 1995) showed that those who frequently gained or lost 11 pounds were at higher risk for death than those who stayed within 2 pounds of the same weight .

Those patients with previous weight loss failures should consider a weight lifestyle change program that includes nutrition and exercise and adds cognitive-behavioral treatment. Some obese patients may benefit from psychotherapy and from consultations for surgical treatments as additional strategies to aid them in lifestyle change.

Currently there are no safe weight-reducing medications available. The fenfluramine-phentermine combination and d-fenfluramine were withdrawn from the market because of reported severe cardiac and pulmonary complications.

EATING DISORDERS. Eating disorders should be suspected in obese patients presenting for any medical care. It is estimated that approximately 30% (Marcus, 1997) of obese patients who attend an obesity clinic have a binge-eating disorder. It is extremely important to screen for this disorder, because nutritional or weight loss interventions in obese patients with an undiagnosed binge-eating disorder are futile endeavors. A physician can elicit a binge-eating disorder by asking the following questions, which were described in *Prime-MD* (Spitzer et al., 1993):

1. Do you often eat, within any 2-hour period, what most people would regard as an unusually large amount of food?
2. When you eat this way, do you often feel you cannot control what or how much you eat?
3. Does this happen as often as twice a week?
4. Has this been occurring for 6 months?

Yes to these four questions confirms the diagnosis.

It is important to address a potential binge-eating disorder first before attempting nutritional or weight counseling. This can best be accomplished by referring the patient to a weight specialist with psychiatric or psychological training.

SEDENTARY LIFESTYLE. Sedentary lifestyle causes 250,000 deaths each year in the United States. The risk of not exercising carries approximately the same cardiovascular risk as hypertension, smoking, and high cholesterol. The National Institutes of Health consensus conference, the U.S. Surgeon General's Office, and the American College of Sports Medicine have found that patients who are sedentary can improve their overall health through moderate exercise (Paffenbarger et al., 1994). Key cardiovascular benefits from exercise include reduction of the risks of premature death, CHD, diabetes, and hypertension; reduction of feelings of depression and anxiety; and enhanced weight control. A moderate level of exercise confers cardiovascular health benefits, improves lipid and glucose profiles, decreases blood pressure, and increases metabolic rate, oxygen consumption, cardiovascular and respiratory efficiency, musculoskeletal strength, and neurological reaction time. It also improves sleep. The Harvard Alumni Health Study (Lee et al.,1995) also revealed that vigorous exercise, above 6 METS (Metabolic Equivalents) of regular conditioning exercise, increases longevity in White men. These results are probably also applicable to women and minorities.

Physicians wanting to plan an exercise program with their patients may want to utilize the Physician-based Assessment and Counseling for Exercise (PACE) Program (CDC, 1987; Long & Wooten, 1992). Alternatively, a physician can do the following:

1. Assess the current level of activity. Is the patient sedentary, or walking and exercising regularly?
2. Obtain a medical history and laboratory testing, with special attention to cardiovascular/pulmonary, musculoskeletal systems, and current medications.
3. Determine the patient's motivation for exercise and educate about health and psychological benefits.
4. In young, healthy patients, some practitioners use the step test to estimate cardiovascular conditioning. For men over 40 and women over 50, or for any patient who has multiple risk factors or CHD, consider formalized stress testing.
5. Set general health goals for exercise.
6. Develop a specific exercise plan that applies the FITT (frequency,

intensity, type of exercise, and time) assessment. Most patients can begin to exercise with a light- to moderate-intensity program. The American College of Sports Medicine and the CDC (Pate, Pratt, Blair, Haskell & Macera, 1995) recommend 20 to 60 minutes of endurance at 60% to 90% of maximum heart rate performed three or more times per week. Exercise heart rate can be determined by:

a. Applying the formula:
   220 – age × 45% to 85 % = target heart range
   Healthy patients can start at 70%, whereas patients with CAD may start as low as 45% in a cardiac rehabilitation unit.
b. Using the Borg Perceived Exertion Scale (Borg, 1982). Patients can rate their own subjective sense of the exercise intensity level on a scale from 0 = nothing at all, to 3 = moderate, 5 = strong, and 10 = maximal exercise.
c. The talk test can also be suggested. Patients should be able to talk while exercising but not able to sing.

7. A step test (Geltman, 1989) for patients with low cardiovascular risk, may be used to assess fitness level (ACSM, 1995). First, obtain the patient's resting heart rate. The patient begins the step test, using a 12-inch-high bench and a stepping rate of 24 steps/min 3 minutes. Heart rate is immediately measured for 1 minute after the test. This heart rate determines a qualitative rating of fitness, which can be correlated with standardized tables (Golding, Myers, & Sinning, 1989).
8. Exercise stress testing, if indicated, will report appropriate exercise levels in METS.

In addition to exercising, stretching should be done three times a week during the warm-up and cool-down periods of aerobic exercise to improve flexibility and reduce injuries. Muscular strength and endurance can be maintained to avoid muscular and skeletal injuries by sessions of free weights, weight machines, or calisthenics two to three times a week. Patients should be educated that they should refrain from exercise under the following conditions: after a meal, after smoking, and after alcohol consumption. During hot, humid weather, the patient should slow down and drink water before, during, and after exercise. If exercising in cold weather at temperatures below 15°F considering the wind chill factor, those exercising should take the special precaution of wearing layers of clothing, wearing hat and gloves, and protecting against dry skin. Advise patients that it is best to exercise 2 to 4 hours after heart medications are taken. Patients should not exercise if ill or with a fever. Exercise injuries should be treated according to the RICE formula—rest, ice, compression, elevation.

Smoking

In the United States, smoking is associated with 20% of all deaths. Approximately 400,000 deaths each year occur from smoking, of which 53,000 are from passive smoke (Bartecchi, MacKenzie, & Schrier, 1994; MacKenzie, Bartecchi, & Schrier, 1994). Smokers not only risk their own health but also increase the health risks of their spouses, children, and coworkers. Approximately 20% of all cases of cardiovascular disease, 85% of lung cancers, and 30% of all cancers have been linked to smoking (Bartecchi et al., 1994; MacKenzie et al., 1994). In addition, smoking is a major factor in the development of chronic lung disease; contributes to gastrointestinal ulcers, gastritis, and reflux; and creates obstetrical complications, including abortion and low birth weight. Secondhand smoke is a major factor in childhood illnesses, especially respiratory conditions, asthma, childhood middle ear infections, and cancers.

The risk of CAD is directly post-myocardial proportional to the amount a person smokes. Lowering the number of cigarettes smoked per day can reduce risk. Smoking cessation in a post-myocardial infarction patient can lower the risk of a second infarction by 50% as well as delay the recurrence of chest pain after the MI.

Smoking cessation is the single most helpful thing a patient and physician can do together, to lower the risk of CAD and to improve a patient's overall health. However, smoking cessation efforts are often frustrating. The average patient will attempt smoking cessation many times before achieving success. It is often helpful to address smoking cessation after a medical event that has an association with smoking. Talking about cessation after pneumonia or an MI can achieve smoking cessation rates as high as 70%. Patients also need to know that the risk of CAD drops quickly over 1 to 2 years after stopping smoking, returning to their baseline CAD risk at 5 years smoke free. The risk of all smoking-related cancers also declines over 10 years.

Efforts at smoking cessation in patients at risk for CAD are often complicated by comorbid psychosocial conditions, such as alcohol and drug abuse, depression, and schizophrenia.

Smoking and Alcohol/Drug Abuse

Fifteen percent to 20% of smokers have current alcohol dependence or abuse, and about 80% of alcohol and drug abusers in treatment are also smokers. About 50% of these patients will attempt smoking cessation (Hughes, 1996). The prevailing clinical wisdom is that smoking cessation, in a drug-abusing patient, should be undertaken simultaneously or immediately after treatment for alcohol and drug abuse. Efforts at smoking cessation during active alcohol or drug use appear to be futile. Patients can decide to quit simultaneously with drug use cessation or after they are drug free (there are no empirical data in this area). About 50% of drug-abusing patients in treatment have no interest in smoking cessation, and they may need to be motivated, through the stages of change, toward cessation.

Smoking and Depression

Approximately 25% to 40% of smokers who seek treatment have a history of major depression or dysthymic symptoms (Hughes, 1996). Quit rates in smokers with a history of depression are exceedingly low. In addition, those patients with a history of bipolar and major depressive disorders commonly will relapse into an episode of depression when smoking cessation is attempted. In one study (Covey, Glassman, & Stetner, 1997), the 3-month incidence of a new, major depression following smoking cessation was 2%, 17%, and 30% in patients with histories of no depression, single depression, and recurrent depression, respectively. This has led to the suggestion that psychotherapy and/or treatment with antidepressants may facilitate smoking cessation in patients with a history of depression.

In clinical trials, nortriptyline, fluoxetine, and bupropion have been shown to increase quit rates compared to no treatment with an antidepressant (Hughes, 1996). When attempting smoking cessation with a depressed patient, it is important to remember that smoking cessation increases blood levels of antidepressants and caffeine, which can produce unwanted side effects from these drugs.

Smoking and Schizophrenia

Smoking cessation in patients with schizophrenia is extremely difficult. Many of these patients are not interested in quitting smoking, and some are comorbid drug users. When attempting cessation with a schizophrenic patient, the physician should be aware that antipsychotic drug levels will increase with cessation and may produce extra pyramidal side effects that can mimic symptoms of nicotine withdrawal.

Smoking Cessation

To facilitate smoking cessation, the physician should assess the patient's readiness to change. Approximately 20% of smokers are ready to quit. The 80% of smokers who have little or no motivation for cessation can be progressed through the stages of change by education and by personalizing the benefits of smoking cessation (Prochaska & DiClemente, 1986). For example, a patient with peripheral vascular disease can be educated that smoking cessation will improve circulation and reduce leg pain. Patients who are most successful at cessation include patients who have quit previously or have a history of prior quit attempts and patients who have progressed from one stage of change to another (e.g., precontemplation to contemplation).

Once a patient is interested in smoking cessation, a physician can facilitate these efforts by assessing the degree of nicotine dependence, stressing motivation and the benefits of cessation, and dealing with patient fears of change (e.g., weight gain, fears of nicotine withdrawal, fears of failure, and fears of developing depression or anxiety). The physician may also utilize nicotine replacement strategies, prescribe bupropion (Zyban) treatment of 150 mg bid for 1 week preceding implementation of the quit date, offering smoking cessation programs, or adding behavioral therapy and psychological treatments (see Table 8, Smoking Cessation Critical Pathway, in chapter 13, A Model for Office-based Cardiovascular Risk Reduction and Behavioral Change).

It is especially important for a physician to recognize a history of depression before having the patient attempt smoking cessation. Smoking cessation can increase the risk of depression, and depression can prevent success in smoking cessation (Covey et al., 1997). It is reasonable to consider pretreatment for depression with antidepressant medications before attempting smoking cessation in patients with a history of prior or recurrent depressions. Bupropion, nortriptyline, and fluoxetine may be logical choices, as these are effective antidepressants that may also foster smoking cessation (Hughes, 1996). The role of other antidepressant medications as an aid to smoking cessation is less clear.

BARRIERS TO LIFESTYLE CHANGE

Facilitating the change of unhealthy behaviors in a patient and fostering self-care and prevention within a health values system are complex, difficult processes. Physicians are often easily frustrated when patients do not make lifestyle changes. Many physicians complain that "patients just don't listen to what we tell them," and they label the patients as "noncompliant."

Noncompliance suggests that patients could comply if they wanted. Rather than being noncompliant, patients may be nonadherent to medical recommendations because of barriers to change. Physicians who understand these barriers can adjust their role with their patients, offering interventions that overcome these barriers and improve patient adherence.

Common patient obstacles to reducing cardiac risk factors include educational barriers, physician barriers, comorbid conditions not diagnosed or treated prior to lifestyle change, timing of lifestyle changes, psychological barriers, social barriers, and systemic barriers.

Educational Barriers

Many patients appear unable or unmotivated to change. For patients to make a lifestyle change, they need to understand exactly what they should change, why they should change, and how they can make the change. Many patients have tried to make lifestyle changes and have failed, because of a lack of proper education or because psychosocial barriers have prevented change.

Providing education about a lifestyle change and helping a patient to overcome a psychosocial barrier are major motivators for most patients to improve their health. Physicians can communicate information about healthy lifestyles in a simple and direct manner and tailor their education to the individual patient. They should avoid technical language and not rely on printed material as the primary educational tool. Explanations that highlight the personal benefits of lifestyle change for a patient are preferable to describing general health benefits. For example, asking a patient to stop smoking because it will reduce the risk of cancer is not as helpful as saying, "If you stop smoking, you will breathe easier, your asthma will improve, and your teeth will get whiter." In addition, physicians can educate patients so that they can progress from one stage of change to another (e.g., moving a patient from contemplation toward preparation for smoking cessation). To make sure that patients have gotten the health message, physicians can ask patients to summarize their understanding of how a lifestyle change can help them and can have patients reflect back on what they can do for their own self-care.

Additional barriers to patient education include language barriers, low literacy, cultural differences, lack of involvement of the patient's family, and lack of available educational material in the patient's primary language.

Physician Barriers

Physician barriers to assisting patients with a lifestyle change arise primarily from the orientation of medical care toward problem solving rather than prevention. Medical education often fails to include training in disease prevention. Physicians may perceive lifestyle changes as ineffective, lack time to provide lifestyle counseling, and even feel that assisting patients with lifestyle changes is not part of their role. Sometimes physicians feel disdain for unhealthy behaviors in patients. Furthermore, many health insurers do not reimburse physicians for time spent on preventive care.

Physicians can overcome some of these barriers by motivating and empowering patients for self-care. The physician can present several treatment options or sequences for change and allow the patient a choice. The more the patient pursues changes in nutrition, exercise, weight reduction, and stress reduction and practices harm reduction from substance abuse, the greater the likelihood that the patient will develop a healthy lifestyle. The physician can also provide hope for a patient to change, acknowledge the long and sometimes painful course of change, and model a nonjudgmental attitude toward the patient's failures, partial efforts, or low motivation for change. A detailed office-based approach for physicians and patients is presented in chapter 13, A Model for Office-based Cardiovascular Risk Reduction and Behavioral Change.

Comorbid Conditions as Barriers to Lifestyle Change

One underrecognized barrier to a patient's lifestyle change is the failure of the physician and/or patient to recognize or intervene in comorbid conditions that prevent such change. The success rate for a healthy lifestyle change may be enhanced if comorbid conditions are treated before attempting a lifestyle change. For example, smoking cessation is likely to fail for those patients who have a history of depression unless depression is also addressed. Weight reduction is very unlikely in a patient who has an undiagnosed and untreated binge-eating disorder. Table 12.5 lists some important comorbid psychosocial factors that influence success rates with lifestyle modification.

Timing for Attempting a Lifestyle Change

It is best to suggest a lifestyle change to a patient during periods of lower life stress. It is often a good idea to suggest that lifestyle changes begin on weekends, during vacations, during periods of decreased stress from work or family concerns, or during the summer or slow months of a seasonal business. Lifestyle changes that begin during a low-stress time need to be integrated into the normal, daily life routine. To do this, flexible routines and practical and attainable schedules need to be developed with each patient.

For some patients, an acute medical crisis offers a new opportunity for the physician to suggest a lifestyle change. For example, smoking cessation occurs at a rate of 70% in the post-MI patient, compared to the 9% cessation rate of the average smoker.

Acute family crises or a traumatic medical event in families can also be used to facilitate a lifestyle change. For example, a patient was finally motivated to make another earnest effort at smoking cessation after the patient's father died of lung cancer and the physician encouraged a new "quit smoking" attempt. Another patient was finally ready to begin to exercise when she learned that her sedentary mother had a bone fracture secondary to osteoporosis. Her physician explained that weight-bearing exercise could help her prevent osteoporosis.

Psychological Barriers

There are many psychological barriers to making a lifestyle change, which can be explored with patients as a way to facilitate change. Some patients will not attempt a lifestyle change because they are afraid they will fail or are afraid about how they will feel about themselves with another failure. Some patients are afraid that failure will bring disapproval from the physician or the patient's family. Other patients are afraid that success in a lifestyle change will reveal other problems. For example, some obese patients fear weight loss, as this means increasing attractiveness and availability for sexual contact. In such a patient, the obesity hides the deeper fear of sex, which is uncovered by the weight loss. Exploration of psychological fears of change can be a great facilitator of change.

Table 12.5 Psychosocial Comorbid Conditions Interfering With Lifestyle Change

Desired lifestyle change	Associated comorbid conditions
Smoking cessation	Depression Alcoholism Caffcinism Schizophrenia Stress Type A/high-hostility profile Anxiety disorders Family member smokes
Nutrition/weight	Binge-eating disorders Mood/anxiety disorders Sexual dysfunction Stress Cultural dietary habits
Exercise	Mood/anxiety disorders Unsafe neighborhoods
Lower blood pressure	Alcoholism Crowded living conditions High-stress occupations

Social Barriers

Social barriers that prevent a lifestyle change include living conditions and economic and cultural factors. Unsafe neighborhoods can make exercise difficult. Crowded living and high-stress jobs can make blood pressure control much more complex. Lack of economic resources can make dietary change and the purchase of needed medications impossible. Cultural attitudes toward smoking and alcohol and culturally diverse dietary practices can be formidable barriers to a successful lifestyle change. Awareness and exploration of these barriers and making culturally sensitive lifestyle recommendations are the best approach to overcoming these barriers.

Systemic Barriers

Systemic barriers to lifestyle change include lack of resources and facilities, lack of a system for preventive services, lack of reimbursement for lifestyle change support, inflexible work schedules that preclude lifestyle change, and institutional inertia that favors acute care medicine over preventive services. These barriers to healthy living are significant impediments that change slowly as new information and research becomes available and as the cost-saving nature of healthy living becomes apparent.

In addition to the traditional risk factors for coronary artery disease, there are less well known psychosocial risk factors. The primary care physician who understands the full range of these risk factors can provide office-based counseling to patients at risk for CAD to reduce their risk, thereby improving their health and reducing the morbidity and mortality associated with these diseases. Intervening for risk reduction necessitates both a physical and a psychosocial approach to patient health, as well as the physician's awareness of the lifestyle changes required to reduce risk and potential barriers to these changes.

REFERENCES

American College of Sports Medicine (1995). *ACSM's guidelines for exercise testing and prescription.* 5th Edition, p. 73. Baltimore, MD: Williams and Wilkins.

Barefoot, J. C., Dahlstrom, W. G., & Williams, R. B. (1983). Hostility, CHD incidence, and total mortality: A 25-year follow-up study of 255 physicians. *Psychosomatic Medicine, 45,* 59–63.

Barefoot, J. C., & Schroll, M. (1996). Symptoms of depression, acute myocardial infarction, and total mortality in a community sample. *Circulation, 93,* 1976–1980.

Barefoot, J. C., Helms, M. J., Mark, D. B., Blumenthal, J. A., Califf, R. M., Haney, T. L., O'Connor, C. M., Siegler, I. C., & Williams, R. B. (1996). Depression and long-term mortality risk in patients with coronary artery disease. *American Journal of Cardiology, 78,* 613–617.

Bartecchi, C. E., MacKenzie, T. D., & Schrier, R. W. (1994). The human costs of tobacco use (Part 1). *New England Journal of Medicine, 330,* 907–912.

Berkman, L. F., & Syme, S. L. (1979). Social networks, host resistance, and mortality: A nine-year follow-up study of Almeda County residents. *American Journal of Epidemiology, 109,* 186–204.

Borg, G. A. (1982). Psychophysical bases of perceived exertion. *Medicine and Science in Sports and Exercise, 14,* 377–381.

Brecht, M. L., Dracup, K., Moser, D. K., & Riege, B. (1994). The relationship of marital quality and psychosocial adjustment to heart disease. *Journal of Cardiology Nursing, 9,* 74–85.

Carney, R. W., Rich, M. W., & Freedland, K. E. (1988). Major depressive disorder predicts cardiac events in patients with coronary artery disease. *Psychosomatic Medicine, 50,* 627–633.

Covey, L. S., Glassman, A. H., & Stetner, M. A. (1997). Major depression following smoking cessation. *American Journal of Psychiatry, 154,* 263–265.

Duke Center for Living. (1995). *How does your diet measure up?* Durham, NC: Duke University Press.

Eliot, R. S. (1994). *From stress to strength: How too lighten your load and save your life.* New York: Bantum.

Eliot, R. S., & Morales-Ballejo, H. M. (1994). The heart, emotional stress, and psychiatric disorders. In R.C. Schlant & R. W. Alexander (Eds.), *The heart, arteries and veins* (8th ed.) (Vol. 2, 2087–2097). New York: McGraw Hill.

Fang, J., Madhavan, S., & Alderman, M. H. (1996). The association between birthplace and mortality from cardiovascular causes among black and white residents of New York City. *New England Journal of Medicine, 335,* 1545–1558.

Follick, M. J., Ahern, D. K., Gorkin, L., Niaura, R. S., Herd, J. A., Ewart, C., Schron, E. B., Kornfeld, D. S., & Capone, R. J. (1990). Relation of psychosocial and stress reactivity variables to ventricular arrhythmias in the cardiac arrhythmia pilot study (CAPS). *American Journal of Cardiology, 66,* 63–67.

Frasure-Smith, N., Lesperance, F., & Talajic, M. (1993). Depression following myocardial infarction. *Journal of the American Medical Association, 270,* 1819–1825.

———. (1994). Depression and 18-month prognosis after myocardial infarction. *Circulation, 91,* 999–1005.

Friedman, H. S. (Ed.) (1992). *Hostility, coping, and health.* Washington, DC: American Psychological Association.

Gettman, L. R. (1989). Fitness testing. In L. Febiger. (Ed.), *Resource manual for guidelines for exercise testing and prescription* (ACSM, p. 73). Philadelphia: American College of Sports Medicine.

Golding, L. A., Myers, C. R., & Sinning, W. E. (Eds.). (1989). *Y's way to physical fitness* (3rd ed.). Champaign, IL: Human Kinetics Publishers.

Goldstein, D. S. (1995). *Stress, catecholamines, and cardiovascular disease.* New York: Oxford University Press.

Goldstein, M. G., & Niaura, R. (1992). Psychological factors affecting physical condition: Cardiovascular disease literature review. *Psychosomatics, 33,* 134–154.

Healthier People Version 4.0 [Computer software]. (1991). Atlanta: Carter Center of Emory University (Health Risk Appraisal Program 1988. Vol 4: Scientific Documentation, July).

House, J. S., Landis, K. R., & Umberson D. (1988). Social relationships and health. *Science, 241,* 540–545.

Hughes, J. R. (1996). Practice guidelines for treatment of patients with nicotine dependence. *American Journal of Psychiatry, 153*(October Suppl.), 263–265.

Jiang, W., Babyak, M., Krantz, D. S., Waugh, R. A., Coleman, R. E., Hanson, M. M., Frid, D. J., McNulty, S., Morris, J. J., O'Connor, C. M., & Blumenthal, J. A. (1996). Mental stress induced myocardial ischemia and cardiac events. *Journal of the American Medical Association, 275,* 1651–1656.

Jonas, B. S., Franks, P., & Ingram, D. (1997). Are symptoms of anxiety and depression risk factors for hypertension? *Archive of Family Medicine, 6,* 43–49.

Kamarck, T., & Jennings, J. R. (1991). Biobehavioral factors in sudden cardiac death. *Psychology Bulletin, 109,* 42–75.

Karasek, R., & Theorell, T. (1990). Healthy work: Stress, productivity, and the reconstruction of the working life. New York: Basic Books.

Kawachi, I., Sparrow, D., Vokonas, P. S., & Weiss, S. T. (1994). Symptoms of anxiety and risk of coronary heart disease. *Circulation, 90,* 2225–2229.

Kawachi, I., Waugh, R. A., Coleman, R. E., Hanson, M. M., Frid, D. J., McNulty, S., Morris, J. J., O'Connor, C. M., & Blumenthal, J. A. (1995). Prospective study of shift work and the risk of coronary artery disease in women. *Circulation, 92,* 3178–3182.

Ketterer, M. W., Lovallo, W. R., & Lumley, M. A. (1993). Quantifying the density of Friedman's pathogenic emotions. *International Journal of Psychosomatics, 40,* 22–28.

Krantz, D. S., & Durel, L. A. (1983). Psychological substrates of Type A behavior pattern. *Health Psychology, 2,* 393–411.

Kubzansky, L. D., Kawachi, I., Spiro, A III, Weiss, S. T., Vokonas, P. S., & Sparrow, D. (1997). Is worrying bad for your heart? A prospective study of worry and coronary artery disease in the normative age study. *Circulation, 95,* 818–824.

Lacy, C. R., Contrada, R. J., Robbins, M. L., Tannenbaum, A. K., & Moreya, A. E. (1994). Coronary vasoconstriction induced by mental stress (simulated public speaking). *American Journal of Cardiology, 75,* 503–505.

Lee, I., Hsieh, C., Paffenbarger, R. S., & Kampert, (1995). Exercise intensity and longevity in men: The Harvard Alumni health study. *Journal of the American Medical Association, 273,* 1179–1184.

Long, B., & Wooten, W. (1992). *Physician-based assessment and counseling for exercise, physician manual.* Atlanta: Centers for Disease Control and Prevention (Cardiovascular Health Branch).

MacKenzie, T. D., Bartecchi, C. E., & Schrier, R. W. (1994). The human costs of tobacco use (Part 2). *New England Journal of Medicine, 330,* 975–980.

Malkoff, S. B., Muldoon, M. F., Zeigler, Z. R., & Manuck, S. B. (1993). Blood platelet responsivity to acute mental stress. *Psychosomatic Medicine, 55,* 477–482.

Marcus, M. D. (1997). Adapting treatment for patients with binge-eating disorder, In D. M. Garner P. E. Garfinkel (Eds.), *Handbook for treatment of eating disorders* (pp. 484–494). New York: Guildford Press.

Meyer, J. M., & Stunkard, A. J. (1993). *Genetics and human obesity* (2nd ed.). New York: Raven Press.

Muller, J. E. Abela, G. S., Nesto, R. W., & Tofler, G. H. (1994). Triggers, acute risk factors and vulnerable plaques: The lexicon of a new frontier. *Journal of the American College of Cardiology, 23,* 809–813.

Ornish, D. (1990). *Reversing heart disease.* New York: Ballantine.

Paffenbarger, R. S., Kampert, J. B., Lee, I., Hyde, R. T., Leung, R. W., & Wing, A. L. (1994). Changes in physical activity and other lifeway patterns influencing longevity. *Medicine and Science in Sports and Exercise, 26*(7), 857–865.

Pate, R. R., Pratt, M., Blair, S. N., Haskell, W. L., & Macera, C. A. (1995). Physical activity and public health: A recommendation from the Centers for Disease Control and Prevention and the American College of Sports Medicine. *Journal of the American Medical Association, 273,* 402–407.

Pratt, L. A., Ford, D. E., Crum, R. M., Armenian, H. K., Gallo, J. J., & Eaton, W. W. (1996). Depression, psychotropic medication, and risk of myocardial infarction. *Circulation, 94,* 3123–3129.

Prochaska, J. O., & DiClemente, C. C. (1986). Toward a comprehensive model of change. In W. R. Miller & N. Heather (Eds.), *Treating addictive behaviors: Processes of change* (pp. 3–27). New York: Plenum Press.

Shekelle, R. B., Hulley, S. B., Neaton, J. D., Billings, J. H., Borhani, N. O., Gerace, T. A., Jacob, D. R., Lasser, N. L., Mittlemark, M. B., & Stamler, J. (1985). The MRFIT behavioral pattern study II: Type A behavior and incidence of coronary artery disease. *American Journal of Epidemiology, 122,* 559–570.

Spiegel, D. (1993). *Living beyond limits.* New York: Fawcett/Columbine, Ballantin.

Spitzer, R. L., Williams, J. B. W., Kroenke, K., Linzer, M., Verloin de Gruy, F. III, Hahn, S. R., & Brody, D. (1993) *Prime M.D.: Primary care evaluation of mental disorders.* New York: New York State Psychiatric Institute.

Summit on Cholesterol and Coronary Disease. (1997). *Proceedings of the 2nd National Conference on Lipids in the Elimination and Prevention of Coronary Artery Disease.* Disney's Yacht & Beach Club Resorts, Lake Buena Vista, Florida. Cleveland, OH: Cleveland Clinic Foundation in cooperation with Disney Institute.

Williams, R., & Williams, V. (1994). *Anger kills: Seventeen strategies for controlling the hostility that can harm your health.* New York: Harper Perennial.

CHAPTER 13

A Model for Office-Based Cardiovascular Risk Reduction and Behavioral Change

Robert E. Feinstein, Peter M. Rabinowitz, Laurel Carey, Joyelle Gallicano, Anne A. Brewer, Abraham Bornstein, Joseph V. Connelly, and Pamela F. LeDeaux

This chapter presents a specific office-based model designed to help the primary care physician facilitate behavioral changes in patients who may need to reduce their risk of cardiovascular disease. It is based on Prevention-Oriented Primary Care, a model developed and implemented at the St. Joseph Medical Center Family Practice Residency Program in Stamford, Connecticut (Rabinowitz et al., 1995–1998). This chapter will discuss the basis of the Prevention-Oriented Primary Care (POPC) model and its application to primary care practice, including the concept of informed shared decision making, a specialized interactional process between patient and physician that integrates prevention and psychosocial care.

OVERVIEW OF PREVENTION ORIENTED PRIMARY CARE (POPC)

Development of the Prevention-Oriented Primary Care model at the St. Joseph Medical Center Family Practice Residency Program (now called The Stamford Hospital Columbia University College of Physicians & Surgeons, Program in Family Practice) originated in an unusual collaboration between Peter Rabinowitz, a family physician and occupational medicine physician with a master's degree in public health, and Robert Feinstein, director of behavioral science at St. Joseph's, who is also a psychiatrist and psychoanalyst. The faculty at our Family Practice Residency Program participated in its development. The authors set out to develop a practical model for office-based care that they call informed shared decision making, which is both prevention oriented and psychosocially sophisticated.

POPC utilizes a host versus environment view point (see chapter 1), which looks at disease as evolving from the interplay between these two forces. The host factor comprises the patient's genetic predisposition, medical conditions, and psychosocial/behavioral makeup, all of which are crucial determinants of a person's immunity or susceptibility to disease. The host is acted upon by the environment, which may include social, biological, physical, chemical, and environmental processes. In this model, disease develops when there is either a weakness in host defenses (such as HIV immunosuppression) or an overpowering deleterious effect from the environment (such as exposure to toxic waste). Informed shared decision making is an integral part of POPC. It is a process and style of working with patients that is geared toward the implementation of prevention-oriented health care. To practice effective preventive care, the doctor and the patient must work collaboratively as equal partners to develop a comprehensive, biopsychosocial view of the patient's health status and realistic possibilities for prevention-oriented care. As the authors developed it, informed shared decision making has eight components: interviewing style; guidelines for physician and patient roles; a prevention-oriented history and a health risk appraisal to develop medical priorities for reduction of risk factors; a patient-health priority list; physician's medical priorities list; a shared priority list for prevention oriented change, which takes into account the chance of success for creating behavioral change; specific intervention plans guided by critical pathways, which include target goals and intervention strategies; and follow-up care with measurable and targeted outcome goals.

Informed Shared Decision Making

Interviewing Style

A recent study (Roter et al., 1997) examined communication styles between patients and physicians and classified them into five approaches: (1) narrowly biomedical (biomedical focus dominated by physician questions and physician information giving), (2) expanded biomedical (same as biomedical but with more patient psychosocial input), (3) biopsychosocial (mixed biomedical and psychosocial talk, lower physician control, and collaborative exchange about patient's health values and preferences with a fostering of patient autonomy and self-reflection), (4) psychosocial (psychosocial focus with patient and physician equally sharing talk; the patient controls talk content, and the physician role is more as therapist or friend), and (5) consumerist (informational focus determined by patient questions with little psychosocial exchange; the physician is the competent expert, and the patient is the consumer).

The Roter et al. study revealed that the predominant physician pattern is still biomedical (66% of visits) and that utilizing a biomedical pattern leads to the physician's having a low level of recognition of the patient's emotional distress. This study also showed that biopsychosocial, psychosocial, and consumerist patterns of communication were no more time consuming than the narrow or expanded biomedical styles. Interestingly, physicians were happiest with the consumerist model, and patients reported the highest satisfaction with the psychosocial pattern.

Because POPC involves a collaborative physician-patient approach, it is heavily tilted toward a mixture of biopsychosocial, psychosocial, and consumerist approaches. Clinically, it appears that these patient-centered approaches are best for modifying risk factors, providing prevention-oriented care, integrating psychosocial issues, and facilitating chances of success for the broadest range of lifestyle and behavioral changes. The POPC patient-centered approach for cardiovascular risk reduction utilizes the informed shared decision-making model.

Physician and Patient Role Within POPC

For POPC to be effective, it is important that both the physician and the patient clearly understand their roles and responsibilities throughout the informed shared decision-making process. In general, the physician and the patient relate with a consumerist role model when sharing information about medical risk, use a psychosocial communication pattern when there are psychosocial problems (such as depression or barriers to lifestyle change), and move to a collaborative biopsychosocial approach when trying to agree on shared prevention plans for a lifestyle change. Table 13.1 describes specific roles and responsibilities for the patient and the physician.

Prevention-oriented History and Health Risk Appraisal

The informed shared decision-making process begins before the first office visit. The patient is given the Prevention-Oriented Primary Care Health History form. This is a prevention-oriented questionnaire, which the patient completes with, or without, the assistance of a member of the office staff. The Prevention-Oriented Primary Care Health History form collects identifying information (age, sex, date of birth, etc.), past medical history, family history, occupational and social history, and prevention history. Within this primary data source is information that is also used as part of a health risk appraisal (HRA).

Ideally, an HRA should be a low-literacy screening instrument, easily completed within 20 minutes, that screens for many of the preventable diseases dealt with in the U.S. Preventive Services Task Force (1996) recommendations. The HRA instrument can provide an overview of the patient's health status and state of wellness, reflect prevention and biopsychosocially oriented primary care, and provide some information about the magnitude and priority of medical risk factors. An HRA should summarize risk factors and assist the physician in setting priorities for the reduction of cardiovascular risk factors.

The optimal use of a prevention-oriented history and HRA is to improve medical data gathering *before* the clinical interview. Accumulating baseline health data streamlines the physician-patient encounter and makes it a more efficient and personalized prevention session that stresses preventive health care as well as intervention with health problems.

There are many HRA instruments available for office use, including the ERIS Clinical Risk Factor Review (ERIS), the Sanford Smart Wellness Questionnaire (ERIS), and the Alaskan Health Risk Appraisal (ERIS). The authors developed their HRA as a component of the Prevention-Oriented Primary Care Health History form.

The ERIS Survey System/St. Joseph Medical Center HRA is a computer-based component of the POPC model for reducing modifiable cardiovascular risk factors in an office practice setting. It measures risk

Table 13.1 Informed Shared Decision-Making Roles

Physician's Role	Patient's Role
Gathering a prevention-oriented history	Providing a detailed biopsychosocial medical history, including: a. describing major health concern, with special emphasis on health problems that are the most troubling b. communicating fears/anxiety related to current or prior medical care
Performing a physical exam, ordering relevant prevention-oriented diagnostic/laboratory testing	
Utilizing evidence-based medicine and/or health risk appraisals to develop with the patient the most important medical priorities for risk factor reduction	Trying to establish a priority list for which health concern should be handled first, second, etc.
Listening to the patient's concerns and health priorities Negotiating with the patient a mutually agreed upon shared priority list for making health changes	Listening to physician's information about medical priorities for health risk Negotiating with the physician a mutually agreed upon shared priority list for making health changes
Educating and informing the patient about the problems and necessary self-care and or monitoring	Asking the physician questions about medical information, treatment plans, side effects of treatments, and self-care options
Mutually developing a prevention plan with a goal, strategies to reach the goal, and an expected time line for accomplishing the goal	Developing with the physician a mutually agreed upon prevention plan and agreed upon time lines
Inquiring about barriers to change	Discussing all issues that are interfering with adherence to the agreed upon prevention plan
Arranging for follow-up with outcome measurements	Following up with scheduled appointments and self-monitoring diaries

factors that are not easily quantifiable (such as dietary fat and fiber); 12 quantifiable, nonmodifiable risk factors (e.g., sex, age, height, and car miles traveled per year, etc.); and 12 quantifiable, modifiable risk factors (e.g., alcohol consumption, HDL, total cholesterol, and blood pressure, etc.). This computer software program uses mortality data to estimate the 10-year future risk of cardiovascular disease and how mortality can be modified by medical risk factor interventions. The physician obtains the 10-year future risk estimate by inputting some basic laboratory information, such as HDL, total cholesterol, and blood pressure. The program then calculates risk. The data source for the ERIS Survey System program uses algorithms and equations that are based on the Framingham studies (Anderson, Castelli, & Levy, 1987; Castelli, Garrison, & Wilson, 1986), the Carter Center studies (Healthier People Version 4.0, 1991), and the recommendations of the U.S. Centers for Disease Control (1987).

The data from the POPC Health History form and the HRA, combined with a physical examination and relevant laboratory/diagnostic testing, are the primary information sources that the physician uses in discussing with the patient a medical priorities list for cardiovascular risk reduction.

Medical Priorities for Cardiovascular Risk Factor Reduction

The ERIS/St. Joseph computer program generates the relative risk data in the form of two reports, which can be added to the patient's chart: the Health Risk Summary of Positive Findings for the physicians and the Clinical Risk Factor Review Personal Report for the patient.

HEALTH RISK SUMMARY OF POSITIVE FINDINGS. The Health Risk Summary of Positive Findings yields the following information about the patient: 12 quantified, modifiable risks; prevention needs, environmental and occupational stressors; and summaries of positive findings in the medical history, drug history, and sexually transmitted disease history. It also lists all current medication, hospitalizations, allergies, and positive family history.

The 12 quantifiable and modifiable risk factors in the HRA are smoking, alcohol consumption, mammograms, Pap smears, blood pressure, total cholesterol, HDL, weight, seat belt use, speeding, smokeless tobacco use, and exercise. Wellness points with a maximal aggregate total of 100 are given for each of these 12 risks according to the magnitude of the risk and the general principle that the lower the risk or the better the health habits for each factor, the greater the wellness points. A score of 100 wellness points equals minimal risk on these 12 measures and no required lifestyle changes, whereas a score of 0 wellness points means risk on all 12 factors and the need to change every risk factor. The ERIS/St. Joseph computer program generates for the physician the Medical Priority List for Cardiovascular Risk Factor Reduction, a component of the program, which is based on 10-year mortality rates from Framingham, Carter Center, and Centers for Disease Control and Prevention (CDC) data sources.

To facilitate patient understanding of the Medical Priority List for Cardiovascular Risk Factor Reduction, the patient receives a report generated by the ERIS/St. Joseph program, the Clinical Risk Factor Review Personal Report.

Clinical Risk Factor Review Personal Report

This report is worded in clear, concise language and gives the patient a wellness score from 100 to 0. It also describes the patient's risk of heart attack, stroke, lung cancer, emphysema, bronchitis, and colon cancer and suggests specific lifestyle changes that would lower risk. For example, to reduce the risk of heart attack, the patient is told not to smoke, to reduce his or her blood pressure, and to exercise. In addition it reviews the patient's health measurements (e.g., the patient's blood pressure, total cholesterol, and HDL) and good habits, makes recommendations to improve the patient's health, and suggests preventive services (e.g., cholesterol testing every 5 years and blood pressure check every 2 years).

Based on the information from these two reports, the physician and the patient can begin the process of discussing the patient's medical priority list for risk factor reduction. The physician explains the risks of high blood pressure, smoking, and low HDL. This is also an opportunity for the patient to ask questions about his or her cardiovascular risk information. Table 13.2 gives an example of a medical priority list generated for a sample patient.

Patient Priority Risk Factors for CVD Risk Reduction

After discussing the medical priorities for risk reduction, it is vital that the physician hears and discusses in detail the patient's major health concerns. It is interesting that there is often a dramatic difference between the patient's assessment of his or her health needs and the physician's assessment. There are various reasons for these differences:

1. The patient's priorities are often based on immediate medical or psychosocial needs that do not focus on long-term risk. For example, a patient may be more concerned about healthy eating (a long-term goal) than blood pressure control (an acute medical goal) because he or she cannot emotionally experience the risk of high blood pressure.
2. The patient may lack sufficient medical information to make a truly informed priority list. For example, a patient may feel that dieting for weight reduction is more important than exercise, whereas medically it is the opposite.
3. Psychosocial variables, of which the physician is not aware, may affect choice. For example, a patient may choose not to lower his or her blood pressure as a first priority, because he or she cannot afford the medication, or the patient may not be able to stop smoking because of a prior history of recurrent depression. Thus the dialogue between the patient and the physician results in two different lists—the medical priority list and the patient's medical priority list. See Table 13.2 for an example of patient health priorities generated with a sample patient.

Shared Priority List for Cardiovascular Risk Reduction

Once the medical and patient priority lists are established, the physician and the patient (usually through a biopsychosocial interviewing style) will collaborate and negotiate to arrive at a shared priority list for cardiovascular risk factor reduction. This shared priority list develops out of the medical priority list, patient priority list, published success rates for change, the patient's stage of change, and the patient's previous history of making desired changes.

In planning a prevention intervention that will be maximally effective, it is important to be aware that there are some cardiovascular risk factors that are easy to change and other risk factors that are more difficult. To guide this process of assessment, the authors use a chance-of-success estimate. The chance of success in modifying a cardiovascular risk factor is a way to estimate with a patient the likelihood that lifestyle change can occur. Chance of success is based on published success rates in creating change (Rabinowitz et al., 1995–1998), the patient's stage of behavioral change assessed using the Prochaska and DiClemente (1986) model, and the patient's past history of success with lifestyle modification.

Published Success Rates for Modifying Cardiovascular Risk Factors. A review of the literature reveals that there are some published success rates for modifying some individual cardiovascular risk factors across a general population. These figures are not necessarily applicable to a specific patient with multiple risk factors or to patients in whom multiple medical conditions may interact with each other. Some published success rates for the chance of modifying a cardiovascular risk factor are cholesterol, 50%; hypertension, 70%; depression, 70%; sedentary lifestyle, 35%; smoking cessation, 9%; HDL, 8%; and weight loss, 5% (Rabinowitz et al., 1995–1998).

Perhaps the concept of published success rates may be more important to the process of behavioral change than the specific accuracy of these numbers for a particular patient. Success rates are intended to remind both the physician and the patient that some cardiovascular risk factors are easier to change than others. Instead of using percentages of chances of success, the authors used a 5-point relative scale. For example, hypertension and depression = 5, cholesterol = 4, exercise = 3, smoking and HDL = 2, and weight loss = 1. Published success rates and the 5-point relative scale for a sample patient are illustrated in Table 13.2.

Patient's Stages of Behavioral Change. When thinking about an intervention for a modifiable cardiovascular risk factor, it is important to assess the patient's interest and motivation for change. The stages of change (Prochaska & DiClemente, 1986) are precontemplation, contemplation, preparation, action, maintenance, and relapse prevention. These stages are reviewed in chapter 19. Using this model, the actual stage of change is important in predicting the likelihood that the patient can make the necessary lifestyle change. The authors' approach has been to rate the patient's stage of change for each cardiovascular risk factor from 1 to 5. Patients who are in precontemplation stage = 1 have the least motivation for change, whereas patients in contemplation stage = 2, preparation stage = 3, action stage = 4, or maintenance stage = 5 phase are more likely to change or sustain change. See Table 13.2 for the rating for stage of change on a sample patient for different cardiovascular risk factors.

Previous History of Change. Often, the best predictor of future success in making a lifestyle change is past history. Those patients who in the past have been able to make lifestyle changes are more likely to be able to do it again (Orleans, 1993). The longer the period in the past that change has

Table 13.2 Calculating Shared Priority List*

Medical priority list	Patient's priority list	Published success rate[a] +	Stage of change[b] +	Prior change attempt[c] =	Chance of success[d]	Shared priority list
1. Smoking	1. Weight	5% (1)	Contemplation (2)	(3)	(6)	1. Cholesterol (11)
2. Cholesterol	2. Cholesterol	50% (4)	Preparation (3)	(4)	(11)	2. Exercise (10)
3. Hypertension	3. Exercise	35% (3)	Preparation (3)	(4)	(10)	3.Hypertension (9)
4. Exercise	4. Hypertension	70% (5)	Contemplation (2)	(2)	(9)	4. Weight (6)
5. Weight	5.Smoking	9% (2)	Precontemplation (1)	(2)	(5)	5. Smoking (5)

* Note: See pp. 338–342 for explanation of numerals and values assigned to each factor.

[a] Published success rates are given relative weights as follows:
weight 5% = 1; smoking 9% = 2; exercise 35% = 3; cholestrol 50% = 4; and hypertension 70% = 5.

[b] The stage of change is given relative weight as follows:
precontemplation = 1; contemplation = 2; preparation = 3; action =4; and maintenance =5.

[c] The prior change attempt is given relative weight as follows:
never changed behavior in the past = 1; changed but relapsed within 1 month = 2; changed but relapsed within 6 months = 3; changed but relapsed within 1 year = 4; and changed but relapsed after more than 1 year = 5.

[d] Chance of success with relative weights = published success + stage of change + prior change attempts.

been sustained, the greater the likelihood that change may occur in the future. The authors' rating scale is as follows: never changed behavior in the past = 1; changed but relapsed within 1 month = 2; changed but relapsed within 6 months = 3; changed but relapsed within 1 year = 4; and changed but relapsed after more than 1 year = 5.

For research purposes only, the authors have attempted to add relative weights for the published success rate, the patient's stage of change, and past history of change to arrive at a single number (listed in the shared priority list) that is a rough estimate of the chance of success (Rabinowitz et al., 1995–1998) for each cardiovascular risk factor. The lowest possible research score is 3, and the highest possible score is 15. For example, if we are looking at a sample patient, as illustrated in Table 13.2, smoking cessation has a published success rate of 9% scored with a relative weight of 2, the patient is in precontemplation stage, scored with a relative weight of 1, and, because he has quit in the past and failed within 1 month, he rates a relative weight of 2 for a prior change attempt. This gives this patient a relative weight research estimate of the chance of success for smoking cessation of 2 + 1 + 2 = 5.

The sample data used, as taken from Table 13.2, show a patient with the medical priority of risk factors listed as follows: (1) smoking, (2) cholesterol, (3) hypertension , (4) exercise, (5) weight. From the patient side (for research purposes), the chance of success in altering the patient's behavior can be estimated by the published difficulty in making a change combined with the patient's motivational stage of change and prior history of successful attempts at change. For example, the patient in Table 13.2 is in the preparation stage to change cholesterol (3), while the published success rate for modifying cholesterol is 50% (4), and he has changed his diet before, for 7 months (4). Therefore, the patient's chances of success for modifying cholesterol levels through lifestyle and/or medications has a relative weight of 3 + 4 + 4 =11. This explains why cholesterol is listed as the number one priority on the shared priority list in Table 13.2. Exercise, which has a research-based chance-of-success estimate of 10 for this sample patient, is therefore the second-highest priority for change. On the other end of the spectrum, the patient has the lowest chance of success at smoking cessation. This is because published rates of quitting are low, estimated at 9% = 2; the patient has a low motivation to stop (e.g., precontemplation = 1); and he has tried to quit before but has relapsed in less than 1 month =2, for a total research estimate of a chance of success of 2 + 1 + 2 = 5. For this reason, smoking is last on the shared priority list.

The other variables of hypertension and weight have shared priorities of 3 and 4, respectively, with corresponding relative weight chance-of-success estimates of 9 and 6, respectively.

Clinically, the physician (either for himself or herself and/or with the patient) can use a pictorial representation of the shared priority list, which can be illustrated as medical risk versus chance of success at modifying cardiovascular risk factors. This process is illustrated in Figure 13.1, Medical Risk Versus Chance of Success. In this figure, the X axis represents the medical risk and the Y axis, the chance of success. Using this paradigm and our sample patient in Table 13.2, we arrive at the illustration in Figure 13.1. The highest medical risk factor with the highest chance of success will be in the "high medical risk/high chance of success" quadrant (locate cholesterol in Figure 13.1). The highest medical risk factor and the lowest chance of success are plotted in the "high medical risk/low chance of success" quadrant (locate smoking in Figure 13.1). In between ratings

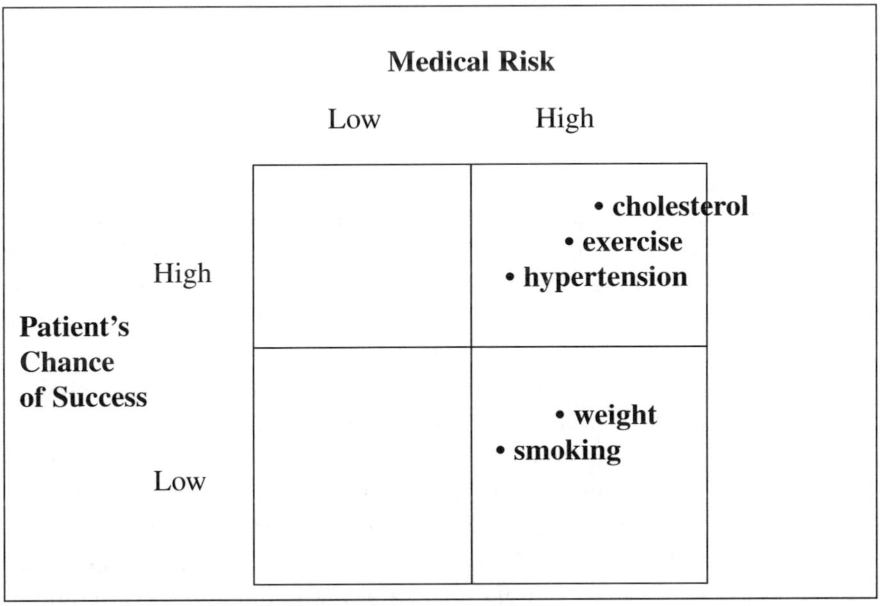

Source: Rabinowitz, P. M., Feinstein, R. E., Carey, L., Gallicano, J., Brewer, A. A., Connelly, J. V., & LeDeaux, P. (1995–1998). Prevention oriented primary care (Advance Grant Section of the Bureau of Health Professionals, U.S. Department of Health and Human Services. Federal Residency Training Grant #5D15PE10297-02 Educational and Prevention Program in Cardiovascular Disease Risk Reduction).

Figure 13.1 Medical Risk versus Chance of Success.

are also plotted and illustrated in Figure 13.1. These plotted variables correspond to the shared medical priority list in Table 13.2.

This process of assessing risk and chance of success combined with a patient-centered interviewing style decides the shared priorities for cardiovascular risk reduction (see the shared priority list illustrated in the last column of Table 13.2). This list represents a summary of all the available clinical information that assisted both the patient and the physician in establishing the priority of risk factors in order to achieve the greatest likelihood of successful behavioral change. The table summarizes the medical priority list, the patient's needs and priorities (patient priority list), the published/graded success rates of change, the patient's stage of change, and the prior history of successful change. The shared decision-making process summarized by the shared priority list guides the intervention sequence.

Intervention Plans

The intervention plan begins with the highest priority for risk factor reduction and is geared toward developing a specific target goal(s), describing the strategy used to obtain the goal/and or a critical pathway, and a timeline for review and modification of priorities. An example of a comprehensive intervention plan for the patient in Table 13.2 is illustrated in Table 13.3.

TARGET GOALS. Target goals for changes in individual modifiable cardiovascular risk factors are clinically established according to cardiovascular risk reduction recommendations from the fifth report of the Joint National Committee on Detection, Evaluation, and Treatment of High Blood Pressure (JNC-V) (1993), the National Cholesterol Education Program (Grudny, 1993), the American College of Sports Medicine (Paffenbarger et al., 1994), the *Physician-based Assessment and Counseling for Exercise Physician* manual (Long & Wootn, 1992), the Centers for Disease Control and Prevention (Pate et al., 1995), the Stop Smoking Program recommended by the American Academy of Family Physicians (1987), *Clearing the Air* (National Cancer Institute, 1995), and other peer-reviewed literature sources. The patient's target goals are often clinically adjusted up or down and are based on the presence of CHD or CAD risk. Target goals need to be both realistic and based on the patient's past history of attempts and successes. The best target goals are achievable within the time frames desired. In general, most patients increase their success at change when they work on only one or two priorities at a time.

Table 13.3 Intervention Plan

Shared priority	Target goal	Strategies	Timeline
1. Decrease cholesterol, LDL, ratio T chol/HDL	≤ 200 ≤ 130 ≤ 4	1. Food diary 2. Record daily saturated fat gram 3. Lovastain 20 mg od	6 months
2. Exercise	Walking 3x/week for 20 minutes, mild intensity	Exercise stress test required. If (–) 1. Begin walking 2. Use Borg Perceived Exertion scale 3. Weekly records of exercise progress	1 month
3. Hypertension	140/90 mm Hg	1. Decrease alcohol consumption 2. Restrict salt 3. Exercise	3 months
4. Depression	Reduce Beck score from 30 to ≤ 20	1. Counseling referral 2. Fluoxetine 20 mg od	3 to 6 weeks
5. Weight	Reduce 2 lb/month 24 lb/year	1. Reduce fats (see #1 priority) 2. Exercise (see #2 priority) 3. Food and mood diary	1 month: 2 lb 1 year: 24 lb

INTERVENTION STRATEGIES. There are many different approaches to choosing the best strategies for reducing a specific risk factor. One approach is to develop a yearlong series of critical pathways utilizing a biopsychosocial prevention plan for specific cardiovascular risk problems. Critical pathways for hypertension, hypercholesterolemia, weight, exercise, and smoking have been developed (see Tables 13.4, 13.5, 13.6, 13.7, and 13.8 respectively). Other critical pathways may be needed for other problems, such as diabetes.

The ideal critical pathways suggest specific office-based interventions at the initial evaluation, a follow-up visit within 2 to 6 weeks, and all subsequent necessary office visits that take place over an entire year. Development of a critical pathway should consider the following:

- A list and method of handling common emergencies (e.g., protocols for the management of hypertensive crises, severely abnormal lipid profiles, or suicidal ideation in a depressed patient with CHD risk)

Table 13.4 Critical Pathway: Hypertension

Quality Outcome: Patient will attain a normal blood pressure, (i.e., under 140/90)

	Visit 1		**Visit 2**	**Visit 3**	**Visit 4**	**Visit 5**	**Visit 6**
	Initial Visit	**Prevention case conference**	**Shared decisions**	**Routine office visit**	**Routine office visit**	**Routine office visit**	**Routine office visit**
Time of visits	30–45 minutes		30 minutes	15 minutes	15 minutes	15 minutes	15 minutes
Timing	Week 1	Week 1	Week 2	Week 3	Week 5	Week 12 response?	1 year
Assessment tools	HRA ERIS/ St. Joseph		Beck scale[a] Hamilton scale[b] Holmes scale[c] GAF[d] PRN	Assess adherence and barriers to change	Assess adherence and barriers to change	Assess adherence and barriers to change	HRA
Lab/ diagnostic test	CBC, UA Chem-7, EKG Lipid profile						CBC, UA Chem-7, EKG Lipid profile
Provider assessments	History and physical Family history	Medical risk priority analysis	Check BP response to treatment	Check BP response to treatment	Check BP response to treatment	Check BP response to treatment	Check BP response to treatment
Primary provider counseling	Discuss patient priorities Diet, exercise, no alcohol		Discuss HRA, chance of success, shared priorities				Discuss new shared priorities

	Visit 1		**Visit 2**	**Visit 3**	**Visit 4**	**Visit 5**	**Visit 6**
	Initial Visit	**Prevention case conference**	**Shared decisions**	**Routine office visit**	**Routine office visit**	**Routine office visit**	**Routine office visit**
Educational materials	Patient education packet on hypertension		Education packet on diet, tobacco, exercise, alcohol				
Other counseling			Stress management, if indicated	Stress management, if indicated	Stress management, if indicated	Stress management, if indicated	Stress management, if indicated
Consultation		Cardiology PRN	Nutrition Exercise			Cardiology PRN	
Medications	Begin medications, if indicated		Adjust dose if indicated	Adjust dose or change/ add	Adjust dose or change/ add	Adjust dose or change/ add	Adjust dose or change/ add

Developed by P. LeDeaux, P. Rabinowitz, A. Brewer, J. Gallicano, R. E. Feinstein, L. Carey, J. Connelly, A. Bornstein (1997).

[a] Beck, A. T. (1978). *Beck depression inventory*. San Antonio, TX: Harcourt Brace.

[b] Hamilton, M. A. (1960). Hamilton Rating Scale for Depression: Physician assessment scale of the patient. *Journal of Neurology and Neurosurgical Psychiatry 23*, 62.

[c] Holmes, T. H., & Raphe, R. H. (1967). Stress scale: Social readjustment scale. *Journal of Psychosomatic Research, 2*, 213.

[d] GAF (Global Assessment of Functioning). American Psychiatric Association. (1994). *Diagnostic and statistical manual of mental disorders* (4th ed., p. 200). Washington, DC: Author.

Table 13.5 Critical Pathway: Hypercholesterolemia Intervention

Quality outcomes: 1. Patient will decrease LDL, increase HDL, decrease total cholesterol 2. Patient will maintain medication adherence and treatment regimen. 3. Patient will demonstrate knowledge in determining low-fat food choices. ("How does your diet measure up?" worksheet)[a]

	Visit 1		Visit 2	Visit 3	Visit 4	Visit 5	Visit 6
	Initial visit	**Prevention case conference**	**Shared decisions**	**Routine office visit**	**Routine office visit**	**Routine office visit**	**Routine office visit**
Time of visits	30–45 minutes		30 minutes	15 minutes	15 minutes	15 minutes	30 minutes
Timing	Week 1	Week 1	Week 2	Week 8	Month 6	Month 9	1 year
Assessment tools	Health risk appraisal (HRA) ERIS/ St. Joseph[b]		1-day food diary eating disorder screen PRN, Beck scale,[c] Hamilton scale,[d] Holmes scale,[e] GAF[f]	2-day food diary assess adherence and barriers to change	Food diaries assess adherence and barriers to change	Food diaries assess adherence and barriers to change	HRA
Lab/ diagnostic test	Fasting lipid profile, Chem-7, EKG (PRN), TFTs, Stress test				Fasting lipid profile	Fasting lipid profile, if indicated	Fasting lipid profile
Provider assessments	History and physical family history	Medical risk priority analysis	Discuss HRA, chance of success, shared priorities				History and physical, family history

	Visit 1		Visit 2	Visit 3	Visit 4	Visit 5	Visit 6
	Initial visit	**Prevention case conference**	**Shared decisions**	**Routine office visit**	**Routine office visit**	**Routine office visit**	**Routine office visit**
Primary provider counseling	Discuss patient priorities		Explain diet and risk factor reduction	Step 1 diet reviewed			
Educational materials	Patient education packet on lowering fat		Cholesterol packet Step 1 diet				
Other counseling			If indicated, assess eating disorder, depression				
Consultation		Cardiology PRN	If indicated, nutrition, exercise	If indicated, nutrition, exercise		Cardiology PRN	Cardiology PRN
Medications					Begin medications	Medications modified?	Medications modified?

Developed by A. Brewer, P. LeDeaux, J. Gallicano, L. Carey, P. Rabinowitz, R. E. Feinstein, J. Connelly, & A. Bornstein (1997).

[a] Duke Center for Living. (1995). *How does your diet measure up?* Durham, NC: Duke University Press.

[b] ERIS Survey System/St. Joseph Medical Center Family Practice Residency Program Health Risk Appraisal. 6363 Hollister Drive Indianapolis, IN 46224.

[c] Beck, A. T. (1978). *Beck depression inventory*. San Antonio, TX: Harcourt Brace.

[d] Hamilton, M. A. (1960). Hamilton Rating Scale for Depression: Physician assessment scale of the patient. *Journal of Neurology and Neurosurgical Psychiatry 23*, 62.

[e] Holmes, T. H., & Raphe, R. H. (1967). Stress scale: Social readjustment scale. *Journal of Psychosomatic Research, 2*, 213.

[f] GAF (Global Assessment of Functioning). American Psychiatric Association. (1994). Diagnostic and statistical manual of mental disorders (4th ed., p. 200). Washington, DC: Author.

Table 13.6 Critical Pathway: Weight Loss Intervention

Quality outcomes: 1. Patient will understand the health risks associated with obesity. 2. Patient will understand the basic food group, calories, and fat content. 3. Patient will understand the relationship between calorie intake and energy expenditure (exercise). 4. Patient will attempt to lose 1/2 to 1 lb/week to reach the target weight 5. Patient will receive instructions and appropriate food and exercise recommendations for maintaining weight loss.

	Visit 1		Visit 2	Visit 3	Visit 4	Visit 5	Visit 6
	Initial Visit	**Prevention case conference**	**Shared decisions**	**Routine office visit**	**Routine office visit**	**Routine office visit**	**Routine office visit**
Time of Visits	30–45 minutes		30 minutes	15 minutes	15 minutes	15 minutes	30 minutes
Timing	Week 1	Week 1	Week 2	Week 4	Week 8	Week 12	1 year
Assessment tools	Health Risk Appraisal (HRA) BMI, % assessed overweight, Food diary/ fat intake		1-week food diary Eating disorder screen, Beck scale,[a] Hamilton scale,[b] Holmes scale,[c] GAF[d] PRN	1-week food diary, assess adherence, and barriers to change	Food diary assess adherence, and barriers to change	Food diary, assess adherence, and barriers to change	Health risk appraisal (HRA) BMI, % overweight, food diary, fat intake
Lab/ diagnostic test profile,	Chem-20, lipid TFTs, stress test PRN		Weight	Weight	Weight	Weight	Weight CBC, UA Chem-7, lipid profile, EKG, etc.
Provider assessments	History and physical family history	Medical risk priority analysis	HRA, chance of success, shared priorities, diet readiness, exercise	Weight change	Weight change	Weight change	History and physical family history

	Visit 1		**Visit 2**	**Visit 3**	**Visit 4**	**Visit 5**	**Visit 6**
	Initial Visit	**Prevention case conference**	**Shared decisions**	**Routine office visit**	**Routine office visit**	**Routine office visit**	**Routine office visit**
Primary provider counseling	Discuss patient priorities/ weight health risks		Review: diary, diet, exercise, set weight goal	Diet and exercise counseling	Diet and exercise counseling	Diet and exercise counseling	Diet and exercise counseling
Educational materials	Weight and exercise handouts	Review weight and exercise handouts	Review weight exercise handouts				
Other counseling			Nutrition or psychiatric				
Consultation			Cardiology PRN Psychiatric PRN Nutrition, exercise			Cardiology PRN	Cardiology PRN
Medications			If indicated	If indicated	If indicated	If indicated	If indicated

Developed by L. Carey, P. LeDeaux, R. E. Feinstein, A. Brewer, J. Gallicano, P. Rabinowitz, J. Connelly, & A. Bornstein (1997).

[a] Beck, A. T. (1978). *Beck depression inventory*. San Antonio, TX: Harcourt Brace.

[b] Hamilton, M. A. (1960). Hamilton Rating Scale for Depression: Physician assessment scale of the patient. *Journal of Neurology and Neurosurgical Psychiatry 23*, 62.

[c] Holmes, T. H., & Raphe, R. H. (1967). Stress scale: Social readjustment scale. *Journal of Psychosomatic Research, 2*, 213.

[d] GAF (Global Assessment of Functioning). American Psychiatric Association. (1994). Diagnostic and statistical manual of mental disorders, (4th ed., p. 200). Washington, DC: Author.

Table 13.7 Critical Pathway: Exercise Intervention

Quality outcomes: 1. Patient will achieve and maintain a level of exercise that will improve health 2. Patient will improve health status, overall health risk, and or depression/anxiety scores. 3. Patient will decrease BMI (body mass index) and improve step test function.

	Visit 1		Visit 2	Visit 3	Visit 4	Visit 5	Visit 6	Visit 7	Visit 8
	Initial visit	**Family practice prevention case conference**	**Informed shared decision making**	**Routine office visit**	**Routine office visit**	**Routine office visit or telephone call**	**Routine office visit**	**Routine office visit**	**Routine office visit**
Time of visits	45 minutes		20 minutes	15 minutes	15 minutes	15 minutes	15 minutes	15 minutes	30 minutes
Timing	Week 1	Week 1	Week 2	Week 3	Week 7	Week 12	Week 16	Week 24	1 year
Assessment tools	Health risk appraisal (HRA), weight, BMI, physical exam		PAr-Q,* PACE* form, step or stress test	Assess adherence and barriers to change	Assess adherence and barriers to change	Assess adherence and barriers to change	Assess adherence and barriers to change	Physical exam weight, BMI step test	HRA, Physical, BMI, weight, step test
Lab/ diagnostic	Lipid profile, Chem-7, EKG	Stress test PRN	Step test PRN						Step or stress Test
Provider assessments	History and physical, family history	Medical risk priority analysis	HRA, chance of success, shared priorities, stress/step test results	Exercise diary, FITT*, physical PRN	Exercise diary, FITT*, physical PRN	Exercise diary, FITT*, physical PRN	Exercise diary, FITT*, physical PRN	Exercise diary, FITT*, physical PRN	Exercise diary, FITT*, physical PRN

	Visit 1		Visit 2	Visit 3	Visit 4	Visit 5	Visit 6	Visit 7	Visit 8
	Initial visit	**Family practice prevention case conference**	**Informed shared decision making**	**Routine office visit**	**Routine office visit**	**Routine office visit or telephone call**	**Routine office visit**	**Routine office visit**	**Routine office visit**
Primary provider counseling	Discuss patient priorities/ sedentary health risks		PACE* Counseling	Exercise Rx PACE* Counseling	PACE* Counseling	PACE* Counseling	Review exercise Rx and change	Review exercise Rx and change	Review exercise Rx and change
Educational materials			FITT* exercise contract, benefits, diary, footwear	Patient education materials, target heart rate, personal exertion, warmup and cool down	Overcoming barriers, and keeping PACE*	Overcoming barriers, and keeping PACE*	Overcoming barriers, and keeping PACE*	Overcoming barriers, and keeping PACE*	Keeping PACE and plan next year's exercise intervention
Other counseling					Nutrition counseling PRN				
Consultation	Cardiology PRN							Cardiology PRN	Cardiology PRN

Developed by J. Gallicano, P. Rabinowitz, R. E. Feinstein, A. Brewer, J. Connelly, L. Carey, A. Bornstein, & P. LeDeaux (1997).

* Long, B. & Wooten, W. (1992). *Physician-based assessment and counseling for exercise, physician manual*. Atlanta: Centers for Disease Control and Prevention (Cardiovascular Health Branch).

Table 13.8 Critical Pathway: Smoking Cessation "Action" Intervention

Quality outcomes: 1. Patient will understand the health risks associated with smoking and the benefits of quitting. 2. Patient will understand his or her personal motivation to stop smoking and learn techniques to help with the urge to smoke. 3. Patient will understand the role of exercise in smoking cessation and learn about the temporary physical withdrawal symptoms that may accompany cessation.

	Visit 1		**Visit 2**	**Visit 3**	**Visit 4**	**Visit 5**	**Visit 6**
	Initial visit	**Prevention case conference**	**Shared decisions**	**Routine office visit**	**Routine office visit**	**Routine office visit**	**Routine office visit**
Time of visits	30 minutes		30 minutes	30 minutes	15 minutes	15 minutes	15 minutes
Timing	Week 1	Week 1	Week 2	Week 4	Week 8	Week 12	Week 16 (q 3mon.)
Assessment tools	Health risk appraisal (HRA), Nicotine dependence[a]		1-day smoke diary, PRN: Beck[d] Hamilton,[e] Holmes,[f] GAF,[g] GARF[h]	Assess adherence, barriers to change PRN	Assess adherence, barriers to change, cognitive-behavior diary PRN	Assess adherence, barriers to change, cognitive-behavior diary PRN	PRN: Beck scale,[d] Hamilton scale,[e] Holmes scale,[f] GAF,[g] diary
Lab/ diagnostic test	Labs PRN, weight	Weight	Weight	Weight	Weight	Weight	Weight, Labs prn
Provider assessments	History/physical, family history, quit attempts	Medical risk priority analysis	HRA, chance of success, shared priorities, depression hx	Cessation/ relapse,weight change, depression hx	Cessation/ relapse, weight change, depression hx	Cessation/ relapse, weight change, depression hx	Cessation/ relapse, History/ physical, weight change, depression?

	Visit 1		Visit 2	Visit 3	Visit 4	Visit 5	Visit 6
	Initial visit	**Prevention case conference**	**Shared decisions**	**Routine office visit**	**Routine office visit**	**Routine office visit**	**Routine office visit**
Primary provider counseling	Discuss patient priorities, health risks, cessation benefits		Set quit date review withdrawal symptoms and cessation benefits	Praise/encourage, discuss weight, exercise, depression, relaxation training	Praise/encourage, discuss weight, exercise, depression, relaxation training	Praise/encourage, discuss weight, exercise, depression, relaxation training	Praise/encourage, discuss weight, exercise, depression, relaxation training
Educational materials	*Clearing the Air*[b] Cessation benefits, Urge to smoke *Why I Smoke?*[c]		Review reducing urges, nicotine patch/gum, bupropion/SSRI, relaxation training	PRN: Review relapse prevention, cessation benefits, relaxation training	PRN: Relaxation response training	PRN: Relaxation response training	PRN: Relaxation response training
Counseling			No smoke contract				
Consultation		Cardiology PRN	Psychiatric PRN	Psychiatric PRN	Psychiatric PRN	Psychiatric PRN	Psychiatric PRN
Medications			Patch, gum, bupropion, SSRI	Adjust PRN	Adjust PRN	Adjust PRN	Adjust PRN

(continued)

Table 13.8 *(continued)*

Developed by L. Carey, R. E. Feinstein, P. LeDeaux, A. A. Brewer, J. Gallicano, P. M. Rabinowitz, J. Connelly, & A. Bornstein (1997).

[a] Fagerstrom, K. O. (1988). Measuring degree of physical dependence to tobacco smoking with reference to individualization of treatment. *Addictive Behaviors, 3*, 235–241.

[b] U.S. Department of Health and Human Services. (1995). *Clearing the air* (NIH Publication No. 95-1647). Rockville, MD: Author.

[c] *The why test*. Stop Smoking Program. American Academy of Family Physicians.Health Education Department Kansas City, Missouri 1993.

[d] Beck, A. T. (1978). *Beck depression inventory*. San Antonio, TX: Harcourt Brace.

[e] Hamilton, M. A. (1960). Hamilton Rating Scale for Depression: Physician assessment scale of the patient. *Journal of Neurology and Neurosurgical Psychiatry, 23*, 62.

[f] Holmes, T. H., & Raphe, R. H. (1967). Stress scale: Social readjustment scale. *Journal of Psychosomatic Research, 2*, 213.

[g] GAF (Global Assessment of Functioning). American Psychiatric Association. (1994). *Diagnostic and statistical manual of mental disorders* (4th ed., p. 200). Washington, DC: Author.

[h] GARF (Global Assessment of Relational Function). American Psychiatric Association. (1994). Diagnostic and statistical manual of mental disorders (4th ed., pp. 758–759). Washington, DC: Author.

- Assessment tools (e.g., instruments for obtaining a dietary history, assessing exercise capacity, detecting the presence of an eating disorder, and screening for depression)
- Physical, laboratory, and diagnostic testing required (e.g., a lipid profile, stress test, or sestamibi scan)
- Time required for each office visit (the initial prevention-oriented office visit may take 30 minutes to 1 hour; the first follow-up visit may take 30 minutes, and subsequent follow-up visits each last 15 minutes)
- Physician counseling interventions that address the patient's needs (e.g., nutritional, exercise, and weight reduction counseling interventions)
- Educational materials for the patient (e.g., a nutritional pyramid or smoking cessation information)
- Criteria for referral/consultation (e.g., when to refer to a nutritionist, exercise physiologist, physical therapist, cardiologist, or mental health professional)
- Patient-oriented diary to track progress of risk factor modification (e.g., a diary of smoking habits or a daily blood pressure diary, exercise diary, or mood-rating diary)
- Specific biopsychosocial interventions (e.g., medications, prevention screenings, lifestyle change, self-care, or other psychosocial interventions)

Our critical pathways are illustrated in Tables 13.4 through 13.8, and the depression and anxiety critical pathways are illustrated in chapter 2, Anxiety Disorders (see table 2.7), and chapter 3, Depression (see table 3.5), respectively.

TIMELINES. In order to create change, it is necessary to create a reasonable timetable for meeting a specific target goal. Timelines help foster reasonable expectations for the patient that change will occur slowly, over a period of months. Timelines are also reminders to physicians about how long to wait before changing an intervention approach.

Office-based Model

The practical application of POPC in an office setting requires planning and training but can be very efficient and provide high-quality care once the process is established at a practice site. We have developed a teaching video describing this process called Prevention Oriented Primary Care, copyright 1998. Training typically involves the use of new forms, training for the uses of an HRA software application, and teaching about the entire informed shared decision-making process. The entire office staff needs to learn about the use of the critical pathways, simple instruments to measure risk factors and/or lifestyle changes, as well as outcome measures that will help to assess the success of efforts to change to a healthy lifestyle.

BEFORE THE INITIAL OFFICE VISIT (20–30 MINUTES). Before the first office visit, the patient is given the Prevention-Oriented Primary Care Health History form, which includes the HRA. The patient fills out the form at home or in the office (with or without the assistance of office staff). This information is given to the physician before the initial visit.

INITIAL OFFICE VISIT (45 MINUTES–1 HOUR). The physician-patient interaction begins with personal contact, which allows an open style of communication and offers a brief introduction to POPC and the process of informed shared decision making. Physician and patient roles in this process are discussed, as in Table 13.1. The physician progresses to the patient's immediate biopsychosocial medical concerns. He or she then reviews with the patient those elements of the Prevention Health Screening form that are either incomplete or require further clarification or questions.

The physical examination is geared to patient concerns and preliminary results from the Prevention-Oriented Primary Care Health History form. The physician begins the discussion with the patient by introducing the concept of a medical priority list and develops with the patient the patient's priority list for health changes. Educational material about the likely priorities for change is discussed and given to the patient. At this visit, the physician suggests relevant laboratory screening or diagnostic tests and schedules a return appointment as soon as laboratory information is available, which allows for the completion of the HRA. This typically means waiting for the results of a total lipid profile and/or the results of other necessary diagnostic tests, such as a stress test.

SECOND OFFICE VISIT (30–45 MINUTES). Before this visit all necessary clinical and laboratory information can be entered into the HRA. The results of the HRA are summarized for the physician in the Health Risk Summary of Positive Findings and given to the patient as the Clinical Risk Factor Review Personal Report. During this visit, the physician reviews with the patient any immediate medical concerns and the patient's reactions to the last prevention visit. In addition, the doctor and the patient review the results from the laboratory and/or other diagnostic tests and the results of the HRA. Using the HRA, the physician describes to the patient the final medical priority list. Because this was roughly sketched out at the first visit before the results of the HRA were available, some modification may need to be made to the final medical priorities list. The physician and the patient discuss the patient's priority list. Together they go through the process of negotiating the shared priority list, which takes into account the chances of succeeding in the desired lifestyle change. Working from the top of the shared priority list, the intervention sequence that addresses the top one or two priorities can begin.

The intervention sequence with the patient typically is guided by a critical pathway for each of the different cardiovascular risk factors. Tables 13.4 through 13.8 are critical pathways for hypertension, hypercholesterolemia, weight loss intervention, exercise, and smoking cessation respectively. See chapter 2, Anxiety Disorders, and chapter 3, Depression, for critical pathways for panic disorder and depression, respectively. Patients are given the summary of the HRA and additional screening or assessment tools, which are used to facilitate change, assist in record keeping, and help follow outcome measurements.

Screening instruments vary depending on the cardiovascular risk factor but can be documents such as the PACE counseling form for exercise, a nicotine dependence test, screening for binge-eating disorder, or the Beck Inventory (Beck, 1978) for depression. In addition, the patient is asked to use a variety of diaries, such as a food, exercise, weight, smoking, relaxation response, and cognitive-behavioral diaries. The initial assessment, which includes the HRA, screening instruments, medical history, and physical and laboratory testing, becomes the baseline from which to measure outcome at the end of 1 year. Patients are also given educational material with a self-help focus and specific information about how to exercise, lose weight, stop smoking, etc. Follow-up visits are scheduled.

FOLLOW-UP OFFICE VISITS. Patients are scheduled according to their need and the specific cardiovascular risk factor for which an intervention is being performed. Typically, there are 2 to 6 follow-up visits over the first year as guided by the critical pathways. In addition, the patient may be referred to paraprofessionals or supportive programs for lifestyle change. For example, some patients should be scheduled with a nutritionist, exercise physiologist, behavioral medicine specialist, or nurse, or referred to a community healthy-lifestyle program.

The Prevention-Oriented Primary Care (POPC) model to cardiovascular risk factor reduction is a patient-centered approach that the authors describe as "informed shared decision making." This approach uses a health risk assessment instrument and takes into account medical risk factor analysis, the patient's health priority concerns, and the chance of the patient's succeeding in changing a particular lifestyle. Informed shared decision making permits the physician and the patient to develop a shared priority list for cardiovascular risk factor reduction. The intervention sequence for lifestyle change is an office-based approach that is guided by critical pathways and office-based interventions. It takes into account target goals, intervention strategy, timelines for expected change, and outcome measurements.

REFERENCES

American Academy of Family Physicians, Health Education Committee. (1987). *Stop Smoking: Physician and office staff manual, patient manual.* Kansas City, MO: Author.

Anderson, K. M., Castelli, W. P., & Levy, D. (1987). Cholesterol and mortality: 30 years of follow up from the Framingham Study. *Journal of the American Medical Association, 257*, 2176–80.

Beck, A. T. (1978). *Beck depression inventory.* San Antonio, TX: Harcourt, Brace.

Castelli, W. P., Garrison, R. J., & Wilson, P. W. F. (1986). Framingham Heart Study: Incidence of coronary artery disease and lipoprotein cholesterol levels. *Journal of the American Medical Association, 256*, 2835–2838.

Centers for Disease Control. (1987). Protective effect of physical activity on coronary heart disease. *Morbidity and Mortality Weekly Report, 36*, 426–430.

ERIS Survey System/St. Joseph Medical Center Family Practice Residency Program. Health Risk Appraisal, 6363 Hollister Drive, Indianapolis, IN 46224.

Grudny, S. M. (1993). *National cholesterol education program. Detection, evaluation, and treatment of high blood cholesterol in adults. Adult treatment panel II* (NIH Publication No. 93-3095). Bethesda, MD: National Institutes of Health.

Healthier People Version 4.0. (1991). Atlanta: Carter Center of Emory University (Health Risk Appraisal Program 1988. Vol 4. Scientific Documentation, July).

Joint National Committee on Detection, Evaluation, and Treatment of High Blood Pressure. (1993). Fifth report of the Joint National Committee on Detection, Evaluation, and Treatment of High Blood Pressure (JNC-V). *Archives of Internal Medicine,153*, 254–83.

National Cancer Institute. (1995). *Clearing the air.* (NIH Publication No. 95-1647). Bethesda, MD: Author.

Long, B., & Wooten, W. (1992). *Physician-based assessment and counseling for exercise, physician manual.* Atlanta: Centers for Disease Control and Prevention (Cardiovascular Health Branch).

Orleans, C. T. (1993). Treating nicotine dependence in medical settings: A stepped care model. In C. T. Orleans & J. D. Slade (Eds.), *Nicotine addiction: Principles and management* (pp. 145–161). New York: Oxford University Press.

Paffenbarger, R. S., Kampert, J. B., Lee, I., Hyde R. T., Leung , R. W., & Wing, A. L. (1994). Changes in physical activity and other lifeway patterns influencing longevity. *Medicine and Science in Sports and Exercise, 26*, 857–865.

Pate, R. R., Pratt, M., Blair, S. N., Haskell, W. L., Macera, C. A., Bouchard, C., Buchner, O., Ettinger, W., Heath, G. W., & King, A. C. (1995). Physical activity and public health: A recommendation from the Centers for Disease Control and Prevention and the American College of Sports Medicine. *Journal of the American Medical Association, 273*, 402–407.

Prochaska, J. O., & DiClemente, C. C. (1986). Toward a comprehensive model of change. In W. R. Miller & N. Heather (Eds.), *Treating addictive behaviors: Processes of change* (pp. 3–27). New York: Plenum Press.

Rabinowitz, M., Feinstein, R. E., Carey, L., Gallicano, J., Brewer, A., Connelly, J. V., Le Deaux, P. & Bornstein, A. (1995–1998). *Prevention-oriented primary care.* [Advance Grant Section of the Bureau of Health Professionals, U.S. Department of Health and Human Services. Federal Residency Training Grant #5D15PE10297-02 Educational and Prevention Program in Cardiovascular Disease Risk Reduction].

Roter, D. L., Stewart, M., Putnam, S. M., Lipkin, M., Jr., Stiles, W., & Inui, T. S. (1997). Communication patterns of primary care physicians. *Journal of the American Medical Association, 277*, 350–356.

U.S. Center for Disease Control (1987). Protective effect of physical activity on coronary heart disease. *Morbidity and Mortality Weekly Report, 36,* 426–430.

U.S. Preventative Services Task Force. (1996). *Guide to clinical preventative services* (2nd ed.). Baltimore: Williams & Wilkins.

CHAPTER 14

Women's Health Through The Reproductive Cycle: Premenstrual Syndrome, Postpartum Disorders, and Menopause

Eve Caligor and Marian Ormont

Reproductive and sexual issues are personal topics for most women. As a result, many female patients are hesitant to discuss complaints related to reproduction or sexuality with their physician. Some patients feel embarrassed, and others fear that they will not be taken seriously if they raise questions or concerns related to their reproductive cycles. These feelings tend to be especially powerful for the female patient who is being treated by a male physician. As a result, when evaluating a female patient, the physician should take the initiative and inquire about premenstrual, postpartum, or menopausal symptoms. Routine inquiry will ensure that treatable conditions are not missed and that all patients receive basic education and reassurance about reproductive issues. In addition, discussion of reproductive issues, when handled tactfully, will help to solidify a positive, collaborative relationship with the female patient and will foster open communication between patient and doctor.

This chapter covers premenstrual disorder, postpartum syndromes, and menopause. Although these three conditions are different, they are all closely linked to the female reproductive cycle.

PREMENSTRUAL SYNDROME

Clinical Presentation and Epidemiology

Premenstrual syndrome (PMS) is an endocrine disorder of the reproductive system of undetermined etiology. PMS is defined by the presence of clusters of certain affective, behavioral, and physical symptoms that occur prior to the onset of menses and remit with the onset of menses or shortly thereafter. The most common symptoms associated with PMS are listed in Table 14.1.

The onset of premenstrual syndrome typically occurs during adolescence, after the menarche. Thirty percent of all women report some premenstrual symptoms; however, only 2% to 10% are severely affected. Fifty-eight percent of women who meet criteria for PMS have emotional and physical symptoms, 37% have emotional symptoms with mild or absent physical symptoms, and 5% have distressing physical symptoms with mild or absent emotional symptoms (Freeman, Sondheimer, Weinbaum, & Rickels, 1985). The diagnosis of PMS is made by prospectively documenting the presence of physical, emotional, and/or behavioral symptoms that are cyclical, recurrent, present in the luteal phase of the menstrual cycle, and remit after the onset of menstruation. Table 14.2 presents diagnostic criteria for PMS.

A diagnosis of PMS requires the presence of luteal-phase symptoms in the majority of cycles as distinguished from the worsening of a chronic physical or emotional disorder. Symptoms must be severe enough to cause significant physical or emotional distress or a deterioration in psychosocial functioning. Most patients do not present for treatment for PMS until their 30s or 40s. PMS follows a chronic course but remits in pregnancy, resolves after natural or surgical menopause, and is not seen in women with polycystic ovarian syndrome. Disturbed circadian rhythms, a history of childhood physical or sexual abuse, physiologic abnormalities such as serotonin deficiency, and poor nutrition all confer vulnerability to PMS.

Table 14.1 Symptoms Commonly Associated With PMS

Emotional	Physical	Behavioral
• Depressed mood*	• Bloating*	• Food craving*
• Mood lability*	• Extremity swelling*	• Increased appetite
• Anxiety*	• Headaches/migraines*	• Increased alcohol intake
• Irritability*	• Abdominal cramps*	• Decreased motivation
• Anger	• Breast tenderness*	• Decreased Efficiency
• Nervous tension	• Weight gain	• Isolative behavior
• Overly sensitive	• Hot flashes	• Sleep changes
	• Palpitations	• Changes in sexual arousal
	• Dizziness	• Decreased cognitive funtion
	• Skin problems	

* The most common symptoms in each category.

Issues for Women

Despite increasing social acceptance of sexual, reproductive, and psychiatric problems, many women still feel reluctant to talk about premenstrual symptoms with their physicians. Women may consider the subject of menstruation private and/or embarrassing, may view PMS as an inevitable part of being a woman, or may consider it a sign of weakness. In fact, PMS can interfere with the patient's functioning for half of every month, can precipitate suicidal thoughts, violent behavior or impulses, and incapacitating depression, and can be frightening to the patient and her family.

Discomfort in discussing premenstrual symptoms can interfere with its timely treatment. In fact, many patients with premenstrual syndrome wait until the situation has become intolerable or delay for years discussing their symptoms with a physician. For this reason, the physician should routinely inquire about PMS as part of a review of symptoms. When a woman does decide to discuss PMS with her doctor, she is likely to be uncomfortable. The patient may be sensitive to the physician's body language, intonation, and choice of words as she tries to gauge the physician's reaction to her complaints.

Issues for Physicians

Physicians may also experience discomfort and/or confusion when evaluating PMS and may share the socially sanctioned attitudes of depreciation frequently directed toward menstrual symptoms. If a woman perceives her physician's bias or experiences the physician as abrupt, disinterested, or uncomfortable, she may minimize the problem or change the subject. She also may become too anxious or embarrassed to hear her physician's recommendation.

The variable diagnostic criteria for PMS can be confusing, as can the fact that the diagnosis relies entirely on patient reporting without objective medical tests for verification. These difficulties can cause the physician to avoid the issue, either by minimizing the patient's complaints or by doing only a cursory assessment.

Discussing PMS With the Patient

The first step in overcoming difficulties in discussing PMS is for the physician to anticipate the patient's discomfort, particularly if the physician is a man. An attitude of attention and concern will reassure the self-conscious patient and let her know that her complaints are being taken seriously. In addition, the physician's familiarity and comfort with diagnosis and treatment of symptoms of PMS will put the patient at ease.

In the clinical interview, the patient may make light of her concerns about PMS with various dismissive comments; however, the physician should take these concerns seriously, inquiring tactfully about symptoms. Normalizing the situation for the patient can be reassuring. For example, to the patient describing premenstrual irritability and affective lability, the primary care physician can explain that irritability is a common symptom of PMS that in no way implies mental instability.

Diagnostic Issues

Although the diagnosis of PMS must be made prospectively, a good history that elicits emotional, physical, and behavioral symptoms can rule out other medical, gynecological, and psychiatric conditions. In taking a history, it is important to clarify which symptoms are most disturbing and disabling and to define these symptoms in terms of their severity, duration, and temporal relationship to the onset of menses. Important areas of inquiry include the patient's sleep patterns, level of occupational and sexual functioning, quality of interpersonal and family life, affective state, and impulsivity. Patients with PMS often report irregular sleep patterns with frequent awakenings, difficulty falling back to sleep, and oversleeping. Disturbed sleep causes fatigue and irritability, which can increase symp-

Table 14.2 Diagnostic Criteria for PMS

1. Cyclical and recurrent physical, emotional, and/or behavioral symptoms:
   - present in luteal phase
   - remit at onset of menstruation
   - present in majority of cycles
   - confirmed by more than two cycles of prospective daily monitoring
2. Symptoms do not represent worsening of a chronic physical or emotional disorder.
3. Symptoms cause physical/emotional distress or a deterioration in psychosocial functioning.

Reprinted with permission from the *Diagnostic and Statistical Manual of Mental Disorders,* Fourth Edition. Copyright 1994 American Psychiatric Association.

tom severity. PMS patients may experience increased levels of social maladjustment in work, problems with interpersonal or parenting roles, decreased sexual desire.

A detailed medical, gynecological, and psychiatric history will also detect other illnesses. In one study, almost 20% of patients who presented for PMS evaluations had undetected medical or gynecological disorders, despite being under medical supervision (Keye, Hammond, & Strong, 1986).

It is equally important to diagnosis chronic psychiatric disorders, some of which have symptoms that overlap or are exacerbated by luteal-phase symptoms of PMS. In fact, 30% to 50% of women presenting for PMS evaluation are found to have a major psychiatric illness rather than PMS, the most common of which are major depressive disorder, atypical depressive disorder, dysthymic disorder, cyclothymic disorder, personality disorders, anxiety disorders (particularly panic disorder), and impulse control disorders. These syndromes must be ruled out before making the diagnosis of PMS. The primary feature for distinguishing PMS from chronic psychiatric disorders is a completely asymptomatic week during the follicular phase of most cycles. This is not seen in chronic psychiatric disorders.

Patients complaining of premenstrual symptoms should undergo a complete physical exam, including measurements of weight and, if the patient complains of bloating, abdominal circumference. Pelvic examination is important because there is a 12% to 50% incidence of gynecological pathology identified in PMS patients. The physician should collect and culture cervical specimens, as there may be an association between pelvic infection and PMS. Symptoms of anemia, thyroid dysfunction, renal disease, and hepatic disease may also resemble those of PMS.

Once the history and medical evaluation is complete, the patient should be asked to record her symptoms prospectively over 2 months (two menstrual cycles). Retrospective reporting is frequently inaccurate. The diagnosis of PMS depends on the temporal relationship between symptoms and menstruation and on symptom severity (see Table 14.2) and is made by examining daily symptom ratings over a 2-month period. A variety of forms have been developed for this purpose. A very useful one is the Calendar of Premenstrual Experiences (CPE) of Mortola, Girton, Beck, & Yen (1990), which successfully distinguishes PMS subjects from controls with a 2.8% false-negative rate and a 0% false-positive rate.

Once the symptom-rating form has been completed and returned to the physician, one of several patterns may be identified:

1. *Patients who have PMS.* These patients are almost completely symptom-free during the follicular phase of their cycles. They develop symptoms after ovulation, which interfere with interpersonal relationships and work.
2. *Patients suffering from a chronic affective disorder with premenstrual exacerbations.* These patients demonstrate affective symptoms throughout the month, with an increase in symptom severity during the late luteal phase. It is important to reassure these patients that their concerns are valid and to explain that although they have very real and distressing symptoms, the diagnosis may not be PMS. The clinician can tactfully refer the patient for a compete psychiatric evaluation to obtain a second opinion or to clarify the diagnosis.
3. *Patients appearing to have intermittent mood and anxiety symptoms with no consistent temporal relationship to the menstrual cycle.* These patients do not have PMS. They may be experiencing a rapid-cycling affective disorder, and a psychiatric referral for diagnostic evaluation may be appropriate.
4. *Patients who suffer from mild luteal phase symptoms.* These patients' symptoms are not severe enough to interfere with psychosocial functioning. As a result, symptoms do not meet the criteria for PMS. These symptoms often respond well to evaluation, education, support, and over-the-counter products.

5. *Patients who suffer from PMS superimposed on a chronic affective disorder.* These patients are differentiated from those with chronic affective disorders because they develop a variety of physical symptoms, such as water retention and pain, that are not present during the follicular phase. Such patients require a coordinated treatment effort between their primary physician and a psychiatrist.

Management of PMS

Early and correct diagnosis is fundamental to the management of PMS. Once the diagnosis is made, the next step is to provide education and support. In addition, stress reduction, exercise, and sleep hygiene are first-line treatments. If these alone are not successful, dietary modification should be attempted. Finally, pharmacotherapy should be considered on an individual basis to address symptoms.

Education

Education, combined with prospective recording of symptoms, has been shown to be satisfactory treatment in 30% of cases of PMS. Patients and their families are relieved to learn that premenstrual symptoms are relatively common and that PMS is a well-described syndrome for which specific treatments exist. The clinician can explain that PMS is a physiological disorder in which hormones interact with neurotransmitters, prostaglandins, and systemic functions to cause physical, emotional, and behavioral symptoms. It is important to emphasize that PMS is not a dangerous hormonal disturbance and that the patient is not imagining her symptoms.

Stress reduction, improved sleep, and exercise are forms of treatment for the symptoms of PMS. It is important to explain to the patient that the treatment goal is to decrease symptom severity and that rarely, if ever, are all symptoms eliminated. This approach will reduce the likelihood of disappointment and doctor shopping. Coherent explanations, concern, an expression of interest in the patient's symptoms, supportive listening, and reassurance on the part of the clinician can help to relieve symptoms and provide support.

Stress Reduction

Stress appears to exacerbate PMS symptoms, and the patient's efforts to reduce or cope more efficiently with psychosocial stresses should be encouraged. There are a plethora of stress reduction techniques that have been found to be helpful in PMS, both in relieving symptoms and in increasing the patient's sense of being in control. These include relaxation response training/meditation (see Tables 2.3 and 2.4 in chapter 2, Anxiety Disorders), yoga, reading, listening to music, hypnosis, and exercise. Behavioral interventions (see chapter 19, Behavioral Counseling and Medical Adherence) can help patients cope with irritability and mood lability. In addition, patients can be encouraged to keep a calendar of their menstrual symptoms and to decrease the number of stressful events on days when they typically are most symptomatic. This will minimize the impact of premenstrual symptoms on a patient's activities.

Exercise

Regular exercise reduces some of the physical symptoms of PMS and may give a PMS patient a greater sense of control over her body and over her life. Although exercise appears to have less effect on emotional symptoms, women who exercise tend to feel better about themselves. (see the exercise section in chapter 12, Cardiovascular and Psychosocial Risk Factors Reduction: Office-based Interventions.)

Diet

The efficacy of dietary change in the treatment of PMS has not been well studied. However, regular, well-balanced, low-fat (less than 50 to 60 grams per day) meals should be recommended for overall health. (For basic low-fat dietary recommendations see chapter 12, Cardiovascular and Psychosocial Risk Factors Reduction: Office-based Interventions). Current thinking is that carbohydrate-rich food may cause temporary improvement in depression, irritability, tension, and fatigue, whereas foods that are high in salt and simple sugars can promote water retention, weight gain, and physical discomfort. Methylxanthine-containing beverages, such as coffee, tea, and cola, should be eliminated from the diet, because they may worsen irritability, tension, and insomnia. After symptomatic control is achieved, small amounts of caffeine can be added to the diet to see if symptoms recur.

Vitamin and mineral supplements may help to relieve PMS symptoms. Pyridoxine's efficacy is controversial. It should be prescribed only in low doses of 50 to 500 mg per day because it often causes neurotoxicity after 6 to 12 months of use. If no improvement occurs after 2 or 3 months, pyridoxine should be discontinued. Calcium supplementation at a dose of 1,000 mg per day has been shown to reduce physical and emotional symptoms of PMS. The effectiveness of magnesium supplementation is controversial; however, doses of 360 mg per day reduce water retention and improve negative affect when used consistently for 4 months (Facchinetti et al., 1991). Alcohol and illicit drugs may worsen the symptoms of PMS.

Medications

If exercise, stress reduction, and dietary modification do not relieve the patient's symptoms, medication management should be considered. When treating a patient's physical, emotional, or behavioral symptoms, it is important to identify specific symptoms and monitor them during medication trials. Medications that do not result in improvement of target symptoms should be discontinued.

It is extremely important to treat severe physical symptoms. Sixty percent or more of PMS patients complain of disturbing physical symptoms, which can cause or exacerbate emotional distress. As a result, treatment of physical symptoms should be reviewed (Smith & Schiff, 1993) and generally should be attempted before medical treatment of emotional symptoms. Mild diuretics, acetaminophen, and nonsteroidal anti-inflammatory drugs are commonly prescribed for specific physical symptoms. Suppression of ovulation with oral contraceptives is another option.

The primary emotional symptoms of PMS that require treatment are depression, irritability, and anxiety. SSRIs have been used successfully to treat depressed mood in patients with PMS. When prescribing antidepressants, it is important to inquire about suicidal ideation and a history of mania to avoid the risk of overdose or inadvertently producing a manic episode. An average dose of an SSRI (sertraline, 75 mg; fluoxetine, 20 mg; paroxetine, 20 mg) for a 6-week trial usually controls mood lability, anxiety, depression, irritability, fatigue, and fluctuations in appetite. Occasionally, higher doses are required in PMS patients. Alternate-day dosing is sometimes used during the follicular phase, with daily dosing during the luteal phase. The patient should be educated about anticipated benefits, side effects, and delayed onset of action. Enlisting the patient as an active participant in the treatment will enhance her sense of control and improve adherence to the medical treatment plan.

SSRIs are usually taken in the morning after breakfast but can be taken at night if the patient experiences drowsiness. For particularly anxious patients or those who are sensitive to any side effect, it is helpful to start with a lower dose of an SSRI (e.g., sertraline, 12.5 mg per day) and to increase the dose at weekly intervals as side effects allow. The effectiveness of SSRIs may diminish after 6 to 10 months of treatment, but this may be offset by increasing the dose during the luteal phase. PMS patients being treated with antidepressants should initially be seen monthly.

Anxiety, excessive worrying, motor tension, restlessness, fatigue, shortness of breath, nausea, and hypervigilance may be predominant premenstrual symptoms in some women. Anxiolytic medications, such as benzodiazepines and buspirone, and behavioral relaxation techniques can be effective in treating these symptoms. For patients who experience time-limited symptoms of anxiety, a benzodiazepine such as lorazepam can be helpful for short-term use only. Women who have a history of alcohol or drug use or women whose activities and/or occupation require that they be especially alert should not receive these medications. A trial of buspirone and use of behavioral relaxation techniques are better options for such patients. The physician should review treatment options with the patient and come to a joint treatment decision with her.

Psychiatric Referral

There will be times when referral for a complete psychiatric evaluation is both necessary and appropriate for the patient with PMS. When a routine psychiatric evaluation is needed, tact and empathy on the part of the physician will preserve rapport and aid patient adherence. The physician should reassure the patient that he or she knows she is not imagining her symptoms, understands that she is suffering, and believes that she will benefit from a second opinion. A patient referred for psychiatric consultation should be scheduled for an appointment afterwards to discuss the consultation and review her treatment plan and progress.

Patients with suicidal, homicidal, or assaultive ideation should be referred to a psychiatrist on an emergency basis to prevent harm to the patient or others (see chapter 7, Violence and Suicide). A patient also should be referred to a psychiatrist in the case of uncertain diagnosis or if there is a suspected history of a bipolar disorder. Psychiatric evaluation will clarify the clinical diagnosis and prevent a potential drug-induced manic episode if antidepressant treatment is warranted.

POSTPARTUM PSYCHIATRIC DISORDERS

Clinical Presentation and Epidemiology

The incidence of depression is higher for women in the postpartum period than at any other stage of life. In addition, the rate of psychiatric hospitalization is markedly increased during the first 3 months after uncomplicated childbirth. As a result, primary care physicians need to know how to recognize and manage the emotional and psychiatric problems that can occur in the postpartum period.

Postpartum psychiatric disorders can be viewed as a spectrum of conditions that present with an onset as early as the first postpartum day and as late as several months after delivery. The three major syndromes are postpartum/maternity blues, postpartum depression, and psychosis.

Maternity blues is the mildest of the postpartum disorders and is often a relatively normal part of the birth experience. It affects 50% to 80% of new mothers in the first week after delivery and usually resolves by the end of the first postpartum month. Maternity blues is characterized by tearfulness, irritability, sleep disturbance, anxiety, fatigue, forgetfulness, and mild confusion. The symptoms usually peak between the third and seventh day after delivery. Risk factors for postpartum blues include primiparous pregnancy and a history of premenstrual syndrome.

Postpartum depression is present in 10% to 15% of new mothers. This is a more severe disorder than maternity blues and is clinically similar to major depressive disorder. Women may present as sad and tearful, may complain of sleep and appetite disturbances, and may have difficulty concentrating. They sometimes experience suicidal ideation and impairment in daily functioning. The diagnosis of postpartum depression is usually apparent by the second or third week postpartum.

Postpartum psychosis is the most severe but the least common of the postpartum psychiatric disorders, affecting 1 to 2 per 1,000 new mothers. It is defined as a psychosis occurring within the first six months after childbirth. Clinical features include obsessive thoughts of hurting the baby or oneself, as well as more classic psychotic symptoms such as auditory hallucinations, delusions, and disorganized thoughts. Postpartum psychosis must be rapidly identified and treated, as the risk of infanticide during an episode of postpartum psychosis may be as high as 4%.

The most important risk factor for postpartum depression and postpartum psychosis is a past history of psychiatric illness. The risk is greatest if the patient has a history of bipolar disorder and slightly lower if she has a history of unipolar depression. Women with a prior diagnosis of an affective disorder have a 20% to 25% chance of a postpartum psychosis. Other risk factors for these disorders include having a first baby, an unwanted pregnancy, environmental stressors during the third trimester or early postpartum period, giving birth by cesarean section, an unstable or absent marital relationship, and a lack of social supports. Women who have a complicated delivery or a premature, abnormal, or sick child are at higher risk for postpartum disorders than are those who have lost the child through stillbirth or perinatal death.

Issues for the Woman and Her Partner

Despite societal expectations that having a baby should be a completely joyful experience, many women are ambivalent about the birth experience. Some women are not prepared for the postpartum blues, nor are they aware of the risk of postpartum depression or psychosis. A woman who unexpectedly develops postpartum blues may find herself experiencing guilt, concern, or fear that having the baby was a mistake. These fears may worsen if the woman's partner is not supportive and if there are no close relatives or friends to give emotional and physical assistance after delivery. A new father may feel worried, frustrated, and helpless in response to his wife's postpartum tearfulness and irritability, which can intensify the mother's sense of inadequacy. Postpartum symptoms can be traumatic for both new parents and may prolong the postpartum syndrome.

Women with a history of affective disorder may become anxious as they approach their delivery date, fearing that their illness will reappear. For those patients who have been advised to discontinue maintenance psychotropic medications during pregnancy, the situation is particularly frightening.

Issues for the Physician

Patients experiencing a postpartum disorder may become demanding of the primary care physician's attention. They may seek constant reassurance, making multiple phone calls and requesting frequent office visits. Patients may present with physical complaints and concerns that are unrelated to their mental or emotional state. When managing a demanding and anxious patient, the physician should avoid speaking abruptly to the patient, acting out irritation, or failing to return the patient's phone calls in a timely manner. These actions may exacerbate the problem.

Women with bipolar disorder who have little insight into the recurrent nature of their illness, who have not taken psychotropic medications during their pregnancy, and who are determined to breast feed present special problems. These patients often refuse to take their mood stabilizer during pregnancy, both because of the potential risk to the fetus and because they lack insight into the risks of discontinuing their medications. For the same reasons, some bipolar patients may refuse to restart medication immediately after delivery and may not recognize or report recurrent symptoms, thus risking exacerbation of their disorder and psychiatric hospitalization during the postpartum period.

Recurrent illness can cause a woman with bipolar illness to become progressively fearful that her husband and physicians are not to be trusted and that she and her baby are in danger. Such a situation can be volatile, even if the primary care physician has a good rapport with the patient and there is close family involvement.

Discussing Postpartum Disorders with the Patient

A patient with affective disorder will do best when she is assured that her primary care physician understands postpartum depression and psychosis and has a plan to manage such problems if they arise. The patient's anxiety may decrease markedly if she and her family are given concrete instructions to observe for new or worsening psychiatric symptoms, such as vegetative signs of depression, suicidal or violent thoughts, and auditory hallucinations. In addition, the physician can help alleviate her anxiety by scheduling frequent follow-up visits, by communicating an understanding of the potential seriousness of psychiatric postpartum complications, and by discussing an action plan with options for psychiatric consultation and physical safety. In addition, the physician may offer a family meeting with the patient's significant others (see chapter 18, Family Counseling).

Diagnostic Issues

The diagnosis of postpartum blues, postpartum depression, and postpartum psychosis is based on the clinical interview and on history from the patient and her family. In treating patients with a history of depression or bipolar disorder, vigilance is essential so that signs of developing postpartum psychiatric illness can be caught early.

Postpartum or maternity blues is a mild adjustment disorder that commonly presents during the first week after delivery in which the new mother has a protracted period of mildly depressed mood with tearfulness, irritability, sleep disturbance, forgetfulness, and mild confusion. Auditory hallucinations, paranoid ideation, obsessive thoughts of harming the baby, or thought disturbances are not present. Reality testing is intact, and the patient is able to function at an adequate level and receive some pleasure from the baby. Symptoms peak by the seventh day and typically last throughout the first 3 to 4 weeks of the puerperium.

Unlike postpartum blues, the symptoms of postpartum depression usually begin in the second week and peak in the third or fourth week after delivery. Women with this disorder generally meet criteria for major depressive disorder (see chapter 3, Depression). Common symptoms are feelings of hopelessness or helplessness, decreased self-care, and inadequate care for the baby. Suicidal and homicidal ideation is not infrequent. The clinician should monitor patients with a prior diagnosis of major depressive disorder or bipolar disorder, as postpartum depression is much more common in these patients.

Postpartum psychosis is an extremely serious condition, with an incidence of about 4% and a high suicide risk. This psychosis is most common in patients with a history of bipolar disorder. Patients with a diagnosis of a psychotic disorder, such as schizophrenia, may experience an exacerbation of their symptoms in the postpartum period, which can be confused with postpartum psychosis. Patients with postpartum psychosis may experience auditory hallucinations and paranoid delusions with impaired reality testing. They also may demonstrate signs and symptoms of delirium, such as a waxing and waning mental state and confusion. The patient may believe that hospital personnel or family members are planning to harm her baby and may attempt to escape from a situation she perceives as dangerous. The combination of auditory hallucinations, paranoid ideation, and intrusive thoughts of the mother/patient harming the baby is extremely dangerous.

If a patient develops psychotic symptoms in the postpartum period and has no prior history of psychosis, the first step is to rule out possible medical causes of psychosis, such as thyroid dysfunction, strokes, CNS tumors, metabolic disturbances, and Sheehan's syndrome, preferably with a work-up during an admission of the patient to a psychiatric unit (see chapter 5, Psychiatric Symptoms Due to Medical Illness).

Evaluation and Treatment

Evaluation and treatment of postpartum psychiatric disorders necessitate a good rapport with the patient and her family. All pregnant women should be educated about the potential risk of developing maternity blues. Framing maternity blues as a frequent event related to hormonal shifts normalizes the experience. This may decrease the shame or guilt that some women feel when reporting depressive symptoms to their physicians.

Pregnant women who have a history of affective illness present a greater management challenge. The primary care physician may find it easier to manage these patients in collaboration with a psychiatric consultant. During pregnancy, these patients, their partners, and their physicians face the dilemma of whether psychotropic medications should be continued. Past pregnancy history, past psychiatric history, patient support system, and the risk the medications pose to the fetus are all factors that must be considered when making this decision. Patients and their partners must be carefully apprised of the risks and benefits, and they must agree to careful physician follow-up.

As the pregnancy nears term, it is important to reinforce the availability of the physician after delivery. Women who have a history of a psychiatric disorder should be seen by their primary physician or their psychiatrist as frequently as every week for the first 2 or 3 months following delivery. Patients and their partners should be treated as a team, educated about the symptoms of psychosis, helped to monitor symptoms, and instructed to contact the physician if they see that the new mother is becoming symptomatic or decompensating.

When a postpartum woman reports emotional complaints, she should be seen as soon as possible. Most of these women will be suffering from postpartum blues. However, missing the diagnosis of postpartum depression or psychosis can be fatal. It is important that the physician assess the patient's self-care and care of the baby, as well as the patient's depressive or psychotic symptoms.

It is helpful to comment on the stressful nature of being at home with a new baby. Questions such as "Sometimes new mothers are so tired and stressed that they have unusual experiences. Have you had any?" will help the patient feel more comfortable. Answering such questions may reveal symptoms. Other statements, such as "It is natural for new mothers to be concerned about their babies' well-being, but sometimes women fear that other people may intentionally harm their child," may encourage her to share any unusual ideas. Nonverbal cues such as hypervigilance, poor eye contact, paucity of speech, pressured speech, and an internal preoccupation should be noted.

Postpartum depression is diagnosed by identifying the symptoms of major depressive disorder (see chapter 3, Depression). Postpartum psychosis is diagnosed by identifying psychotic symptoms such as auditory hallucinations, paranoid ideation, persecutory delusions, ideas of reference, and diminished self-care. Any depressed or anxious postpartum woman must be asked about intrusive or frightening thoughts of hurting her baby.

Women who appear to be suffering from postpartum blues respond well to reassurance and increased emotional support from her clinician and family. Adequate home support is crucial to avoid chronic sleep deprivation, which exacerbates the symptoms of postpartum blues. A new mother needs sleep and some time for herself. Exercise may diminish depressive symptoms. A healthy diet low in simple sugars may diminish the intensity of dysphoria.

A patient who meets the criteria for major depression but who is able to care for herself and her baby often can be treated in a primary care setting. However, psychiatric consultation is helpful to strengthen the patient's safety net and improve the early recognition of emerging psychotic, suicidal, or homicidal symptoms. Patients who do demonstrate suicidal, homicidal, or psychotic symptoms or are neglecting care of themselves or their baby need emergency psychiatric treatment. Such a mother should be referred for psychiatric evaluation immediately (the same day) and should not be permitted to be alone with her baby until she has undergone the evaluation. If a psychiatrist is not readily available, the patient should be escorted to a hospital emergency room.

Postpartum patients tend to resist hospitalization, because they do not want to be separated from their babies. The patient's family may also resist her hospitalization. Despite this difficulty, outpatient treatment is not appropriate in cases in which the patient presents a potential danger to herself or to the baby. On most general psychiatric units, patients can have frequent visits with their partners and babies in the presence of a staff member. Stabilization of the patient often occurs quickly, so that early discharge is possible.

The patient suffering from postpartum depression who is not suicidal or homicidal can be managed as an outpatient; however, this requires the involvement of the patient's entire support system. The patient's significant other will probably have little or no experience in dealing with his partner's depression and will need to be educated about the disorder. He will need to understand that postpartum depression is a psychiatric disorder caused by temporary chemical imbalances in the brain and that the mother is not to blame. If a depressed mother is not able to take care of her infant, home care can help protect the infant from adverse sequelae of maternal depression. Such assistance also enables the patient to feel less pressured and less guilty during the illness and can enable her to have some quality time with her baby.

Antidepressant medications generally are prescribed in the treatment of postpartum depression. However, as most antidepressants are secreted in breast milk, pharmacotherapy often precludes breast feeding. Although many women and their partners may choose breastfeeding over treatment with antidepressants, treatment should begin without delay. This is because maternal depression in the postpartum period can interfere significantly with mother-infant bonding, and severe maternal depression is associated with infant depressive symptoms, failure to thrive, delayed infant development, and behavioral problems.

When antidepressants are necessary, patients should be educated about their side effects, delayed onset of action, duration of treatment, and drug interactions. SSRIs have become first-line treatment for depressive disorders because of good side effect profiles and relative safety with overdoses. If a patient has responded previously to an antidepressant such as nortriptyline, she generally should resume the drug.

One of the most serious potential adverse effects of all antidepressants is mania. Patients with a history of bipolar disorder should be treated with antidepressants only after they are on a therapeutic dose of a mood stabilizer, such as valproate, lithium, or carbamazepine. It is very important to involve a psychiatric consultant in the care of such patients.

Patients without a past history of psychiatric disorders may experience postpartum depression as a first manifestation of bipolar disorder. Such patients may have a greater tendency to become manic on antidepressants and should be monitored closely for manic symptoms. If pressured speech, increasing insomnia, racing thoughts, or psychotic symptoms develop in a patient on an antidepressant medication, the medication should be discontinued and the patient referred immediately for an emergency psychiatric consultation.

MENOPAUSE

Definition

Menopause is defined as the permanent end of menstrual periods. The perimenopause refers to the 5 to 10 years before the cessation of menses. During the perimenopausal years, ovarian and neuroendocrine changes lead to menopause.

Clinical Presentation and Epidemiology

Menopause usually occurs between ages 48 and 55, with an average age of approximately 51. Shortening of the menstrual cycle usually is the first clinical manifestation of the perimenopause. Many women subsequently experience prolonged cycles interspersed with shorter ones. Vasomotor symptoms occur in approximately 75% of all menopausal women in the United States (the incidence in surgical menopause is roughly 90%) and occur with the highest frequency during the first 2 years after menopause. Nocturnal hot flushes are common and can cause sleep disturbances. Decreased estrogen levels can cause osteoporosis and atrophy of vagina and urethra. These conditions occur gradually over several years following menopause, and the incidence of symptoms increases with advancing age. The cardiovascular protection that estrogen confers is gradually lost from menopause onward unless hormone replacement therapy is initiated.

There has been significant controversy and misinformation about psychological and sexual changes associated with menopause. Scientific studies do not support the commonly held belief that menopause is associated with depression. In fact, the incidence of depression during the menopausal years is lower than in earlier life. However, women with a previous history of depression or severe psychosocial stresses or who have a negative attitude about menopause are at risk for depression.

One major effect of menopause is sleep deprivation caused by nocturnal vasomotor flushing. Women experiencing frequent night flushes may suffer from daytime fatigue, irritability, decreased concentration, and dysphoria.

While there is no increased incidence of affective disorder associated with menopause, there may be an increased incidence of depression during the perimenopause in women who have a long, symptomatic perimenopausal period. This probably reflects a complex interaction of psychological, physiological, and social factors. In addition, some women may experience sudden mood shifts during the perimenopausal period. It is important (and relatively easy) to distinguish these sudden, transient, and relatively minor mood fluctuations from symptoms of depression.

The belief that menopause results in loss of sexual interest and pleasure is also unfounded. Sexual responses tend to slow and change in men and women with advancing age, but this is not specifically related to menopause. Dyspareunia due to vaginal dryness, menopausal vaginitis, and/or vaginal atrophy may be an issue, but these can be treated with vaginal estrogens, lubricants, or hormone replacement therapy (HRT).

Although there is no increased risk of depression accompanying menopause, this period of life frequently brings a variety of psychological and social stresses, including children leaving home, aging and dying of parents, and an increased frequency of medical problems for the woman, her spouse, or loved ones. In this setting, menopausal symptoms present yet another physical and psychological stressor for women. The psychological impact of menopause for a given woman will be closely tied to her attitude toward aging, her physical health, her social supports, and her general satisfaction with her life.

Issues for the Patient

There is wide variation in the information and attitudes women have about menopause. Some women look forward to freedom from menstruation and the need for contraception. Others fear menopause as a time of aging, loss of sexual pleasure, or the passing of physical attractiveness. Despite these concerns, most women make the transition to menopause without difficulty, although perimenopausal women may experience greater emotional distress about menopause than do menopausal women.

The most common causes of perimenopausal and menopausal distress are lack of accurate information about the physiological changes and symptoms accompanying menopause and the tendency to displace more general concerns about aging onto the anticipated loss of menses. Menopause can raise general questions about personal vulnerability, the possibility of chronic illness, and the inevitability of death. For many women, the perimenopausal years bring concerns about loss of sexual and physical attractiveness. Some women experience the loss of reproductive capacity or sexual attractiveness as a loss of power. In general, women who typically cope poorly with stress and change are likely to experience greater distress. Those who are optimistic, satisfied with their lives, and cope well are likely to respond to menopausal symptoms in a positive fashion.

A woman's emotional reactions to menopause will be affected by the reactions of her spouse and/or other loved ones. For a middle-aged man, his partner's menopause will confront him with his own anxieties about his sexual potency, attractiveness, aging, and death. How he copes with his own fears will have an impact on his partner's experience of her menopause. For example, an admiring and sexually interested partner who responds to his wife's hot flashes with tender humor can go far to help a woman cope with the menopausal transition.

Issues for the Physician

Physicians have a broad array of psychological reactions to perimenopausal and menopausal patients. Younger physicians who place high value on their own youth, sexual attractiveness, or reproductive capacities may find it difficult to be empathic to the needs of the perimenopausal patient.

They also may find it difficult to talk explicitly about sexual practices and sexual problems with older patients, because older patients may be cognitively associated in younger physicians' minds with their own parents. However, to appropriately evaluate, educate, and treat the menopausal patient, it is necessary to talk about sexual matters.

Older physicians are often more comfortable discussing menopausal and sexual symptoms with their female patients. Male and female physicians who are enjoying midlife and successfully navigating midlife transitions can usually maintain a collegial relationship with the menopausal patient. In contrast, physicians who are having personal difficulties in this area are more likely to avoid discussion of menopause or discuss menopause in a way that is not supportive.

A common pitfall for physicians is to "medicalize" the menopausal transition, viewing menopause as a chronic illness rather than a normal physiological and psychological milestone. Taking this type of "illness" approach to menopause distances the physician from his or her own feelings about menopause and from the patient.

All of the difficulties mentioned above can be surmounted. The first step is to become aware of one's feelings and attitudes and learn what women commonly experience, both physically and psychologically, as they go through menopause. For physicians who tend to avoid discussing sexual matters with patients, it is helpful to develop a standard approach to taking a sexual history (see chapter 10, Sexual Disorders and Sexual Trauma).

The Clinical Interview: Assessment and Diagnosis

When evaluating the perimenopausal or menopausal patient, the physician should make a series of assessments: (1) ascertain whether the patient is perimenopausal or menopausal; (2) clarify what symptoms she is having and how they affect her, and (3) assess how the patient is coping with the symptoms of menopause and the psychological challenges presented by the menopausal transition. Most women appreciate the invitation to discuss their symptoms, questions, and concerns related to menopause.

For many women, the menopausal transition becomes a time to begin taking better care of themselves. For the primary care physician, the perimenopause provides an opportunity to review with a patient lifestyle factors that influence her general health, psychological well-being, and risk of developing chronic illness. Lifestyle issues include exercise, weight, dietary fat and cholesterol, cigarette smoking, and intake of calcium, caffeine, and alcohol. Assessment of the patient's social circumstances, sexual life, and psychological well-being should be a routine part of the evaluation. Education, advice, and appropriate interventions can follow.

Patients who are coping well with the menopausal transition typically are relaxed in relating medical history and feel comfortable voicing their questions. Women who are having greater difficulty are likely to be more reticent during the interview. These women may answer questions only briefly or incompletely or may change the subject. It can be helpful to say something like "Sometimes menopausal changes can be stressful, but most people find they feel more comfortable and less worried after going over things with their physician."

Some women will present with overtly anxious or depressive reactions to menopause. In this setting, it is important to determine if the patient's emotional state is a reaction to menopause or a displacement of distress relating to other life issues (e.g., empty nest, aging parents, or marital problems). After obtaining a history of the patient's menopausal and psychological symptoms, the physician can inquire about any stresses she is facing. If there are significant marital or psychosocial problems, or if the situation is unclear, the patient's partner may be helpful. If it becomes apparent that the patient is experiencing significant psychosocial impairment, evaluation for a major psychiatric disorder is indicated. Affective and anxiety symptoms should be evaluated as described in chapter 2, Anxiety Disorders, and chapter 3, Depression.

Treatment

Most women do not require any formal treatment to manage the psychological challenges of menopause. However, all will benefit from education, reassurance, and support in the context of a routine primary care visit. The physician should allot enough time to allow the patient to ask her questions and air her concerns.

For women who are having great difficulty coping with the menopause, there are a number of options. Clarifying how the menopausal transition is causing her distress allows the physician to offer specific information and support. It is often helpful to bring in the patient's partner as well. A follow-up visit should be scheduled within a month's time, and the patient should be encouraged to seek out support and advice from friends, especially older women who have already made the transition. Self-help groups also can be helpful.

A variety of psychosocial problems can present to the primary care physician under the guise of menopausal symptoms. This frequently happens when a patient wants help but is reluctant to discuss a psychosocial problem. In other cases, the patient may be unaware that her distress about menopausal symptoms is a manifestation of a psychosocial problem. Marital problems, substance abuse, affective or anxiety disorders, and the exacerbation of long-standing psychological problems may present in this fashion. These problems should be fully evaluated and treated in the routine manner.

When a woman becomes menopausal, hormone replacement therapy (HRT) becomes an important question. For some women, this decision can be confusing and anxiety provoking. The decision to initiate HRT is complex and may be clouded by emotional issues. For example, a patient whose previously independent mother sustained a hip fracture and died in a nursing home 6 months later is likely to have a very different attitude toward HRT than the woman who watched her mother painfully waste away with metastatic breast cancer. In general, patients tend to weigh symptom-related benefits relatively heavily when deciding to initiate HRT, whereas physicians place more weight on prophylaxis of chronic disease. The decision to undertake HRT must weigh the benefits and risks (see Table 14.3) and must be made on an individual basis. The decision-making process should be a collaborative effort between patient and primary care physician.

Before making a decision about HRT, a complete medical, gynecological, and breast exam should be performed, as well as a Pap smear and mammogram. Liver function tests and lipid profiles should be obtained, and an EKG and bone densitometry may be indicated. In addition, the patient's personal and family history of cardiovascular disease, osteoporosis, and cancer should be reviewed.

Because the decision about HRT involves so many complex scientific and emotional decisions, it is best to begin discussion about menopause and HRT early in the perimenopause. This approach leaves time for the patient to do research, ask questions, and make an informed decision. Shared decision making may improve adherence to HRT as well. A recent study demonstrated that 20% to 30% of prescriptions written for HRT are never filled (Ravnikar, 1990). Although most physicians currently favor HRT for women who have no contraindications, patients as a group remain less enthusiastic.

Table 14.3 Potential Risks and Benefits of HRT

Benefits—Estrogen	Benefits—Progestins
• Relief of vasomotor symptoms • Prevention/reversal of urogenital atrophy • Risk reduction for coronary artery disease • Prevention of osteoporosis	• Prevention of estrogen-induced endometrial cancer • May have synergistic effect with estrogen on bone metabolism
Risks—Estrogen	**Risks—Progestins**
• Endometrial hyperplasia and endometrial cancer • Gallbladder disease • Breast cancer (controversial)	• Adverse effects on serum lipids

Medications

Women who decide against HRT can be treated for vasomotor and atrophic symptoms if they cause subjective distress and functional impairment.

Treatment of insomnia related to vasomotor flushing is no different from treatment of insomnia due to other causes. An initial approach is to advise the patient to abstain from alcohol and caffeine, improve sleep hygiene, and discontinue medications that can cause insomnia. Wearing layered cotton clothing can also be of help. Hypnotic medications are effective but should only be prescribed on a short-term basis. Zolpidem, 5 to 10 mg, lorazepam, 0.5 to 1.0 mg, or temazepam, 15 to 30 mg, have favorable side-effect profiles and do not result in the accumulation of active metabolites. Another option is the antidepressant trazodone, which can be prescribed at a dose of 25 to 75 mg hs.

Persistent insomnia may represent an underlying depression. Although the menopausal years carry a decreased incidence of depression, women who have long-standing depression may present to the primary care physician with depressive symptoms at the onset of perimenopausal symptoms. Depressive disorders should be treated aggressively (see chapter 3, Depression).

Referrals

In general, the primary care physician can effectively manage menopausal symptoms and associated psychological distress. Any patient who has difficulty coping with menopause, despite the interventions described, should be referred to a support group of peers. These groups function as effective sources of information and psychological support. Menopausal patients who have serious marital, sexual, or psychological problems may benefit from referral to a mental health specialist for counseling. Menopausal patients with a history of bipolar illness and those who do not respond to an SSRI, or are suicidal, depressed, or anxious, should be referred to a psychiatrist.

REFERENCES

Facchinetti, F., Borella, P., Sances, G., Fioroni L., Nappi, R. E., & Genazzani, A. R. (1991). Oral magnesium successfully relieves premenstrual mood changes. *Obstetrics and Gynecology, 78,* 177–181.

Freeman, E. W., Sondheimer, S., Weinbaum, P. H., & Rickels, K. (1985). Evaluating premenstrual symptoms in medical practice. *Obstetrics and Gynecology, 65,* 500–505.

Keye, W. R., Hammond, D. C., & Strong, T. (1986). Medical and psychological characteristics of women presenting with premenstrual symptoms. *Obstetrics and Gynecology, 86,* 634–637.

Mortola, J. F., Girton, L., Beck, L., & Yen, S. S. (1990). Diagnosis of premenstrual syndrome by a simple, prospective, and reliable instrument: The calendar of premenstrual experiences. *Obstetrics and Gynecolog, 76*, 302–307.

Ravnikar, V. A. (1990). Compliance with hormonal therapy. *American Journal of Obstetrics and Gynecolog, 156,* 1332–1334.

Smith, S., & Schiff, I. (Eds.). (1993). *Modern management of premenstrual syndrome.* New York: Grune and Stratton.

CHAPTER 15

Death and Dying

Anne A. Brewer and Joseph V. Connelly

Death and bereavement are universal experiences; however, working with the bereaved and dying challenges the innate denial of mortality that most people, including physicians, maintain. Furthermore, the very essence of the physician's work is healing to prevent suffering and death. For this reason, physicians may view the death of a patient as a personal failure and may distance themselves from the dying patient. Nonetheless, physicians are in a unique position to accompany their patients through these final, very painful experiences, particularly the primary care physician who has been the principal health care provider (often for many years) to many members of the patient's family.

Dealing with the dying and the bereaved is as emotionally and professionally challenging for the primary care physician as it is for everyone involved in the death. Because of the influential role the physician plays in the patient's life, he or she is in a unique position to bring comfort, understanding, and emotional support to the patient and the patient's family during this most difficult and painful period. This chapter will attempt to help physicians deal compassionately and competently with bereaved and dying persons. It provides an overview of attitudes and techniques that may be helpful in this challenging part of medical practice. Because some situations will warrant special psychosocial support, the chapter will offer guidelines to assist the physician in determining when a referral to a mental health professional may be appropriate.

COMMUNICATING BAD NEWS

One of the more difficult tasks for a physician is communicating bad news: the death of a loved one, the diagnosis of a life-threatening illness, or a grave prognosis. The way in which the physician handles this demanding task may influence how a family copes and adapts to grave news or grief or how a person copes with a life-threatening or terminal illness. The primary care physician is often the best person to convey this news because of the continuity and closeness of the physician-patient relationship. Even if the patient learns of the bad news from another source, the primary care physician may need to provide education, care, and support.

The physician must be adequately prepared to deliver bad news. Also, he or she must be attentive to the setting in which the news is conveyed, how the news is to be delivered, and the necessary follow-up care to the patient or family members. For example, communicating with a family after a sudden or unexpected death requires an approach that may be somewhat different from that used to convey a diagnosis of terminal or grave illness.

Physician Preparation for Delivering Bad News

Physicians need to prepare for conveying bad news in several ways. They first need to gather all the available facts. In the case of a sudden death, data collection includes reviewing prehospital and hospital care, assembling diagnostic information, and being prepared to answer family questions about the patient's care and the last moments before death. In cases in which a terminal or grave illness is suspected or diagnosed, the physician should review available data on the patient's condition and research treatment options.

Physicians also should be prepared for the various ways in which patients and family members respond emotionally to bad news. Some people react in a numb way, particularly at first. Others may be stoic or hostile, whereas others may be very distraught. In allowing patients and families time to express strong feelings that may be present, the physician may facilitate their assimilation of the bad news and their coping. On some occasions, the family or individual emotional responses may be so strong as to constitute a crisis, and the physician will need to employ techniques described in chapter 17, Crisis Intervention in Office Practice. Patients or families with a history of substance abuse or other antisocial features may be particularly volatile. The physician should be prepared for the rare occasion when a severe emotional reaction or physical violence is a possibility. If such reactions are anticipated, the physician should arrange in advance for assistance from other staff members or even police or security officers. See chapter 7, Violence and Suicide, for strategies for managing such violent encounters.

The physician may also have to go through his or her own psychological preparation to deliver bad news in the most effective way. When possible, physicians should plan to deliver bad news when they are rested and are not pressured for time. Physicians have to decide their own comfort level of personal emotional expression and should mentally rehearse what, where, when, and how they will convey the bad news.

The Setting

The setting in which bad news is conveyed is important. A location that is quiet, private, and comfortable is preferable, one in which physicians, patient, and/or family are seated at the same level with no barriers such as a desk between them. Delivering bad news in a hallway or in the middle of a crowded, busy emergency room adds stress to an already difficult situation. It is essential to allow adequate time and to schedule a convenient time for the discussion with the patient and family. In an office setting, it may be best to see the patient or family before a lunch break or at the end of the day to allow more time for discussion and care. In many situations, having the family accompany a patient or drawing together the family's support network (extended family, close friends, or clergy) may facilitate the discussion and provide support. In cases in which the physician is not fluent in the language of patient or family, he or she should arrange to have an interpreter present.

Delivering Bad News

The manner in which bad news is conveyed is extremely important. It is not unusual for patients or families to recount, years later, bitter tales of how a physician delivered bad news in an offhanded or callous manner. The beginning of the discussion, except in an emergency situation, should explore what the person and/or family wish to know and what they already know and fear. The physician should attempt to soften the bad news by revealing information in stages. This can begin by asking the patient what he or she suspects. The physician can then express concern about how the patient has been feeling and/or concern about the results of a diagnostic test. For example, a verbal warning shot such as "I'm concerned about your biopsy report . . . it suggests a tumor " is preferable to the bluntness of "You have cancer." Information should be provided in an honest, straightforward, and realistically hopeful manner, including acknowledgment of uncertainties that may exist. When giving bad news, the physician should also convey empathy and warmth while reassuring the patient and family that he or she will not abandon them in this grave situation. When it is appropriate, the physician can provide hope to the patient and family in terms of possibilities for further diagnostic workup or other treatment options. In this case, the physician needs to maintain hope while discussing the uncertainty about the diagnosis and the plans for further evaluation. When there is little hope for survival, the physician can offer continued care and support and reassurance that death will be as painless as possible.

During the discussion, the physician should encourage questions and answer them honestly. However, many patients are too overwhelmed with the news of a serious diagnosis to have many questions during the initial discussion. Physicians may need to schedule follow-up visits or phone calls to deal with questions that arise as people gradually assimilate the diagnosis and prognosis.

Near the end of the meeting, the physician should attempt to assess the understanding of the patient and the family and should review the information and plans for follow-up care. For some patients and their families, providing written information and instructions may be necessary to promote understanding. Physicians should anticipate that patients will not retain much of the information they receive at the first discussion. Having the family present may improve comprehension somewhat, but the emotional reaction to bad news may lessen everyone's ability to absorb information.

Conveying the news of the death of a family member or loved one encompasses many of the same elements as giving news of a terminal illness to a patient. However, some factors are different. Death may be sudden, or it may be expected. In either case, in the United States, it is most likely to occur in a hospital or nursing home. Whenever possible, news of a death in the family should be conveyed in person by the physician who has cared for the patient. If covering physicians, emergency room physicians, or nursing staff have been directly involved in the patient's care, delivering the news of a death may become their responsibility. In all these situations, attention to setting and method of delivering bad news is just as important as in the case of advising of terminal illness.

Follow-up

Patients and their families may require additional support following the delivery of bad news. The physician should make arrangements for necessary follow-up care or referrals. In most situations, particularly when the patient or the family is distraught, physicians should assume responsibility for arranging after care. Otherwise, the patient's or family's denial or strong emotional reactions may delay necessary ongoing medical care. Where there is hope, the physician should reinforce that message. Where death is the likely outcome, the physician should reassure the patient and family of his or her ongoing support and involvement and offer the hope of death with dignity.

STAGES OF COPING WITH TERMINAL ILLNESS

Elisabeth Kubler-Ross, in her seminal work *On Death and Dying* (1969), outlines five stages of dealing with terminal illness and death: denial, anger, bargaining, depression, and acceptance. She describes these stages based on her experiences in interviewing many terminally ill patients at a time when physicians generally regarded death as the ultimate enemy to be combated. Kubler-Ross characterized the movement of patients through these stages, not as a linear progression, but as a process in which patients may move back and forth between stages or experience several stages simultaneously during the course of their illnesses. Moreover, not all patients experience all five stages; some may remain in one stage until death.

Denial is the first experience of most people when they are confronted with the news of a terminal illness. Denial is characterized by the statement "This cannot be happening to me." It is usually present to some degree and can be damaging or helpful. If denial prevents reasonable medical care, pursuit of potentially beneficial treatment options, or causes the patient isolation from his or her social supports, it may be necessary to attempt to help a patient work through this maladaptive behavior. In some of cases of denial, referral for psychiatric consultations may be helpful. In other circumstances, such as sudden bad news, denial serves an important coping function. It temporarily protects the person from a reality that may be overwhelming, allowing additional time for other defenses to mobilize.

Anger usually surfaces when denial lessens, is no longer necessary, or cannot be maintained any longer. It is characterized by the statement "Why me, why not someone else?" Anger can be very intense, and it can be difficult for families and health care providers to manage it. It is often directed toward the self, the family, staff, clergy, or God. Expression of rage and resentment can alienate those close to a person at the very time that they are most needed. If the family or physician reacts to anger defensively, the patient may become angrier or more isolated. If, however, the patient can express the anger to a receptive listener, the anger may dissipate over time.

Bargaining often follows anger. It is characterized by the statement "What can I do, how can I behave, or what can I trade that will give me back my life?" Bargaining is often directed toward God. It is an attempt to postpone death, either as a reward for good behavior or to achieve a specific goal. Bargaining may progress to guilt if terminally ill patients feel they did not keep promises or if they regret past actions, for example, if they feel they should have loved their children more or expressed that love more readily.

Depressive symptoms are a normal experience of people facing terminal illness. These symptoms may involve grieving for losses caused by the disease (e.g., loss of physical beauty, energy, finances, and activities). Depressive symptoms also may involve anticipatory grief for the losses that the disease will cause for loved ones and loss of life itself. Both of these forms of grieving may be alleviated by receptive listening and psychological work with letting go and accepting the inevitability of death.

In some cases, depressive symptoms become a major depressive disorder. This form of clinical depression is not uncommon in the terminally ill; however, it should not be considered a normal part of the death and dying landscape. If a major depressive disorder occurs, it should be treated aggressively (see chapter 3, Depression), as it can adversely affect medical treatment, prognosis, and ultimate outcome of many terminal illnesses, including terminal heart disease, HIV infection, and many cancers.

Acceptance is the final stage of dealing with terminal illness. It is characterized by the statement "I am prepared to die and accept dying and death as a part of the natural order of living." Full acceptance of death is probably rare, but in some it is accompanied by a reaching out to loved ones, a heightened sense of spirituality, and a peace and contentment that come from a life well lived. In actuality, acceptance is often a combination of exhaustion and/or a delirium that appears as a resignation to death. Acceptance often can be characterized as "Leave me alone; I can't fight anymore." Resignation to death can be acceptance and may occur when a patient suffers with worsening weakness, chronic pain, overwhelming exhaustion, or withdrawal from interest in activities or people. However, it is important not to mistake the signs of untreated depression and a total loss of hope for acceptance.

These five stages are descriptive rather than prescriptive. Every person who deals with terminal illness is an individual with a unique history and web of relationships. Most people with terminal illnesses move in and out of the various stages over the course of the illness, and only some patients will ever attain true acceptance of death.

CARE OF THE DYING PATIENT

Care of the dying patient and the suffering associated with terminal illness can be very difficult for both patients and families. Effective care of the dying seeks to relieve suffering, ameliorate symptoms, and ease the transition for dying persons and their families. The suffering of a dying person can be physical, emotional, social, and spiritual, and care for the dying must address all these realms. A multidisciplinary approach, such as that employed in the hospice program, is often the most effective one.

The hallmark of hospice care is the focus on care and relief of symptoms instead of on cure. One of the most difficult aspects of caring for the dying, particularly with the powerful medical technology now available, is discerning when it is appropriate to shift from an emphasis on cure to an emphasis on care and relief of symptoms. Physicians, patients, and families struggle with this discernment, and conflicts often arise when different parties to the decision have different views of the situation.

Since Kubler-Ross published her book in 1969, there has been a resurgence of interest in palliative care. Hospice programs, mostly outpatient but some inpatient, have been organized in many communities. Laws have been passed to allow people to execute advanced directives for their care in a terminal situation. However, it is still not uncommon to see deaths in the intensive care unit, where the patients' pain and suffering was not optimally managed and medical interventions prolonged their dying without providing clear benefit.

Physical Aspects of Palliative Care

The physical suffering that accompanies terminal illness is often the most feared aspect of dying. Yet many physicians, concerned about addiction or audits from agencies that regulate controlled drugs, undermedicate pain in terminal illness. Concerns about addiction should not deter physicians from treating pain. The development of concentrated oral morphine, transdermal narcotic patches, and narcotic infusions that can be delivered in the outpatient setting have allowed many patients with severe pain to be cared for out of hospitals. Aggressive treatment of nausea, dyspnea, anorexia, itching, skin breakdown, and constipation can improve the quality of life of dying patients.

Psychological Aspects of Palliative Care

Attention to emotional and psychiatric issues is central to care for the dying patient. Although depressive symptoms are a common experience as persons journey toward death, treatment of major depressive disorders often improves the quality of life for dying patients. It is not always easy to distinguish between depression, which is one of the stages of moving toward death, and major depressive disorder, which warrants treatment. However, depression that is accompanied by such vegetative signs as insomnia and anorexia or by atypical signs such as hypersomnia and weight gain or by suicidal ideation usually responds to treatment with antidepressants and/or psychotherapy. (See chapter 3, Depression, for a fuller discussion). Physicians sometimes do not treat depression in terminally ill patients, believing that the patient has good reason to be depressed. They thus miss the opportunity to improve the quality of life for the dying person and in some cases overlook chances to extend life.

Other psychiatric conditions that occur frequently during the dying process are anxiety and insomnia. These should be treated aggressively with no concern about possible habituation (e.g., to anxiolytics). Stress reduction and relaxation techniques may provide additional benefits (see chapter 2, Anxiety Disorders).

Delirium may occur during the course of terminal illness, and this may be distressing for both the patient and the family. As in any other situation in which delirium occurs, the physician should undertake a vigorous search for the medical causes of delirium. An exception to this precept is the final phase of terminal illness in which use of psychotropic medications may be appropriate without an exhaustive medical evaluation (see chapter 5, Psychiatric Symptoms Due to Medical Illness).

Social Aspects of Palliative Care

Care of the dying patient must address the needs of the family or social unit in which the person lives. Terminal illness places a great deal of stress on those who are caring for the dying patient. If this stress exceeds the capacity of the family, the caregiving system will break down. Many caregivers feel guilty if they take time for themselves, and some terminally ill persons resist receiving care from outsiders. However, if a terminal illness is lengthy, caregivers may not be able to sustain the care that is needed, and a crisis may arise as a result. Respite care, whether through home nursing agencies, hospice volunteers, or short-term hospital or nursing home placement, may allow families to continue to care for the ill family member. Physicians need to discuss self-care with families, especially the primary caregivers, and offer family support and counseling when indicted (see chapter 18, Family Counseling).

Early in the course of a terminal illness, after the patient and the family have assimilated the diagnosis and before physical and psychological deterioration is far advanced, it is appropriate to address the issue of end-of-life care. Advance directives offer patients a way to make their wishes known and to facilitate their care at the end of life or if a crisis arises. Patients may execute documents giving family members durable power of attorney for health care decisions as well as for financial affairs. These discussions, though often difficult for patients, families, and physicians, can prevent inappropriate interventions that are contrary to the person's wishes and prevent future family disagreements about end-of-life care. It is not uncommon for families to panic if the dying person becomes severely dyspneic, for example. If clear do not resuscitate (DNR) orders are not in place, which may include special bracelets for persons who request DNR, the emergency medical system is obliged to transport the person to a hospital and apply advanced life support measures. Instead of a peaceful death, the patient and family are subjected to a chaotic transfer and emergency room experience.

The issue of advanced directives may need to be discussed with the person and the family repeatedly during the course of an illness. When there is a major change in the person's condition, the type of care that is appropriate may change as well.

An 87-year-old man was admitted to a nursing home with a primary diagnosis of Alzheimer's dementia. He had discussed advanced directives with his daughter early in the course of his illness, so DNR orders were written when he was admitted. Six months later, he had an episode of pneumonia for which he was hospitalized and treated with intravenous antibiotics. One month later, he was rehospitalized and treated for pneumonia after having aspirated food. After this hospitalization, the physician discussed with his daughter the change in his condition. She decided not to have a feeding tube inserted and not to rehospitalize him again. A few weeks later, he developed recurrent aspiration pneumonia and died peacefully in the nursing home.

The setting in which death occurs has changed over the course of this century. At the turn of the century, many deaths occurred at home. After World War II, most deaths occurred in hospitals, particularly with the advent of more powerful medical technology. In the last 20 years, there has been a shift back to the home or nursing home as the setting for death. The hospice movement has strongly influenced this shift by providing programs and support that make it possible for families to care for dying persons at home. Hospice also provides respite care in a nursing home or hospital to assist families. The hospice approach provides the option for hospitalization for terminal care if the patient's symptoms become unmanageable at home.

Hospice care, whether in the home, the nursing home, or the hospital, focuses on comfort and relief of symptoms. Medical and nursing interventions that are usually routine, such as vital signs and blood drawing, are often omitted when they do not directly contribute to the person's comfort. The focus of care is shifted to relief of symptoms such as pain, nausea, dyspnea, and anxiety. If a person has been cared for in a nursing home, it is often appropriate for the patient to be cared for in a familiar environment during the terminal phase of an illness. Many nursing homes have developed expertise in terminal care. There are also free-standing hospice facilities that may be options for some patients.

Spiritual Aspects of Terminal Care

From the beginning, the hospice movement, with its focus on the care of the whole person, has included spiritual care. Recent interest in spirituality within the medical profession has widened this focus. Some terminally ill patients have a strong connection with a spiritual community, which may provide support and participation in religious rituals. Dying persons can be encouraged to maintain their spiritual practices, reconnect with their religious community, or enhance or develop a new spiritual connection. Other patients may have no present or past religious or spiritual connection and may prefer a psychological approach to dying. Terminal illness raises profound questions about the meaning of life and death, what happens after death, and the purpose and accomplishments of one's life. These spiritual issues often affect a patient, and reconnection with the spiritual aspects of living can be a source of comfort.

> A man with terminal cancer was receiving care from a hospice team in his home. He had been estranged from his church for many years. The hospice nurse noted that he was extremely anxious and seemed to feel guilty about events in his past. He was encouraged to contact the priest in his parish, and the hospice nurse spoke with the priest before he visited the patient. After the priest's visit, the man was much less anxious and died peacefully a few weeks later.

Hospice Care

Hospice care has benefited many terminally ill patients. Although it is usually associated with cancer, the principles of hospice care can be applied to most terminal illnesses. Hospice care addresses the physical, emotional, social, and spiritual needs of terminally ill persons. Most programs have an interdisciplinary team, including physicians, nurses, social workers, mental health professionals, pharmacists, chaplains, and volunteers. The team works with the patient, the family, and the physician in the care of the patient.

Most hospice programs offer care to persons with terminal illnesses whose life expectancy is limited (usually less than 6 months). The Medicare hospice benefit requires a physician's statement that the prognosis is less than 6 months, although patients may remain on the hospice benefit if they survive longer than 6 months. Most hospice programs require that patients have chosen not to pursue aggressive therapies for their disease, although therapy for symptom relief is considered part of hospice care. This may include radiation and chemotherapy for some oncology patients.

Referral to a hospice program is appropriate for any patient with an illness that is expected to cause death within a limited time. Diagnoses for which hospice care may be indicated include cancer; AIDS; cardiac, pulmonary, cerebrovascular, renal, and liver diseases; and dementia. Hospice care can be most helpful to patients and families if it is begun early in the terminal phase of a patient's illness. Early referral allows the hospice team to assess needs, develop plans of care, and build relationships with the patient and the family.

For many patients and families, hospice care allows a better quality of life during the dying process. Not only does this relieve the suffering of the patient, but it also aids the family in caring for the patient and in the bereavement process, which may prevent pathological grief reactions.

Ethical Concerns in the Care of Dying Patients

Ethical issues in the care of the dying have been publicly debated, particularly in the areas of euthanasia and physician-assisted suicide. These issues sometimes have obscured broader ethical issues that are relevant to care of the dying. Issues include withdrawing and withholding care, futile care, physician-assisted suicide, and euthanasia. It is important to distinguish among them, because some of the debates have lumped all ethical issues under the rubric of euthanasia. This lack of distinction may push families, patients, and physicians into actions that may not be desirable or beneficial to the patient.

> A 78-year-old woman resided in a nursing home after a series of cerebrovascular accidents had left her aphasic, unresponsive, and hemiparetic. Because of her inability to swallow, a gastrostomy tube was inserted for feeding. She was hospitalized repeatedly for recurrent episodes of aspiration pneumonia despite the feeding tube. Her sister requested that she not be rehospitalized when another episode of pneumonia occurred. The physician replied that by not hospitalizing her he would be killing her. He said he would continue to treat the patient only if the family agreed to hospitalize her if she again developed pneumonia. During the next hospitalization, the feeding tube fell out and the sister refused permission for reinsertion. Under the physician recommendation, the original nursing home refused to readmit her unless the feeding tube was reinserted. The patient was eventually discharged to another nursing home without a feeding tube, where she died uneventfully 2 weeks later.

This case demonstrates the confusion in the physician who equated withdrawal of care (no feeding tube) with euthanasia. It also demonstrates the negative consequences to a family when this distinction is not clearly made.

One of the principles of medical ethics is autonomy, the right of an individual to accept or refuse treatment. Any competent patient may decline treatment even when medical personnel believe that treatment would benefit the patient. If a patient is unable to make decisions, a family member or other close person may be deputed to make those decisions in the patient's stead. Direction can be given to decision makers through the instruments known as living wills, health care proxies, or advance directives.

During the course of many illnesses, the time arrives when aggressive medical care is not likely to bring a cure or further benefit the patient. This point in the care often occurs either because the side effects of treatment are too severe or because the disease will not respond to further treatment. In patients with chronic debilitating illnesses, intercurrent illnesses, such as aspiration pneumonia, often precipitate the need for this decision-making process, as described in the case above. In many of these situations, withdrawing or withholding care, even when death may eventuate, may be in the patient's best interest. Withdrawing or withholding care is not the same as euthanasia. Physician-assisted suicide or euthanasia causes a death that otherwise would not have occurred at that time. Withdrawal of care is ceasing combat against a disease and allowing the disease process to follow its natural course. Many common medical treatments, including antibiotics, intravenous fluids, feeding tubes, dialysis, surgery, ventilators, and CPR, may be withdrawn or withheld if they do not offer benefit to the patient.

Physician-assisted suicide and euthanasia have been the subject of much debate in recent years. Many advocates of these measures regard them as the ultimate expression of patient autonomy, particularly in situations where suffering is extreme. Opponents of these measures consider them unjustified killing or murder. Many practitioners of palliative care view the debate as a distraction from other issues. The ethical, political, and legal debate undoubtedly will continue. The consensus of most physicians is that physician-assisted suicide and euthanasia generally conflict with another principle of medical ethics, nonmaleficence (not causing harm).

Regulatory and Administrative Issues for Physicians

Physicians are charged by the state with the task of determining death and the cause of death. Cause of death, which is recorded on the death certificate, helps public health authorities track patterns of disease to improve the health of the community. Death certificates generally list immediate cause of death, the chain of events that led to the death, and other illnesses that existed but did not immediately cause death.

Determination of death is the physician's responsibility. In many states, this responsibility may be delegated to nurses, especially for deaths that are anticipated to occur outside the hospital (nursing homes and hospice patients). In general, the determination of death is made by noting absence of pulse and respiration. In some instances, death may also be determined by absence of EEG activity, usually in cases of an accident or cerebral catastrophe or when organ donation is contemplated.

In some situations, the cause of death may be unclear to the physician or the family. In such cases, an autopsy may be helpful. An autopsy may be mandated by state law in certain situations, such as sudden, unexpected deaths and deaths where there is a question of homicide or suicide. These autopsies, which may have legal ramifications, are performed by the medical examiner.

BEREAVEMENT

Bereavement, the loss of a loved one, is the most powerful stressor that most people ever experience. It affects all aspects of functioning: physical, emotional, spiritual, and social. The emotions produced by bereavement are among the most painful known to human beings. Although the expression and social organization of bereavement vary across cultures, bereavement is a universal phenomenon.

Normal Grief

Although bereavement has been experienced and described from biblical times, the systematic study of grief began with the work of Lindemann (1944). Uncomplicated, or "normal," grief, begins with shock, numbness, and disbelief at the news of a death (Osterweiss, Solomon, & Green, 1987). These normal grief responses occur whether a death was expected or unexpected. At this point, the reality of the loss has not yet set in, and the bereaved may appear to be functioning well. As the reality of the loss is felt, numbness gives way to intense waves of painful emotions of loss. The bereaved may experience physical symptoms with somatic distress, fatigue, exhaustion, insomnia, changes in appetite, gastrointestinal symptoms, somatic pain, and involuntary sighing. Bereaved persons frequently present to a primary care physician with illnesses, such as bronchitis or gastric pain, that may be slow to resolve. They may experience an altered mental state described as numbness, shock, unreality, or a distance or depersonalization from the world. Behavioral symptoms may include sobbing, screaming, and/or periods of intense sadness that are often experienced in waves of great intensity. These mood swings are often accompanied by anger, irritability, anxiety, and guilt. Some patients experience intense dreams or sensations of seeing the deceased, which may represent the attempt to find or reconnect with the lost person. In most patients the physical manifestations of grief are resolved in approximately 6 weeks (Lindemann, 1944). Psychological symptoms with or without depressive mood swings may last from several months to more than a year.

Eventually, except in cases of pathological grief, the bereaved are able to resume normal behavioral functioning quickly and to incorporate the loss into their lives. Many survivors describe a "hole" in their lives that never goes away, although the acute pain of the loss abates.

The process of grief, like the process of dying, is not linear. Bereaved persons move in and out of the various stages of the process for many months, even years. The time course of normal grief varies, from a few months to years, depending on the circumstances of the loss, the ambivalence in the relationship, and/or the closeness of the relationship.

Bereavement in children and adolescents differs in some ways from bereavement in adults. Young children, who do not understand the finality of death, may not express grief verbally but may demonstrate somatic or behavioral manifestations, such as sleep or eating disturbance, enuresis, and aggressive or withdrawn behavior. School-age children and adolescents may react with school problems, depression, aggression, or withdrawal. The presence of a reliable caregiver and social supports may assist children and adolescents in coping with their grief.

Pathological Grief

It is not always easy to distinguish between normal and pathological grief. The time course of grief varies, and the feelings that surface may be intense. However, if any of the stages of grief remain unresolved over a period of time and there is persistent social or occupational dysfunction, the grief reaction may be pathological. For example, depressed mood, tearfulness, difficulties with concentration, and sleep disturbances occur in normal grief. If these symptoms do not lessen over time, or if suicidal ideation, psychosis, intense somatic preoccupation, or progressive withdrawal and loss of function occur, a major depressive disorder may be present.

Management of Grief

Primary care physicians who care for many or all members of a family may provide assistance to families experiencing grief. Physicians can explain that the patient's physical symptoms are grief related and reassure them that an acute grief reaction is not "going crazy." Other sources of support for bereaved persons are friends, family, clergy, support groups, and mental health professionals. A referral for psychiatric consultation is warranted if the patient requests it, if the physician suspects pathological grief, or if there is evidence of suicidal ideation or psychosis.

Physicians are often asked to provide medication for bereaved persons, especially those in the midst of acute grief. Often the request is made by other people who are distressed by the acute pain of the bereaved. Sleep medications, such as zolpidem tartrate (Ambien), 10 to 20 mg hs, may be utilized judiciously. Overmedication with other sedative-hypnotic medications may blunt the acute grief reaction or may interfere with grief resolution. If symptoms are persistent or if the patient is dysfunctional and headed toward depression, antidepressant medication may be used to prevent severe social or occupational dysfunction.

For many bereaved people, referral to a peer support group can be helpful, particularly in the later stages of the grief process when the bereaved person is facing the task of reconstructing his or her life. Access to others who have "been there" may provide reassurance, emotional support, and practical advice in dealing with bereavement. Most hospice programs and other agencies, hospitals, and mental health professionals offer bereavement support groups. Some bereaved persons also benefit from books that describe experiences of grief (Cain, 1974; Curry, 1990; Lewis, 1961).

DEATH OF A CHILD

The death of a child raises all the issues of grief described above, as well as particular issues for bereaved parents. Pregnancy loss, whether through miscarriage or stillbirth, can result in profound grief. The grief is usually proportional to the duration of the pregnancy and/or the amount of bonding that has already taken place. Even early miscarriages, particularly of desired pregnancies, can be experienced by parents as a very traumatic loss. It is often helpful to caution women who have miscarried to ignore the acute advice often given by well-meaning friends or relatives: "You can always have another child." Once mourning has occurred, a new attempt at childbirth may again be possible.

The death of a child from Sudden Infant Death Syndrome (SIDS) or by other means represents an acute trauma for parents and may also represent the potential loss of the future of being a parent. SIDS deaths are particularly distressing, as parents are often under suspicion or investigation for the child's death. Referral to a SIDS support group or mental health professionals may assist parents in coping with their grief. This is particularly important if the parents are temporarily dysfunctional or if there are other children in the family whose needs may be overlooked during the parents' grief.

UNNATURAL DEATH

Compared with natural death, "unnatural" death often produces more prolonged and complicated bereavement. Unnatural death is characterized by violence, violation, or volition (Rynearson 1987). Violence can be the result of accident, natural disaster, or human action. Violation involves disfigurement or other severe damage to the human being. Volition can be directed toward self (suicide) or other (homicide) or may be the result of human error or negligence. These unnatural deaths are usually sudden and involve a disproportionate number of young people.

Physicians who care for survivors of unnatural death should be alert to the likelihood of complicated or pathological bereavement, PTSD, major depression, or other anxiety disorders. When appropriate, referrals should be made to mental health specialists. Support groups may also provide benefit for survivors. Many survivors also become involved in political or social action to prevent future deaths (i.e., advocating gun control after a loved one has been killed by a firearm or working against drunk driving after a child has been killed by a drunk driver).

PHYSICIAN REACTION TO DEATH AND BEREAVEMENT

Medical education generally focuses on mastery of medical and technical information, with less attention paid to psychological reactions to illness, death, and bereavement. Detachment, which may be a necessary part of clinical decision making, may be misinterpreted by patients as impassiveness or lack of caring. Excessive physician detachment may defend against the fear of death that most people experience, medically trained or not.

Physicians risk burnout or being perceived as cold or lack of caring if they do not recognize their own grief, touch the emotional experience of their patients, and find appropriate ways to deal with their own emotions.

Few physicians can care for a patient, particularly for long periods of time, without feeling a sense of connection with him or her. When a patient dies, the physician experiences a loss and should expect to feel some grief. Attending wakes or funerals of patients who have died is one way of expressing that grief. Most families feel honored when a physician attends a funeral or wake. Writing sympathy letters or sending cards can also express the physician's grief and help families in their bereavement.

The universal experiences of death and bereavement challenge physicians to care for patients and families in an empathic manner and to appreciate our common humanity. As physicians accept their own mortality, they have the opportunity to form close ties with patients and families at pivotal times in their lives.

REFERENCES

Cain, L. (1974). *Widow.* New York: William Morrow.

Curry, C. L. (1990). *When your spouse dies.* Notre Dame, IN: Ave Maria Press.

Kubler-Ross, Elisabeth (1969). *On death and dying.* New York: Macmillan.

Lewis, C. S. (1961). *A grief observed.* New York: Seabury Press.

Lindemann, E. (1944). Symptomatology and management of acute grief. *American Journal of Psychiatry, 101,* 141–148.

Osterweiss, M., Solomon, F., & Green, M. (1987). Bereavement reactions, consequences, and care. In S. Zisook (Ed.), *Biopsychosocial aspects of bereavement* (pp. 3–18). Washington, DC: American Psychiatric Press.

Rynearson, E. K. (1987). Psychological adjustment to unnatural dying. In S. Zisook (Ed.), *Biopsychosocial aspects of bereavement* (pp. 77–93). Washington, DC: American Psychiatric Press.

PART 3

Psychosocial Treatments in Primary Care

CHAPTER 16

Consulting and Counseling in Primary Care

Leslie Prusnofsky and Robert E. Feinstein

This chapter focuses on the nonpsychiatric patient entering the primary care physician's office for treatment of a medical complaint. The etiology of a medical complaint can be primarily biological, psychological, or social, or most commonly, a mixture of all three. The purpose of this chapter is to provide an aid to the primary care physician who seeks to incorporate some sophisticated techniques in counseling as a portion of his or her primary care role. The chapter will provide an overview of (1) patient-physician interaction utilizing a Balint (1964) model, (2) physician readiness for psychological counseling, (3) counseling goals for the primary care physician, (4) practical aspects of office-based counseling, (5) performing a psychological assessment, and (6) a description of four office-based counseling approaches.

THE PATIENT, THE PHYSICIAN, AND THE PATIENT'S SYMPTOMS

The patient comes to the primary care physician with the expectation of treatment and relief from medical symptoms and suffering. The patient has a conscious wish for the physician to accomplish this task; however, there may also be an unconscious fear or wish on the part of the patient that this will not happen. The patient rarely presents expressing his or her underlying emotional pain. The physician has to elicit this. Without realizing it, the patient ultimately relies on the ability of the primary care physician to recognize his or her psychological difficulties adjusting to or coping with a medical illness or its sequelae. Patients may also be suffering and seeking help for unrecognized problems, such as affective, anxiety, personality, and psychotic disorders, as common comorbid entities that can present simultaneously with medical complaints. It is important for the physician to remember the maxim that if you do not think of psychological issues or psychiatric conditions, you cannot diagnose or treat them.

The psychological interaction between doctor and patient was described by Balint (1964) as a four-step process:

1. *Patient offers an illness.* The patient presents to the physician with symptoms or complaints for which the patient has a tentative explanation. Often the patient has a fear of some horrible illness, such as cancer or AIDS, or perhaps a belief that he or she has a hereditary illness. The patient begins his or her encounter with the physician with certain core beliefs as to the cause and meaning of the symptoms.
2. *Physician's view of the patient's illness.* The physician has his or her view of the patient's complaints and symptoms and brings to the interaction his or her core beliefs (based on the physician's medical knowledge and personal bias) about the nature of the patient's medical complaints.
3. *Compromise.* One of the many roles of the primary care physician is to offer a compromise between the patient's and physician's views of the problem. One conception of this process has been described as informed shared decision making (see Chapter 13, A Model for Office-based Cardiovascular Risk Reduction and Behavioral Change). If the patient and the doctor reach a common understanding of the problem, the doctor-patient interaction proceeds smoothly. However, more often than not, the patient and the physician either partially agree or do not agree as to the cause of the symptoms. This discord is especially likely when the doctor finds no clear physical illness. The physician may either tell the patient nothing is physically wrong or, alternatively, tell the patient there is a psychological component to the illness or an undiagnosed psychiatric problem causing the medical symptoms. Patients who are

psychologically inclined either already suspect this or are willing to proceed with further exploration into the psychological component of their symptoms. Other patients may be offended by the suggestion that psychological issues are either important or predominantly responsible for their symptoms. In this group of patients, the process of working with the mind and body together is precisely the function of counseling in primary care.

4. *Consequences*. The consequences of the patient/physician agreement or disagreement as to the cause of the patient's symptoms are well known. Agreement often leads to improved patient-physician interaction and satisfaction, improved medical care, improved adherence to medical diagnostics or treatment recommendation, and better medical outcomes. Disagreement between patient and the physician can lead to patient and physician dissatisfaction, malpractice lawsuits, poor diagnostics and treatment, and less than desired outcomes.

PHYSICIAN READINESS FOR CONSULTING AND COUNSELING

Many primary care physicians do not see counseling as part of their daily office practice work, yet they often perform these functions without formal education in advanced psychotherapeutic techniques. Formal preparation for primary care counseling begins with an acknowledgment that counseling tasks are valuable and require skills that need to be learned, just like other medical procedures. The physician has to be prepared to work to develop and improve these skills to counsel effectively and should be prepared to spend additional time with some patients to be able to perform patient assessment and counseling.

In addition to acquiring counseling skills, the physician needs to be aware that his or her attitudes affect his or her ability to empathize with patients. Nonverbal as well as verbal communication can affect the work. Facial expressions reflecting emotions other than those being verbalized can be disconcerting to a patient who expects the physician to be forthright in his or her feelings. Preparedness for transference and countertransference reactions with the patient is also essential when counseling patients. This is especially helpful when doing more interpretive work (described later in this chapter) and when deciding if referral to a mental health specialist is indicated.

Physician attitudes toward the time pressure of counseling are important in a busy office setting. Physicians often feel that open-ended questioning can make an office visit prohibitively long. However, it has been shown that taking the time to allow patients to more fully express themselves, without being overly directed, does not lead to longer meetings. In fact, a period of open-ended questions can save time in the long run by providing the primary care physician with more accurate and patient-specific information, leading to earlier planning and better problem resolution (Frankel, Morse, Suchman, & Beckman, 1991). Self-reflection and the use of one's staff as auxiliary cotherapists can be helpful in the refining of one's counseling skills. It takes time and experience to develop the skills necessary to form a therapeutic alliance and to negotiate with difficult patients, as does obtaining and delivering information, which can include clarifications, confrontations, interpretations, and education. As one becomes more experienced, ease and facility in using these skills will allow for more expedient office interactions with patients. (See chapter 8, Personality Disorders in Office Practice, for definitions and an application of these psychotherapeutic interventions.)

PHYSICIAN ROLES: CONSULTANT OR COUNSELOR?

Physician as Consultant or Patient Educator

Does the physician see himself or herself as a consultant and patient educator with a particular patient, or does the patient need a counselor to foster psychological intervention? When a physician assumes the role of consultant, the patient primarily owns and controls the process of patient-physician interaction. The patient uses the physician as an expert consultant in what has been called a consumerist type of interaction. When consulting, the roles of patient and physician are equal and limited, but they are different. The patient seeks information about his or her illness or wants help with a specific medical concern. The patient will receive information, is not obligated to accept it, may not attempt to achieve a specific goal, and may not want or seek to continue a therapeutic relationship. The physician encourages the patient to discuss the problem, makes clear what the patient needs to know, and explains what he or she can offer to the patient (Street & Downey, 1996). The physician supplies the patient with medical information and may set out diagnostic treatment options, discuss long-term prognosis, or offer psychosocial opinions or advice. The consultation model can stand alone for one office visit, can be a prelude for other consultations, or may progress to counseling.

Physician as Counselor

As a counselor, the primary care physician's perspective is to help the patient achieve goals in a more open-ended process. In the counseling model, the process is initiated by the client, but the counseling process is jointly shared and controlled. The primary care physician assumes the role of the expert, and the patient is in a dependent role (Street & Downey, 1996) as the one seeking help. The physician needs to decide if he or she can experience satisfaction in counseling in the primary care setting, or, alternatively, if he or she prefers simply to identify the need for psychological intervention and refer the patient to a mental health specialist.

The primary care physician who feels interest, satisfaction, and comfort in a counseling role must accept flexibility in the patient's participation. Ultimately, each physician must decide what type of role he or she can play as a counselor. Do the physician and the patient prefer a biomedical, narrowly biomedical, biopsychosocial, psychosocial, or consumerist role in counseling? (See chapter 13, A Model for Office-based Cardiovascular Risk Reduction and Behavioral Change, for a discussion of these models.) Each physician has to be aware of his or her own counseling style and preference but, at the same time, must be able to utilize all styles to be better able to counsel a variety of patients. The physician also has to be intuitive regarding the patient's preference for interviewing style, as this may affect how a patient can best accept counseling. A recent study (Roter et al., 1997) revealed that patient satisfaction was highest with a psychosocial style of interviewing, whereas physician satisfaction was highest with the consumerist model. Physicians pursuing optimal counseling effectiveness will have to make this clinical decision on a case-by-case basis.

Different patients will need different counseling styles, and sometimes the same patient may need a different approach. Depending on the nature, severity, and immediacy of the problem, the primary care physician's flexibility in being more or less active or directive will help determine the therapeutic alliance with the patient. The physician needs to have clear goals for counseling sessions and should decide individually his or her goals for what is acceptable counseling in the office setting.

Consulting and Counseling Goals for the Primary Care Physician

The general goals of consulting and counseling in a primary care setting are listening, understanding, and having a therapeutic impact that creates the desired change. Each physician must make a personal choice as to what is acceptable consulting and counseling in the office setting and should determine in advance how flexible he or she wants to be when offering help to a patient. Following are some patient-specific goals for consulting (numbers 1 to 5 below) and counseling (numbers 1 to 10 below).

1. Learn about the meaning of the patient's symptoms.
2. Understand the patient's medical illness from his or her point of view.
3. Assess the patient for psychosocial problems that are interfering with medical care.
4. Explore in greater depth the possibility of psychiatric diagnoses and/or suggest psychological treatment and/or psychiatric medications when appropriate.
5. Discuss treatment options.
6. Focus with the patient on the solution to one specific psychological or psychosocial problem at a time.
7. Work through the problem in a limited number of sessions.
8. Discuss the success, partial success, or failure of the counseling.
9. Decide whether or not to continue the counseling to work through a second problem.
10. Decide when to end counseling or when to refer to a mental health specialist.

Practical Aspects of Consulting and Counseling

Time

There is limited time for consulting and counseling in the primary care physician's office. Sessions generally run in multiples of fifteen minutes. 15 minutes is often adequate for patient assessments or consulting, and even limited counseling can sometimes be accomplished in this period. For more extensive counseling, the physician can exercise an option to double-book a patient for a 30-minute session or can schedule a longer counseling meeting during the last time slot of the morning or afternoon session. Some primary care physicians with a real interest in counseling can set aside additional counseling time on a once-per-week or monthly basis, which is structured into the weekly or monthly office schedule. Office-based counseling with any complexity is practically impossible if scheduled during a regular office session.

Setting

Patient assessment, identification of the psychological problem, and consulting or counseling require an interactive setting conducive to this process. The physician needs to greet the patient in a professionally friendly manner, making good eye contact. If possible, any chart material should be read before seeing the patient to avoid physician distractions of writing or glancing at the chart and to maximize a conducive atmosphere for psychological exploration. The interview should be conducted in the physician's consultation room, not the examination room. Interviews should be face to face with few barriers (e.g., a desk) between patient and physician to give the patient a sense of concern, attention, and interest on the physician's part. Whenever possible, avoid interferences during the meeting by taking only emergency telephone calls. It is important to inform office staff not to interrupt these brief sessions.

Psychological Assessment

Identifying the Problem

Using all forms of observation to help identify the patient's problem is very important. As the patient attempts to communicate his or her history of present illness, the physician should take note of what is said; what information is omitted; the patient's affect, body language, and discrepancies among these; speech pattern and voice tone; gesticulations; and other verbal and nonverbal cues. This will help the physician assess the patient's emotional state (e.g., whether the patient is anxious, depressed, dissociated, or psychotic). Using a formal mental status examination may further improve the physician's observation skills.

The physician can use facilitating comments and gestures to encourage the progression of the assessment. Gentle, open-ended questioning, clarifying comments and questions, repeating back to the patient the assessed affect and tone, and simple nods of recognition show interest and communicate empathy to the patient while simultaneously facilitating the development of a therapeutic alliance.

The nonpsychiatric patient enters the primary care physician's office with a problem, usually describing medical symptoms. Using the above techniques, the primary care physician can seek out additional information and encourage the patient to describe the problem in his or her own words. Is this a medical problem creating emotional problems? Is this a medical problem due to emotional problems? What, if any, are the environmental issues: family, workplace, social settings, relationships? During the typical 15 to 30 minute meeting, these issues require only several minutes to ascertain. Depending on how the patient responds, the physician should determine the urgency of the situation and manage the case accordingly (see Figure 16.1)

Crisis or Emergency Situations

In a crisis situation (see chapter 17, Crisis Intervention in Office Practice), the primary care physician may be involved in temporary emergency management and may have to assume an authoritative role, using a narrow or expanded biomedical approach to obtain vital emergency information (e.g., pills taken in an overdose, source of pain, or investigation of other potential or immediate dangers). A medically ill, actively suicidal, or potentially violent patient usually requires crisis intervention by a mental health care provider to determine the patient's potential for self-harm or potential for harming others (see chapter 7, Violence and Suicide). If the patient can participate actively in his or her own care, the primary care physician may be able to proceed with a consultation, taking an advocacy position utilizing a biopsychosocial, psychosocial, or consumerist approach (Roter et al., 1997).

Acute Situation

The patient may present with an acute situation or problem without a sense of life-or-death emergency. This may be an acute but not immediately life-threatening medical problem or an acute emotional reaction to a new medical situation. The capacity for patient involvement in his or her care will help the physician determine the best intervention options for the patient. The patient may present with new symptoms, an acute change in health, a diagnosis of a severe or terminal illness, or acute, vague medical com-

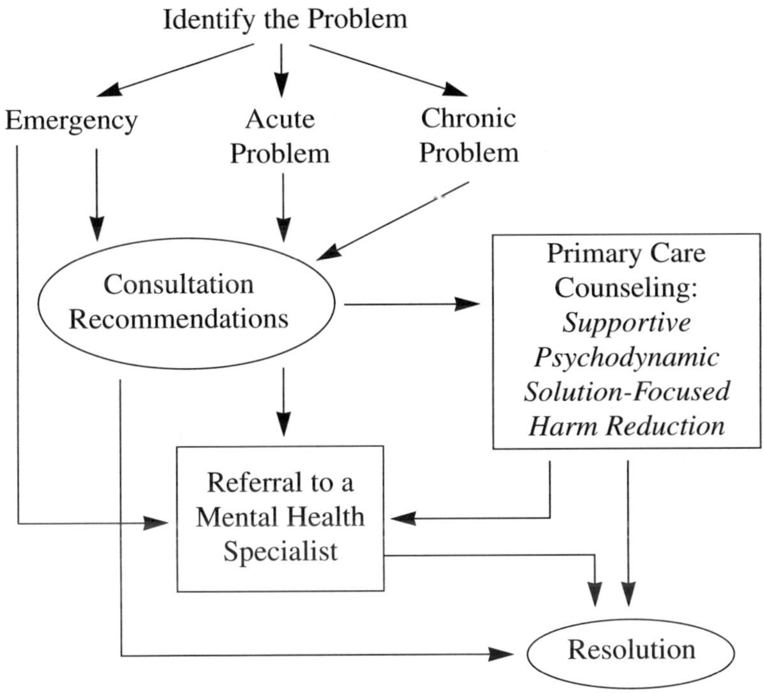

Figure 16.1 Evaluation and Treatment Options.

plaints with underlying worries about illness or impending loss of a loved one. He or she may need assistance with health-related lifestyle changes, a work or financial problem, changes in the home environment, or marital, child-rearing, or social problems. Medical problems can stir up fears about anticipated changes in one's internal or external environment. Emotional issues relating to dependency, separation anxiety, and loss may be at the core of many internal conflicts. Through counseling, the primary care physician may be able to alleviate emotional suffering and improve the overall health status of the patient in acute distress.

Chronic Problems

Often a patient suffers with a chronic medical condition and all the associated emotional and psychosocial sequelae. Chronic disorders such as coronary artery disease, diabetes, chronic obstructive pulmonary diseases, hypertension, chronic depression, renal failure/dialysis, HIV infection, breast or prostate cancer, and intractable pain are all conditions that may benefit from brief counseling by the primary care physician. Problems such as physical handicaps and disabilities; substance abuse, alcoholism, and other addictive behaviors; eating disorders; and gambling may also present the primary care physician with the possibility for psychological intervention.

Brief psychological interventions for chronic problems can focus on the following issues: (1) current symptoms; (2) updates and new information about changes in medical care or treatment; (3) understanding the patient's current adaptation to the chronic illness; (4) diagnosing, treating, or referring for treatment any comorbid psychiatric conditions that may be exacerbating the medical problem (depression, anxiety, eating disorders, somatoform disorders, etc.); (5) working psychologically with the patient to improve daily functioning by clarifying what is a medical limitation for the patient versus a psychological limitation; (6) developing an understanding of psychological conflicts affecting daily functioning; (7) working with the patient to improve his or her social support by involving family, friends, or a religious organizations; and (8) working with the patient to encourage him or her to accept external support from visiting nurses, social service agencies, or a community organization.

Gathering Psychological Data and Determining the Patient's Needs

The need for psychological interventions becomes apparent as the physician identifies the presence of an emergency, acute, or chronic emotional problem in the patient. The physician should collect preliminary psychological data via open-ended questions. Through this process the patient will offer valuable information. The physician may also have additional information about the patient from previous contacts or from prior contact with the patient's family or friends. The physician should try to gather psychological information that is most relevant to the patient's current problem. If the patient is seen only for brief office visits , it may take months or several years of such visits for the physician to gather the entire scope of a patient's psychological history and functioning. Alternatively, additional information may be obtained quickly if the physician is willing and able to have several longer assessment meetings.

The full scope of information that the primary care physician can obtain includes the following 12 domains:

1. What is the here-and-now experience of the patient's problem?
2. How much is this problem affecting the patient's current life?
3. How does the patient see himself or herself in the problem (e.g., contributing to it, victimized by it, or in control of it)?
4. Is the patient self-destructive, or is there a risk of violence?
5. What is the patient's history of problem solving? How has the patient handled similar problems before?
6. How does the patient typically deal with stress?
7. What is the nature of the patient's interpersonal relationships? Can the patient maintain relationships? How close, distant, dependent, or interdependent are they?
8. What is the developmental phase of the patient's current emotional functioning? Child, adolescent, and adult developmental levels present different psychosocial issues. For example, childhood/latency developmental issues may invoke conflicts about trust, autonomy, initiative, and self-esteem; adolescent developmental issues may focus on identity development and separation; adult developmental issues focus on intimacy, competition, productivity, and integration; late-life issues may revolve around the integrity of one's life, despair, and/or decline (Erikson, 1980).
9. What is the defensive structure of the patient? Does the patient use the high-level functioning of a neurotic personality structure or the more primitive defense mechanisms of a borderline or psychotic personality organization? (See chapter 8, Personality Disorders in Office Practice, for a discussion of personality levels.)
10. What is the patient's support system (spouse, family, friends, etc.) and his or her interactions within that system? Are the main support members aware of the patient's problem and empathic, angry, or psychologically attuned to helping the patient?
11. What is the quality of the patient's interaction with others (e.g., dependent, in need of the sick role, fearful of separations, or needing to isolate and withdraw)?
12. What is the transference reaction (see chapter 8, Personality Disorders in Office Practice) to the primary care physician? Is the reaction to the primary care physician developing positively with a working alliance, or is there a negative reaction to the primary care physician, with a corresponding sense of defiance, rebellion, or resistance?

Therapeutic Sequence

The flow of therapeutic assessment and treatment options are outlined in Figure 16.1. After the first brief psychological assessment, a preliminary treatment plan should be made. Emergencies or crises should be handled first (see chapter 7, Violence and Suicide, and chapter 17, Crisis Intervention in Office Practice). The next decision is whether to take a consulting or counseling approach. Often the consulting approach is chosen initially and may or may not progress to counseling. The consulting approach results in problem identification, education about the problem, an understanding of the patient's efforts to date to solve the problem, and a discussion of treatment options for resolution of the problem. After the consultation, the physician's role with problem solving may be complete. Some patients may want to progress to brief counseling sessions, in which the physician is an active participant with the patient in problem resolution.

Brief Counseling: Overview

Brief counseling is time-limited psychotherapy (usually 2 to 20 sessions) that the primary care physician can use when the need for psychological intervention has been agreed upon (Flegenheimer, 1982). In primary care settings, the workup of a medical problem or a troublesome medical diagnosis can create an acute emotional response that will precipitate the need for counseling. Fear of losing one's ability to function, one's independence and mobility, and one's relationships with loved ones may require rapid physician intervention (Druss, 1995). Understanding the patient's history of handling stress, at what level and the extent to which psychological defensive structures are used, the quality of past and present relationships, and the ability for psychological insights can lead the primary care physician to useful counseling approaches that can help the patient have a better outcome and prognosis or can allow for a less tumultuous, emotionally painful life experience.

In brief counseling one is dealing with the release of feelings, both conscious and unconscious. The primary care physician can help the patient explore ambivalent feelings and the duality of these feelings. The patient may express one feeling, whereas the opposite feeling is suppressed or is unconscious. For example, a patient who has just lost a loved one may present to the physician with vague medical complaints, intense conscious sadness, or an acute bout of psychological turmoil that may lead to anxiety, reactive depression, or pathological grief. Not uncommonly, in addition to helping the patient deal with the sadness, the physician needs to help the patient find hidden anger that the patient feels toward the lost loved one in reaction to abandonment. Both the patient's anger and sadness need to be addressed to help the patient. The empathic physician counselor can help the grieving patient cope with these dualities by promoting mourning, preventing pathological grief (caused by self-directed anger), and helping the patient to work through the anger at the deceased. Unresolved anger could lead to self-effacing, guilt-ridden, even self-destructive behaviors.

Patients often express other conflicting feelings. For example, a patient may experience a desire for autonomy but have an unconscious need to be dependent, or the action-oriented patient may be unconsciously fearful of his or her passive tendencies.

Brief supportive and psychodynamic therapies are organized around psychological work in a triad of domains: the patient's past, the present situation, and the patient's relationship with the physician (Davanloo, 1980). Treatment is primarily concerned with supporting the patient's efforts to manage the current situation and maintaining a relationship with the physician. Psychodynamic work tries to help the patient develop insight by examining all sides of the triad using patterns in each domain to problem solve in the other domain. For example, the past affects how you handle the present, or a new learning experience with the physician can affect the present and how you understand the past.

The psychological work of counseling begins with trying to identify the patient's feelings by the use of empathic interest, clarification of the situations presented, and gentle confrontation of contradictions (nonjudgmental connections), all aimed at helping the patient become more aware of his or her emotional state. The patient with chronic somatic complaints, for example, needs a medical work-up as well as a psychological evaluation. It is common for patients with chronic psychosomatic disorders to be unable to recognize, experience, or even acknowledge the presence of feeling states (see chapter 6, Somatoform Disorders). Once the somatic symptoms or feelings are assessed and identified by the primary care physician as a psychological process, plans for intervention can be made (Lemkau & Smith, 1986).

This process can be supportive counseling, in which the primary care physician supports the daily functioning of the patient, or it can be psychodynamic counseling (also called exploratory or interpretive), in which the primary care physician is a more neutral counselor fostering insight. There may be a need at times to use elements of both forms of brief intervention. The primary care physician must determine what to emphasize during part of a session, an entire session, and throughout the entire treatment.

The style of individual counseling used is determined by a combination of the patient's need and type of problem and the physician's expertise in the treatment modality. Many different counseling modalities are helpful. Four counseling options that will be discussed in some detail are brief supportive counseling, brief psychodynamic counseling, solution-focused counseling, and harm reduction counseling.

Brief Supportive Counseling

Once a decision to counsel is made, the primary care physician has to determine the extent to which the patient can actively participate in the treatment. Brief supportive counseling focuses more on life situations and adaptation. The intent is to restore equilibrium, decrease symptoms and stress, and prevent psychological deterioration. The supportive counseling technique is often helpful for patients with difficulty in daily functioning who may have certain additional characteristics (see Table 16.1).

When conducting brief supportive therapy, the physician creates more gratification in the session, offers praise when needed, and is more directive. The physician avoids exploration of uncomfortable emotions and instead provides guidance and advice. He or she can use structured problem solving and may occasionally offer personal disclosures and information to teach the patient by example. The physician tries to facilitate a positive transference and redirect a negative transference by focusing on external relationships, not on the patient's relationship with the physician.

In supportive counseling, the physician encourages the patient to use mature defenses and discourages immature ones. The supportive treatment focuses on conscious rather than unconscious processes and is facilitated when the physician offers reflection, awareness, questioning, and clarification while using little or no interpretation (Piper, 1996).

Based on the patient selection criteria and the physician's role in the counseling process, the supportive counseling approach can be either authoritative with support or supportive and nondirective. Supportive authoritative counseling may be helpful when the patient needs a rapid life change (e.g., dealing with acute medical management of an illness), needs to stop smoking or make other healthy lifestyle changes, has family stress or job difficulties, or needs direction to facilitate health care or medical adherence as part of the treatment of a chronic medical problem. Supportive

Table 16.1 Patient Characteristics for Supportive Counseling

- Poor daily functioning
- Poor self-care
- Disturbed sense of reality or disturbances in reality testing
- Impaired judgment and/or impulse control
- Lowered pain tolerance
- Less psychological-mindedness or insightfulness
- Primitive defense mechanisms (e.g., projection and projective identification)
- Alexithymia (e.g., somatoform disorders)
- Poor interpersonal relations
- Decreased motivation for change
- Poor achievement in school or work
- Inability to deal with chronic environmental stress

nondirective counseling may be indicated to foster coping with medical illness, to prevent depression or anxiety associated with chronic medical problems, to support medical stability and daily functioning, or as part of palliative medical treatment for terminal illnesses. A supportive approach is usually combined with problem-solving techniques, "psychoeducation," and harm reduction techniques and might be coordinated with family treatment (see chapter 18, Family Counseling).

Brief Psychodynamic (Interpretive or Exploratory) Counseling

The primary care physician can attempt to relieve symptoms and solve problems using a psychodynamic approach, which is designed to help the patient to develop insight into his or her problems. The treatment focus is on conscious levels and on unconscious levels that are easily accessible to the patient's conscious awareness. Consistent in the literature of brief dynamic psychotherapy is the need for the patient to have both capability and interest in his or her own psychological life. The earlier assessment of the patient, as described above, will help in this determination. The physician should also look for strong patient motivation for this type of intervention. Druss (1995) has written about how severe illness and "reality crises" have motivated resistant or defended patients to explore their inner selves. Other important inclusion/exclusion criteria (Rockland,1992) for considering psychodynamic counseling are listed in Table 16.2.

Some patients are helped by insight development, an approach in which the primary care physician assumes a role as neutral counselor, interpreting the patient's psychodynamic conflicts. In brief psychodynamic counseling, the neutral counselor uses interpretation to integrate the conscious, immediate situation with other emotional (usually unconscious) material derived from clarifications and confrontations (see chapter 8, Personality Disorders in Office Practice, for a review of these techniques). The interpretive technique helps to promote the patient's psychological insight about his or her emotional functioning and helps the patient to see current problems in the light of recent or past experiences. Brief psychodynamic counseling is also helpful when the patient has conflicting fears and wishes, needs to improve adaptations and minimize maladaptive coping, wants to understand how present problems relate to the past, and is seeking insight into unsuccessful past relationships to foster successful future relationships.

Not infrequently, a brief psychodynamic treatment may require the use of several techniques at various times during the counseling process. Of significant importance in determining the use of this counseling modality is the matching of the patient's needs, goals, level of functioning, and desire with the needs, goals, and ability of the primary care physician to conduct this form of brief treatment.

Case Illustrations

A middle-aged man feeling "under the weather" noticed a swollen nontender nodule in his neck. During the assessment, the primary care physician established that the patient had no recent history of physical or psychological problems, had been functioning well in a midlevel corporate position, had been happily married for 12 years, and had been experiencing a fulfilling social life. The patient asked questions about occult malignancies in an educated manner, indicating his worry about his diagnosis. The primary care physician was appropriately willing to answer questions while offering realistic hope to prevent a premature escalation of fear. The physician elicited some background about the patient's current and past functioning around illness. She discovered that during his early teens, the patient had been placed in a body cast for 6 months for the treatment of scoliosis. With this history of incapacitation, the physician was alerted to the possibility that this patient might have underlying fears about a new loss of function, incapacitation, and dependency on others if

Table 16.2 Inclusion/Exclusion Criteria for Brief Psychodynamic Counseling

Inclusion criteria

- Patient demonstrated ability to negotiate major stress in his or her past
- Capacity for handling age-appropriate tasks
- History of good interpersonal relationships, including those with family members
- Ability to function well at work
- Ability to use leisure time well
- Ability to use higher levels of defense mechanisms such as intellectualization, sublimation, rationalization, and humor
- A low risk of regression during the introspective process (this may not be entirely apparent during the first couple of sessions)
- A higher level of intelligence and a reasonable capacity for psychological-mindedness (which some believe can be taught during therapy)
- Desire to understand present problems
- Ability to recognize and understand the effect of his or her past experiences on the present problems

Exclusion criteria

- Severe character pathology
- Severe affective disorders
- Borderline personality organization (some authors feel that psychodynamic work can help some borderlines)
- Substance abuse
- Somatization
- Psychotic illnesses

he were to become ill. The physician arranged for an appropriate work-up including a biopsy of the node. During the next three meetings, while the biopsy results were pending, the physician facilitated dialogue about the patient's fears. She encouraged him to recall how he had dealt with his scoliosis treatment, thus enabling the patient to focus on his prior ability to cope with uncertainties while waiting for results and answers. They examined the concrete things he had accomplished during his teenage years and also explored his concerns about asking others for help. This assisted the patient in coping with the time waiting for the biopsy results.

The biopsy diagnosis was lymphoma of the Hodgkin's type. The appropriate oncologic interventions were made, and periodic office visits for medical care and brief counseling were continued. The physician combined supportive and interpretive techniques around the issues of incapacity. In addition, she provided the patient with information and a referral to a support group. The patient's wife was included in some of the meetings, giving her an opportunity to participate in the overall psychological intervention for her husband. The physician facilitated open expression for both about their fear and pain regarding the diagnosis and prognosis. This helped the couple work with the physician to explore all medical options while preventing anxiety or depression from escalating to dysfunctional levels. Between sessions, the patient was able to maintain his connections with work, family, and community. He was able to receive their support without feeling overwhelmed and guilty. His treatment on all levels was successful, and he sustained a complete remission.

A psychological diagnosis need not always be exact in order to determine a counseling approach, as in this case. The patient's current functioning and an understanding about his history through brief assessment allowed the primary care physician to help this patient on medical, psychological, and social levels, an approach essential for each patient.

A middle-aged man with tense demeanor presented with bouts of abdominal/gastrointestinal distress. The primary care physician used open-ended questions to learn the medical history and facilitate the retrieval of the patient's current psychosocial situation. For years, the patient experienced gastrointestinal upset when stressed. Currently, the patient's marriage was in danger, because his employer had asked him to relocate. The primary care physician assessed the patient medically and simultaneously set up several office visits for brief supportive counseling. During the first 15-minute meeting, the physician felt it likely that the patient was suffering with irritable bowel syndrome, which was exacerbated by recent stress. He further diagnosed intense separation issues and acting-out, adolescent-phase behavior with his wife. The patient seemed unable to use insight from interpretations. This led the physician to conclude that brief supportive counseling with this patient might yield behavioral change and break the vicious cycle of his acting-out, adolescent behavior against his wife. The physician kept open the possibility for interpretive work should the patient show some receptivity at a later time. The physical exam and medical tests confirmed the diagnosis of irritable bowel syndrome. The physician's brief counseling enabled the patient to become acutely aware of his fears and wishes and his conflict between loyalty to his wife and his need to relocate to maintain his job. The ability to identify his anxiety about change and identify and express his fear of losing his job or wife allowed him to stop his threats and provocation of his wife. When he expressed his fears to her, she became more empathic about his worries. This lowered his overall anxiety, reduced his somatic gastrointestinal pain, and allowed the couple to collaborate and calmly discuss realistic options.

The patient who presents with acute issues but upon evaluation also has chronic problems should have the acute disruptions attended to first. The "first things first" approach can help the patient deal with immediate problems (Lemkau & Smith, 1986).

A 70-year-old, widowed woman had a consultation with her doctor for right upper quadrant abdominal pain radiating to her right shoulder. During her first medical consultation, the primary care physician took 5 minutes to get a brief psychosocial history, which included past medical history and personal, social, and family background. The physician learned that her new patient was a Holocaust survivor who had been rescued from a German concentration camp at age 15. Several members of her family were killed in the camps. During the interview, the physician noted the patient's constricted affect and stoic life philosophy and how she expressed her medical problem in a business-like, aloof manner.

The medical assessment indicated cholelithiasis. A surgical consultation, arranged by the primary care physician, confirmed that a cholecystectomy was the preferable treatment. The day the patient was admitted, the surgeon saw the patient at bedside and outlined the details of the next day's surgery. The patient developed acute panic attack symptoms, including shortness of breath, palpitations, a feeling of dread, and light-headedness. After the surgeon ruled out any medical cause, he paged the patient's primary care physician and explained what had just transpired. Knowing her patient's history and current level of functioning, the primary care physician gently discussed the patient's fears. The patient described her fear of losing control and dying while under anesthesia. The physician gently raised the possible connections between her concentration camp experiences and the loss of family members with her current panic and fear. The patient wept with memories of watching people, including relatives, being herded off to gas chambers disguised as bathhouses. She talked about how she had never fully mourned her losses nor dealt with the full impact of her Holocaust experiences. The physician combined clarification and interpretation, bringing together her fears of the current surgery and anesthesia, which were associated with the "gas" at the concentration camps. The patient felt understood and reassured. The primary care physician consulted with the surgeon to request the use of spinal anesthesia instead of general anesthesia. The surgeon agreed, and her entire medical team discussed her option of being fully awake for the procedure. The patient was offered and accepted a mild anxiolytic medication and agreed to the surgery, which was uneventful and without a recurrence of panic.

After the surgery, the patient followed up with the primary care physician for two additional 15 minute meetings. These office visits enabled the patient to begin grieving. During these sessions, the physician became aware of her own sadness and identification with the patient, as she was the oldest daughter of Holocaust survivors. The doctor, fearful of her own sadness (physician countertransference), discussed with her patient a referral to a psychiatrist specializing in Holocaust survivors. The physician, sensing the patient's hesitance, reassured the patient about her availability and encouraged her to call after the initial psychiatric consultation. The patient had a brief course of therapy with a psychiatrist that helpful mobilize the patient's healthier defenses. She joined a Holocaust survivor's group and her synagogue's Holocaust education program.

This case describes how a patient's acute emotional problem was managed so that it did not interfere with necessary treatment of her medical problem. The physician used a crisis format at first, then a brief therapeutic intervention. The physician also recognized her own excessive countertransference feelings and the limitations of her time and expertise. She tactfully referred the patient to a psychiatrist. The physician was successful in managing the acute disruption and panic in her patient. Her interpretive and supportive work provided this patient with an uneventful surgery and opened the door to interventions for her chronic psychological traumas.

Solution-Focused Counseling

Assessment of patients can lead to other counseling interventions. An alternative brief counseling approach is called solution-focused counseling (Walter & Peller, 1992). The basic idea of this approach is to help the patient do more of what has worked in the past or alternatively, to encourage the patient to do things differently to create new solutions. The focus in therapy is not to look for the cause of the problem (which is part of supportive and psychodynamic thinking) but to focus on what maintains a problem within a system and, based on this, to focus on solutions that can be constructed for future change. The solution-focused approach looks at circumstances in which the problem is absent (life experiences that are exceptions to the problem when things have gone well) and past functioning that has been effective but is not currently being used. The patient is asked to repeat old successful behaviors and learns how to be proactive in creating new solutions to current problems. The patient works along with the primary care physician as his or her own "expert," doing and behaving differently to create new solutions. The physician focuses with the patient on the here and now, utilizing patient strengths with a focus on positive change (Stuart & Lieberman, 1993). The physician offers an empathic acceptance of the patient's situation, thus giving the patient "permission" to feel what he or she is feeling, maintaining a positive alliance from the beginning, and encouraging exploration of all options for change. The physician's active stance provides new information, helping the patient think about new options and act in new ways. He or she provides hope for future change, counsels the patient to postpone premature decisions that have led to past failures, and facilitates the patient's expressions of his or her needs to a support system. The people who make up the support system can be brought in as active problem-solvers. Table 16.3 outlines this approach.

> A recently promoted corporate executive, a married man in his early 50s, sought consultation with his primary care physician for the recent onset of headaches. During the assessment and review of systems, the physician learned that the patient had been under a lot of new-job stress. The physician quickly recognized that the man was a "no-nonsense" person, using defenses of intellectualization and isolation of affect, and that he had an obsessive-compulsive, or Type A, behavior pattern. The patient showed no interest in exploring his issues but wanted headache relief. While the physical exam showed no obvious organic etiology, the physician's brief questions and an expressed desire to help enabled the patient to discuss his history of headaches during final exams in college. The physician encouraged the patient to recall anything that had helped him during those times (finding a past solution to apply to the present situation). The patient recalled that his headaches were helped by his taking brief "time-outs" and periods for exercises. He was asked to think about how he could accomplish this now. When the full medical and neurologic work-ups were negative, the patient began to wonder if his headaches might be related to what he was now "allowed" to identify as stress/tension. He realized that he could take brief breaks from work and exercise at the company's gym in his office building. At a follow-up visit, the patient had instituted an exercise regimen that had already decreased his headaches. He and the physician talked about other solutions to his stress. They decided that he could involve his wife in his stress relief by jogging with her more often. At a 1-month follow-up, the patient reported less frequent and less intense headaches and commented that he was spending more leisure time with his wife. The ability to identify his headaches as real and as stress-related enabled him to find practical solutions to his medical complaints.

Table 16.3 Problem-Solving Approach

Select a Problem
- What do I want to change?
- Where am I now?
- Where do I want to go?

Analyze the Problem
- What maintains the status quo?
- What are the barriers to change?
- How have I solved similar problems in the past?

Generate Potential Solutions
- What I can change in myself, in others, or in the environment?
- What can I do **differently**?

Plan the Solutions
- Set priorities for change: (What do I do first, second etc.?)

Implement the Solution
- Am I following the plan?
- Evaluate the solution
- Did I solve the problem?
- Do I need to solve other problems?
- Can I solve a new problem?
- Do I need additional help?

This case shows how problem solving and focusing on the here and now in brief counseling, can assist patients who may not be interested in, nor appropriate for, more interpretive forms of counseling.

Harm Reduction Counseling

Support, insight, or solutions to problems are not always possible. Helping patients find options and take increasing responsibility for their health and reducing harm to patients are also very important aspects of counseling. Helping patients find reasonable compromises when extreme, dangerous health-related behaviors exist can be a goal in itself. Patients who smoke, who abuse alcohol or other substances, who ignore HIV precautions, who speed when they drive or do not use seat belts, can benefit from harm-reducing interventions. Negotiating harm reduction requires physician flexibility commensurate with what the patient needs and can tolerate. For example, psychoeducation and referral to 12-step programs are important but often are not accepted by patients. Abstinence from alcohol, even though the preferable goal, is often unrealistic, given the limitations of certain patients. "Harm reduction" techniques (Marlatt, Somers, & Tapert, 1993) are geared toward reducing harmful consequences of a problem behavior. Asking an alcoholic or smoker to reduce consumption by a third can be more helpful than trying for abstinence and failing. Harm reduction interventions, such as methadone maintenance for opiate addiction and nicotine replacement for smokers, are helpful alternatives. In reducing the extremes of behavior, the patient is reducing self-harm.

Harm reduction approaches are controversial for many physicians, but flexibility with different patients may allow broader and improved health-related change for a greater number of patients. Being empathic to patients' efforts at change and setting a nonjudgmental harm reduction goal can help a patient find a middle ground that reduces harm and keeps the patient in a collaborative relationship with the physician. Education about the benefits of harm reduction can facilitate the patient's progression through stages of change (see chapter 19, Behavioral Counseling and Medical Adherence). Regular follow-ups are necessary to sustain changes at harm reduction levels.

> A 68-year-old divorced man who lived alone had a long history of alcohol abuse. His routine physical exams revealed signs of liver inflammation consistent with the long-term effects of chronic alcoholism. Set in his ways, he informed his doctor that at this point in his life the pleasure he had from the use of alcohol outweighed the possible medical risks. The use of alcohol was a major part of his social life. He refused referral to a 12-step program or alcohol counseling. The doctor straightforwardly informed the patient about his alcohol-related liver problems. In collaboration with his physician, the patient agreed to reduce his alcohol consumption in social situations. This coupled with close medical follow-up helped keep the alcohol-related liver problems from escalating for the next several years.

For this patient, a more rigid approach with a demand for abstinence would have created a patient-physician stalemate or an abruption in the doctor-patient relationship.

Referral for Counseling

Primary care physicians who offer consultation and counseling will often be faced with a decision about when to refer patients to a mental health specialist. Referral should be made immediately when there are psychiatric emergencies of suicide or the potential for violence or for any other problems requiring psychiatric hospitalization. A referral is also indicated if the patient requires interventions that are beyond the limits of the physician's ability or are impractical in an office-based practice. Sometimes the need for a psychiatric referral may not be recognized until a brief course of counseling has already been attempted. More severe character pathologies underlying the presenting problems may first be recognized after some intervention has been made. Longer term, more intense, or psychopharmacological treatment may be additional reasons for referral to specialists. Adjunctive referrals, such as the addition of a support, self-help, or 12-step group, may provide invaluable assistance to both the patient and the physician. Other concurrent treatment modalities, such as hypnosis and acupuncture for certain somatic complaints, may offer further relief in addition to the primary care physician's counseling (Druss, 1995).

Helping the patient to understand the need for the referral is important in reducing the risk that the patient may feel rejected. A referral is also a support for the physician who may not be able to treat a particular patient or handle certain kinds of psychological problems. As Lemkau and Smith (1986, p. 234) have suggested: "Sometimes the best help the physician can provide involves referring the patient to another professional. Other times the physician may be called upon to accept the reality that for some patients, being ill is better than being well and that chronic conditions are best managed without an aspiration to cure."

Consultation and counseling are a regular part of the everyday practice in a primary care setting. Many patients can be reached to help them better cope with their medical problems and their conscious and unconscious emotional pain. The primary care physician has many alternatives from which to choose in order to accomplish such goals. The interest and determination of the physician, added to the patient's desire for relief of suffering, can lead to counseling interventions that are often very successful in the context of the primary care setting.

REFERENCES

Balint, M. (1964). *The doctor, his patient, and the illness* (2nd ed.). New York: International University Press.

Davanloo, H. (1980). *Short-term dynamic psychotherapy.* Northvale, NJ: Jason Aronson.

Druss, R. G. (1995). *The psychology of illness: In sickness and in health.* Washington, DC: American Psychiatric Association.

Erikson, E. H. (1980). *Identity and the life cycle.* New York: Norton.

Flegenheimer, W. W. (1982). *Techniques of brief psychotherapy.* New York: Jason Aronson.

Frankel, R. M., Morse, D. S., Suchman, A., & Beckman, H. B. (1991). Can I really improve my listening skills with only 15 minutes to see my patients? *HMO Practice, 5,* 114–119.

Lemkau, J. P., & Smith, C. W., Jr. (1986). Back to basics: A psychosocial primer. *Family Medicine, 18,* 232–234.

Marlatt, G. A., Somers, J. M., & Tapert, S. F. (1993). *Harm reduction: Application to alcohol abuse problems* (NIDA Research Monograph Vol. 137). Washington, DC: National Institute for Drug Abuse.

Piper, W. E. (1996). Psychodynamic psychotherapy. In L. J. Dickstein, M. B. Riba, & J. M. Oldham (Eds.), *Review of psychiatry* (Vol. 1, pp. 109–1218). Washington, DC: American Psychiatric Press.

Rockland, L. H. (1992). *Supportive therapy for borderline patients: A psychodynamic approach.* New York: Guilford Press.

Roter, D. L., Stewart, M., Putnam, S. M., Lipkin, M., Jr, Stiles, W., & Inui, T. S. (1997). Communication patterns of primary care physicians. *Journal of the American Medical Association, 277,* 350–356.

Street, E., & Downey, J. (1996). *Brief therapeutic consultations: An approach to systemic counseling.* New York: Wiley.

Stuart, M. R., & Lieberman, J. A. (1993). *The fifteen minute hour: Applied psychotherapy for the primary care physician.* Westport, CT: Praeger.

CHAPTER 17

Crisis Intervention in Office Practice

Robert E. Feinstein and Laurel Carey

Routinely, primary care physicians are faced with requests from their patients to solve a wide range of biopsychosocial problems. Many physicians do not consider themselves competent to work with their patients to formulate the problem in a way that practical solutions can be developed within the time limitations of a general office medical practice. Crisis intervention provides a theory and treatment model that can be readily applied to helping patients with their biopsychosocial problems.

DEVELOPMENT OF CRISIS THEORY

During World War I Thomas Salmon (1917), a British military physician, was asked to evaluate severe "shell shock," which was producing a psychological paralysis in Allied soldiers. He discovered that the French suffered fewer psychological casualties from the horrors of wars than did the British soldiers. The factors that seemed to account for the French advantage were that French soldiers were told that they could expect to recover

Reprinted with permission from Feinstein, R. E., and Carey, L. (1995). Crisis intervention in office practice In R. Rakel (Ed.), *Textbook of family practice* (5th ed., pp. 1502–1509). Philadelphia: W. B. Saunders.

from their psychological trauma. They received immediate psychological treatment for these traumas close to the front and were returned to battle as quickly as possible. These principles became the cornerstones of modern crisis treatment. Patients entering crisis treatment can expect that they will be treated immediately, recover from the crisis, are generally treated while living in their natural environment, and are returned to normal life as soon as possible.

Eric Lindemann (1944) applied and expanded on Salmon's theories. He studied the acute grief reactions of many individuals who had lost family members in the Coconut Grove fire, a disaster in Boston that claimed approximately 500 lives. Lindemann discovered that normal people, surviving such a horrific experience, develop an emotional crisis of pain, confusion, anxiety, and temporary difficulty in daily functioning. He found that these reactions are natural states that last for about 6 weeks. He also noted that the psychological trauma caused by the crisis had little relation to preexisting psychiatric illness. Instead, the outcome of the crisis was more closely related to the severity of the stressor, the personal reaction to the trauma, and the effect the trauma had on the person's support network of family and friends. Lindemann found that most survivors recovered spontaneously, and a smaller group seemed to decline to a low level of functioning.

Eric Erickson (1959), a sociologist, introduced the idea of a life cycle comprised of developmental stages and crises. He described eight periods throughout the life span that involved age-specific psychological issues. For example, he described adolescence as a period in which a normal individual seeks an adult identity with social roles that eventually permit autonomy, away from parents. Those who cannot successfully traverse this crisis period do not progress from their child-like dependence on parental figures. Erickson described normal developmental crises throughout the life cycle that must be worked through and resolved if a person is to be able to progress successfully into the next life phase. His basic concept of "developmental crises" has been expanded to include crises such as leaving home for the first time, midlife crisis, and parents experiencing the "empty nest syndrome." For many patients, a crisis is experienced at transitional points between life phases, such as the crises of marriage, divorce, retirement, and death.

Gerald Caplan (1961, 1964) synthesized many of these earlier ideas into modern-day crisis theory and treatment. He defined the crisis state as a brief personal psychological upheaval precipitated by a stressor, or "hazard," that produces emotional turmoil such that persons are temporarily unable to cope, adapt, or function in their daily activities. Caplan demonstrated that a crisis implies both a potential for danger and an opportunity for growth. He subscribed to Lindemann's theories that how a crisis evolves depends on the severity of the trauma or precipitant, the personalized meaning of the event, and the effects of events on the support network of family and friends. He added that a crisis might also be based on failure of a person's individual coping style and ability to adapt. Unlike Lindemann, he thought that the preexisting personality may also affect the development, evolution, and resolution of the crisis. Caplan confirmed that most crises resolve in about 6 weeks with four possible outcomes: (1) improved functioning; (2) functioning restored to precrisis levels; (3) incompletely restored functioning with a susceptibility to the development of future crises; and (4) a severely impaired, but stable, level of lower functioning. He confirmed Lindemann's findings that some individuals coped with a crisis by spontaneously and flexibly developing novel coping or problem-solving styles and developed a crisis treatment that focused on developing better coping mechanisms and adaptations to life's traumas. An overview of a modern crisis theory is represented in Figure 17.1.

EVALUATING THE CRISIS

When a crisis develops, it may be evaluated and treated by understanding the interplay of the elements or the dynamics that contributed to its formation. These elements are the normal equilibrium state, precipitant or stressor, the personalized interpretation or meaning of the events to the individual, the crisis state, the selective history, the system of social supports, and the preexisting personality or psychiatric condition.

Normal Equilibrium State and Stressors

Under normal circumstances, an individual has a sense of internal psychological equilibrium and environmental support that generally permits daily activities of living, working, and having pleasure. Psychological equilibrium is determined by a delicate balance between the individual's internal wishes and fear, skills and capacities, and values and ideals. Environmental equilibrium refers to a stable balance between the basic

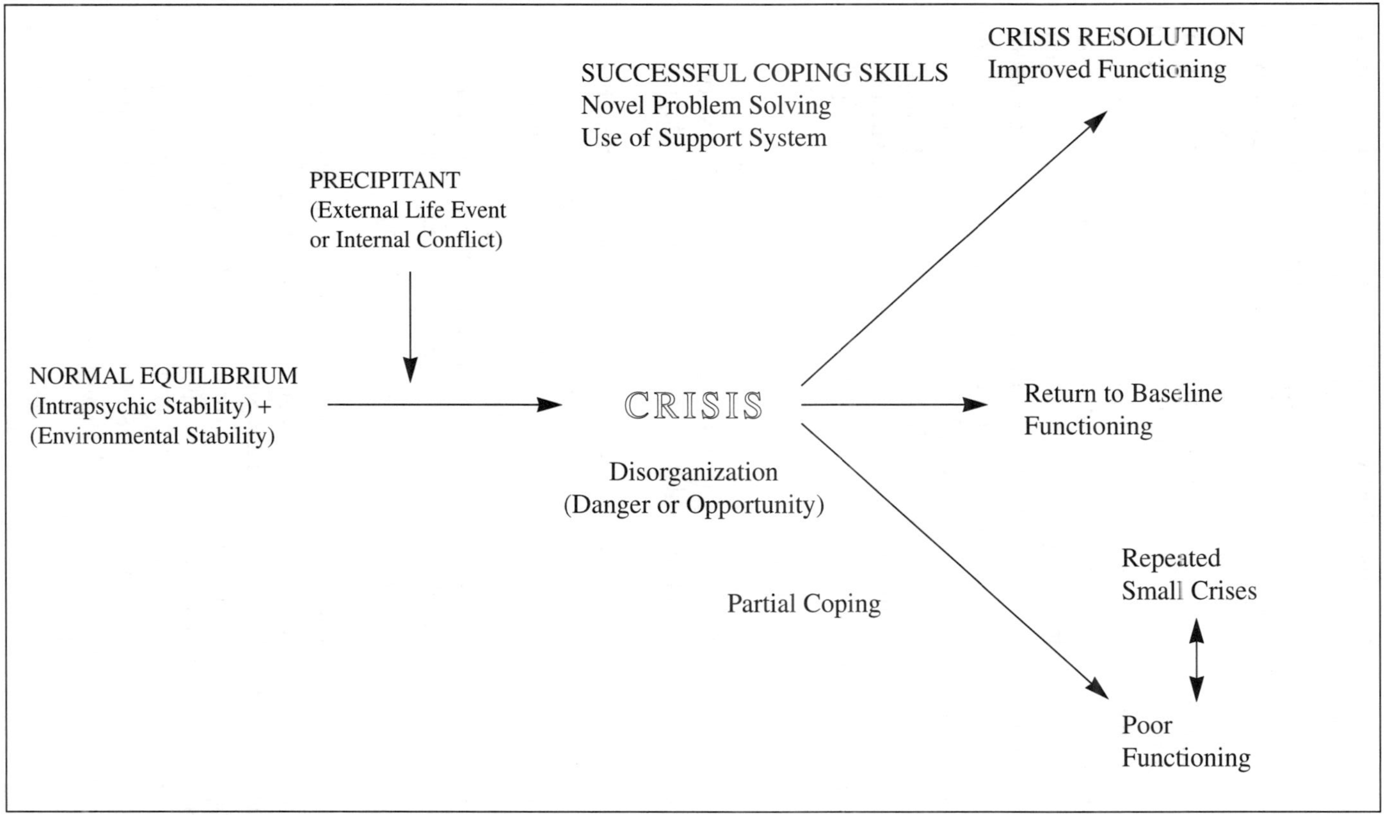

Figure 17.1 Crisis Intervention Theory.

need for food, shelter, and physical comfort and the social supports of job, family, religion, and society. A patient typically enters the emotional storm of a crisis after a stressor or acute precipitant disturbs the normal equilibrium. Stressors can be external life events, psychological events, such as a disturbing dream or sudden anger, and developmental problems, such as adolescence and midlife crises. Reality stressors frequently seen in a physician's office include loss of health due to disease and the stress of coping with a death, divorce, marital separation, job loss, or financial loss. Holmes and Rahe (1967) developed a Social Readjustment Scale that lists 43 external life stressors that precipitate stress in most people. The events range in severity from death of a spouse (1), to divorce (2), through change to a different line of work (18), to change in social activities (36), to Christmas (42). Some common psychological stressors include loss of self-esteem, loss of love, sexual dysfunction, and sudden overwhelming emotions, such as fear and rage. Common developmental stressors include latency, puberty, adolescence, marriage, birth of a first child, midlife crisis, chronic medical illness, and retirement.

Generally, most precipitants causing a crisis have components from a real-life event and an internally disturbing idea or feeling. These precipitants produce emotional turmoil and a transient inability to adapt during the early stages of a crisis.

Most patients who seek treatment are surprised to discover that there has been a major unrecognized stressor either the same day as or several days before the onset of the crisis. Less commonly, the stressor had occurred some time during the previous 6 weeks. Generally, events that have occurred more than 6 weeks previously are not acute stressors. Instead, these important past events may represent a previous crisis that was incompletely resolved and may be linked to the current crisis.

> Susan is a 40-year-old woman who presented to the Family Medicine Center with worsening headaches and feelings of "shakiness" all over. Exploration of the precipitant of the crisis revealed that Susan's symptoms began 3 weeks ago, when her only daughter, Jennifer, left for an out-of-town college. With questioning, Susan began to realize that since her daughter's departure she has been tearful and upset over the tiniest things. In fact, she recalled suffering the "worst migraine of her life" two nights ago, when her daughter informed her that she was so happy, loving school and meeting new friends, that she was not coming home for Thanksgiving.

Interpreting the Meaning of the Stressor

Whether precipitated by an external life event or an internal psychological thought or feeling, a stressor is interpreted by each individual. For some people, as with Susan, an external life event may seem minor, yet, because of the special meaning of the stressor to the individual, it may produce a crisis.

Susan's perceived loss of her only child was a stressful precipitant that triggered a crisis. This initial precipitant gains significance because of the particular meaning she ascribed to this normal developmental crisis of leaving home. Susan became pregnant with Jennifer, her only child, before Thanksgiving of her first year in college. This event had "forced" Susan to marry Jennifer's father, drop out of school, and abandon her dream to be a teacher. Although she willingly had devoted her life to Jennifer, Susan became panic stricken and developed "shakiness" and migraines out of a fear that her daughter was about to make this same mistake. Her daughter's departure for college was a painful reminder of Susan's lost career and triggered feelings of jealousy and anger toward Jennifer. "I began shaking with anger when Jennifer told me she wasn't coming home for Thanksgiving," Susan said. This crisis was inadvertently heightened by her husband, who had recently been talking with her about her developing some outside interests. Susan felt angry and betrayed by her husband, who had originally asked her to stay home.

This sequence of events—her daughter leaving home, her fear that her daughter might make the same mistake and become pregnant, her anger and jealousy over the daughter's opportunity to have a career, the missed chance for her own teaching career, and her unresolved anger at her husband—formed the personalized meaning that created this crisis for Susan. Once these events were formulated as precipitants with a personalized meaning, Susan could be helped to see that her life was not over. She was encouraged to speak with her daughter about the risk of pregnancy and discuss contraception. Susan also acknowledged jealousy of Jennifer's promising career and her residual blame and anger toward her husband. This recognition led to Susan's considering the idea that it was not too late for her to return to school to become a teacher. Her husband backed this idea, which helped her to see him as supportive. She resolved her crisis with improved functioning and the potential for a new career.

Crisis State

The crisis state has been defined as a brief psychological upheaval that is precipitated by a stressor. This upheaval produces an intense state of inner turmoil or disorganization that overwhelms a person's ability to cope and adapt. Patients who seek help while in a crisis have impaired normal functioning and may be in obvious psychological distress and pain. Typically, the pain of a crisis is so intense it is denied, unconsciously perceived as overwhelming distress, and may lead to an inability to cope. As with Susan, a crisis can be heralded by somatic complaints, or it may be expressed by crying, by becoming hysterical or mute, or by appearing confused, bewildered, severely anxious, depressed, suicidal, violent, or even occasionally psychotic. Typically, patients cannot explain why they are in crisis. A family physician can assist in such cases by becoming the detective of the "Why now?" aspect of the crisis. Answering this question initiates the crisis treatment and begins to facilitate resolution.

For example, a son, who brought his dead father to the emergency room after a car accident, appeared completely normal without any apparent emotional awareness of the tragedy. The family physician asked the son to describe the specific events of the father's death, the "Why now?" This exercise produced brief hysteria in the son, moving him into an emotional crisis state and enabling him to cry and begin grieving. Frequently, people in crisis do not seek help by themselves but, instead, are brought in by concerned family members, lovers, friends, or perhaps the police, ambulance, or other municipal personnel. In these cases, the crisis can be so intense that it may take hours until the specific causes and problems of the crisis can be identified.

Successful resolution of a crisis can be growth promoting and can lead to improved functioning. For most patients, however, crisis resolution means a return to their normal baseline functioning. Other patients may "seal over" or deny any meaning of their behavior. For example, a patient who swallows pills, then denies any suicidal feelings, has sealed over the crisis. Denial of the crisis and its causes can lead to partial crisis resolution and continuing poor adaptations. These patients then have a latent weakness, called a missed or unresolved crisis. Unresolved crises predispose a patient to future crises caused by even less stressful precipitants. In addition, these patients' stable functioning subsequently remains at a lower level. This group of patients may still have a future opportunity to be helped if the next crisis opens up the "sealed over" or unresolved crises, which can then be resolved in a more adaptive way.

Selective History

From a crisis point of view, the patient's history is relevant only insofar as it can be utilized to help explain and resolve the current crisis. This telescoping and inquiry about how the patient's history relates to the current crisis may be difficult to untangle and understand. Many patients, wishing to avoid the pain of the current crisis, lead the physician "down the garden path" to chronic complicated problems that cannot be helped in a single office visit. To avoid this situation, the physician must first try to understand the dynamics of the current crisis, then look for similar events in the patient's past that are the same as, or have a configuration similar to, that of the current situation. For example, a selective history that relates to a current suicide attempt might include the timing, circumstance, and effects of past suicide attempts or hospitalizations, or the past precipitants of such suicidal behavior. This selective history can then be utilized as a clue to making the current suicide attempt intelligible. Additional history, helpful for understanding a current suicide attempt, might be considered with prior deaths, separations, severe medical illnesses, depression, alcoholism, or family suicides. Selective history that might be relevant for violent crisis could include the timing and circumstances of past episodes of violence, childhood experiences of abuse or neglect, prior hospitalizations for violence, prior incarcerations, other legal problems, and past neurological or medical history.

Social Systems

Every individual lives within a network of social interaction and social support. Most of our daily social interactions are with spouses, family, friends, lovers, work colleagues, neighbors, landlords, and so on. Each individual also lives in a social network or society that enables him or her to obtain housing, food, clothing, work, education, finances, and medical care. In general, a stable, interested, helpful, available social support system tends to prevent crises. Sometimes a dysfunctional support system produces or contributes to the crisis. When a patient is in a crisis, a family physician can help the patient choose, then mobilize the most helpful people in the support network. Such actions may include calling in a specific family member, speaking to a difficult boss, helping the patient obtain an attorney, and helping a patient access cost-effective medical care, economic assistance, food, clothing, or shelter.

Relative damage to a support network can have profoundly different effects. For example, an earthquake results in a catastrophic destruction of the fabric of a society, which produces a sustained and prolonged crisis from which many never recover. The death of a spouse produces a more severe crisis if the deceased was also the sole financial provider. Even a minor disturbance in a small or dysfunctional support network can produce a major crisis. For example, an elderly woman, who is housebound, without family, friends, or telephone, experienced a major crisis when her home health aide missed her appointed visit. To assess the support network, a family physician must consider if the network members are capable of helping, are interested, and are available.

Previous Personality or Psychiatric Disorder

For most people, there is no correlation between a previous personality or psychiatric disorder and their capacity to deal with a crisis. A schizophrenic may be just as able to handle an acute crisis as others who do not have psychiatric problems. How well an individual handles an acute crisis depends primarily on the variables previously discussed: the precipitant, the meaning of the events, the crisis situation itself, the patient's coping skills and styles, and the effect on the patient's support systems.

There are some cases in which a preexisting psychiatric disorder may cause or influence the development of a crisis. Consider the case of a mentally retarded boy who became severely violent after his breakfast food was not available to him. This situation would be a minor stressor for most people, but for him, disruption of his daily routine and loss of his favorite food was perceived as catastrophic. His low intelligence and lack of verbal skills, specifically related to his psychiatric condition, predisposed him to the development of a crisis of violence.

Those with severe personality disorders who have rigid coping styles are at risk for developing a crisis. They have less adaptive capacity to develop new coping styles to aid in the resolution of a crisis.

CRISIS INTERVENTION TREATMENT IN THE OFFICE SETTING

Basic Approach

The focus of a crisis treatment is the evaluation of the precipitants of the crisis, the personal meaning of the events, the crisis state itself, the selective history, the support network, and if relevant the current psychiatric illness. This information is used to formulate the causes of the crisis, so that specific problem-solving interventions may be used for crisis resolution.

A crisis treatment, consisting of a therapeutic contract for three to five sessions, can be offered to any patient with a biopsychosocial crisis. The time required for each session depends on the complexity of the case and the physician's skill. A primary care physician may begin the crisis therapy by exploring the "Why now?" (acute precipitant) of the crisis. If the crisis involves suicide, violence, or a life-threatening medical illness, these factors take priority over everything else and become the focus of the crisis treatment. The next priority level involves the immediate crises of a lack of food, clothing, shelter, or adequate medical care. Finally, the physician must examine the crises of everyday living.

The crisis treatment should focus on the dynamic interplay of recent events over the last few days to 6 weeks that have contributed to producing the crisis. Important aids that can guide identification of the crisis components and treatment of these specific elements are the timeline, support network map, and wheel-and-spoke formulation of the crisis. Assessment and development of more adaptive coping styles follow. These elements lead to a general crisis resolution strategy.

Timeline

A timeline is a pictorial representation of recent and past events that have led to the crisis. A primary care physician can build a timeline of events with the patient by discussing the immediate crisis and working backward over the last 6 weeks, looking for precipitants, contributing events, and the selective history that relates to the current crisis. Use of the timeline is illustrated in the following case:

> John, a 35-year-old obese man who lives with his mother, presented to his primary care physician with depression and anxiety. He had been anxious for the last month since his company announced the possibility of layoffs. He had become increasingly sleepless over the last week when thinking a job loss would create severe financial strain. He believed his job loss would also result in his having to postpone his marriage and would make it impossible for him to leave his mother's home. This patient had made a serious suicide attempt (by overdose) 1 year ago, after a job loss and an argument with his mother, in which she humiliated him as an "inadequate provider." After his suicide attempt, he was briefly hospitalized, then placed on an antidepressant for 3 months. He did not seem to fully recover until he got his current job 6 months ago. Five months ago he became engaged and made plans to be married 8 months later.

A timeline representing this case is shown in Figure 17.2. Developing such a timeline with a patient helps focus on recent events and begins the process of formulating what can be done to help.

Support Network Map

A support network map can be organized around the patient's genogram and immediate environmental supports. This map includes the patient's immediate family, the family of origin for three generations, and all the people who are in the patient's immediate living environment, such as neighbors, landlord, and physician. In addition, it is helpful to include close friends and the religious or social agencies that are (or could be) involved for the benefit of the patient. With this map of the patient's support network, a physician can help decide who needs to be more involved in the patient's care, who should be excluded, and what social, religious, legal, or economic agencies can be mobilized to assist the patient in crisis. To choose the most helpful participants, look for individuals and agencies that are interested, available, and capable of assisting. Such a support network map is shown in Figure 17.3 with the case example from above.

> John's support system reveals the potential resources that may be mobilized to help him in the resolution of the crisis. His fiancee, mother, grandmother, best friend, and boss could be called upon to assist John or to help develop a plan for crisis resolution. His church, the employee assistance program at work, and unemployment insurance are potential additional resources that could be utilized. The decisions about which support system elements to use should be negotiated in collaboration with the patient. John and his physician decided that his fiancee and the employee's assistance program would be the best choices for additional help. John also agreed to inquire about obtaining unemployment insurance should he be laid off.

Suicide attempt, job loss; fight with mother; hospitalized	Anti-depressant D/C'd	Got current job	Engagement; marriage set for 8 months later	Threatened job layoff	Sleepless	Depression; anxiety; suicidal?
1 year ago	8 months	6 months	5 months	1 month	1 week	office visit

Figure 17.2 Crisis Time Line.

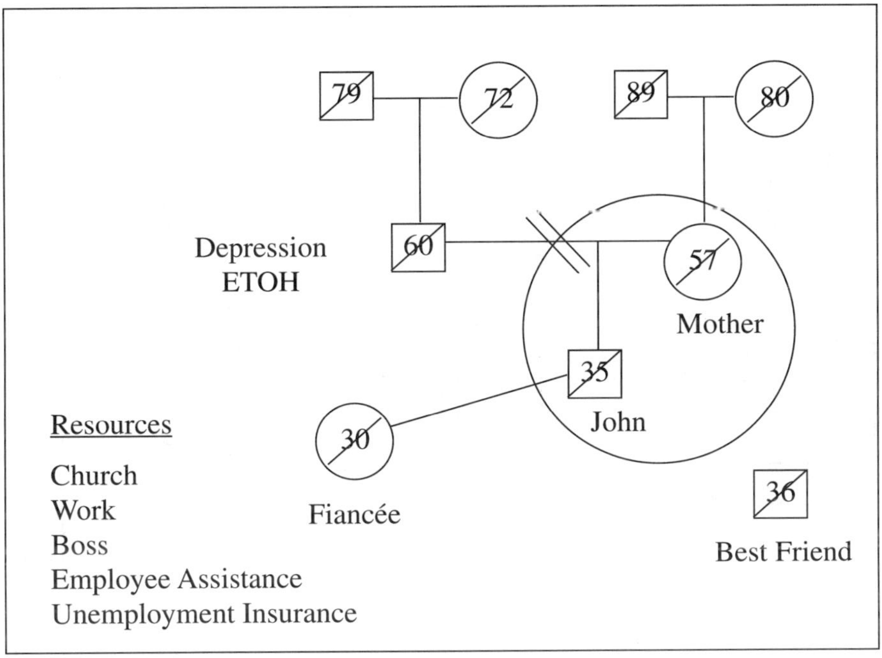

Figure 17.3 Support Network Map.

Wheel-And-Spoke Formulation of the Crisis

It is important to develop a formulation that specifies the multiple causes of the crisis. The wheel-and-spoke format helps the clinician and patient identify and formulate the crisis, as well as focus on setting the priorities for problem resolution. This format can also be used to suggest any required specific acute treatment. A pictorial way to represent a case is to think of the acute crisis at the center of a metaphorical wheel. The spokes of the wheel are the problems that are thought to be causing, contributing to, or feeding into the crisis. The physician can establish the priorities regarding the problems that are to be solved and in what order. This list of priorities can be indicated by numbers. For each problem listed, the family physician can recommend a specific assessment or evaluation, tests, or treatment approach that would be most helpful to the patient. Application of the wheel-and-spoke diagram for the case of John is shown in Figure 17.4.

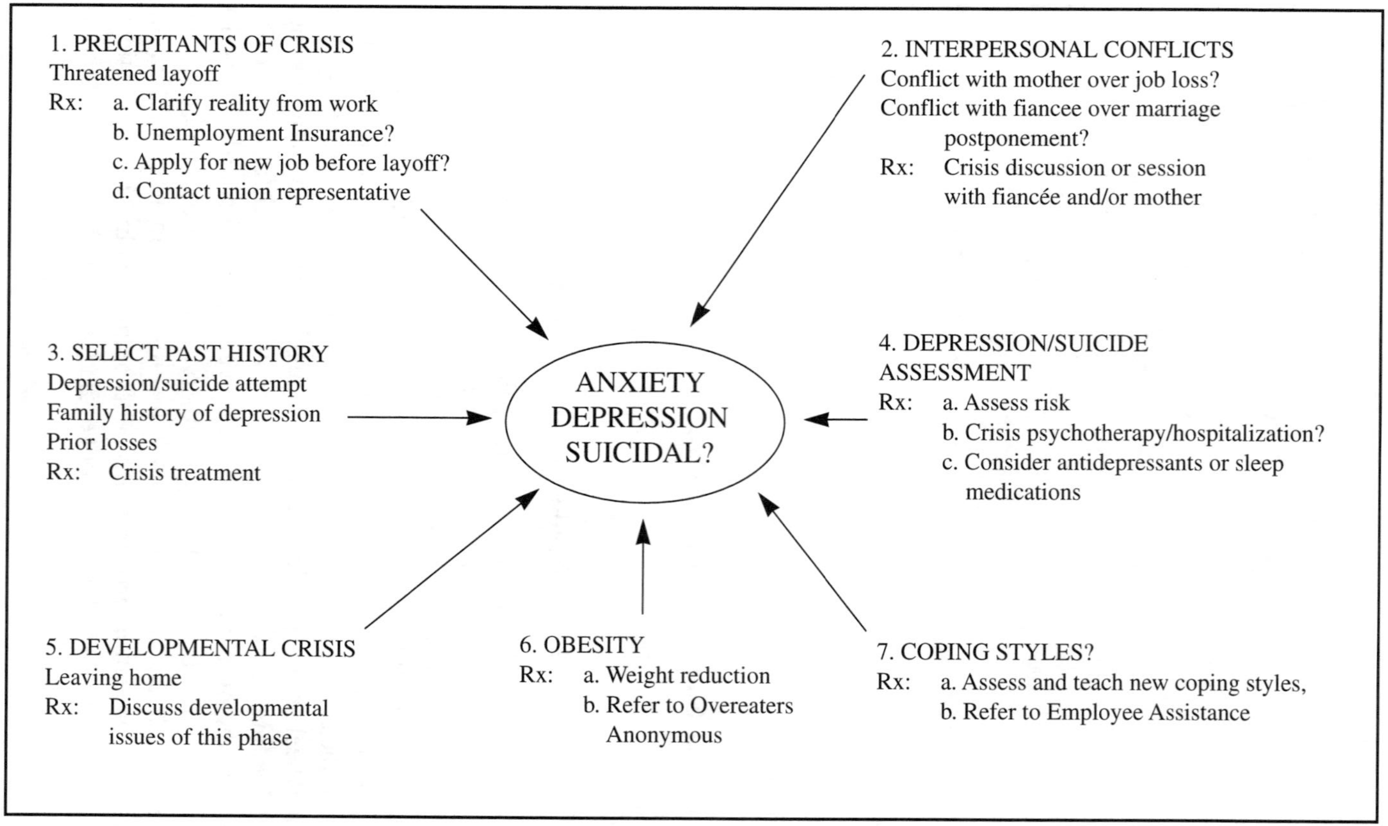

Figure 17.4 Wheel-And-Spoke Crisis Formulation and Treatment Plan.

COPING SKILLS, NOVEL PROBLEM SOLVING, AND ADAPTATION

Fortunately, most individuals find ways to handle or cope with a crisis within 6 weeks. Crisis resolution can be promoted by evaluating a patient's coping style and, when necessary, suggesting to the patient alternative or novel coping styles. These new skills facilitate a patient's adaptation to the stressful life circumstances that produced the crisis.

Coping styles are the unique way patients deal with stress. Everyone has a repertoire of coping styles. For example, some cope with a stressful crisis by analyzing it, asking others for help, and gathering additional information that might suggest a solution. It is generally found that some coping styles work better in certain situations than others. Table 17.1 lists some typical and some pathological coping styles.

Those who can use multiple coping styles are the most successful at crisis resolution and problem solving in general. Many patients in crisis rely too heavily on a single coping style, which may not be the most adaptive for a particular situation. Patients who lack the capacity for developing a novel coping style, when confronted with a crisis, may become dysfunctional.

To illustrate coping styles and novel coping skills, we return to the case of John. John has a history of coping with job loss by suicidal manipulation. In his current situation, it is a major concern that he not revert to this pathological style of problem solving. By discussing again his prior maladaptive style and by suggesting he could use a help-seeking and informational-coping style, John came to believe he had new options. Using a help-seeking style, he asked his fiancee for her aide. She was interested, willing, and able to pursue finding a job to help relieve the possible financial crisis. John used an informational style of coping to find out that he was eligible for unemployment insurance. This new information partially relieved the crisis. Furthermore, he began looking for new job opportunities.

CRISIS RESOLUTION STRATEGY

In addition to coping styles and coping skills, a family physician can teach a general strategy of crisis resolution. This crisis resolution strategy (Feinstein, 1995) is based on the crisis principles previously outlined and is summarized in Table 17.2. The family physician must walk through the

Table 17.1 Coping Styles

Adaptive Coping Styles

Intuitive: using imagination, feelings, and perceptions to solve a problem

Logical/rational: employing carefully reasoned, logical, deductive approach

Trial and error: trying a random solution and, if it fails, modifying it and trying again

Help seeking: asking others for help

Informational: gathering information, then deciding

Wait and see: allowing time or circumstances to determine the outcome

Action-oriented: taking an action to immediately rectify the problem

Contemplative: quietly thinking over the problem before action

Spiritual: asking for God's direction

Emotional: using emotion such as anger or fear to help problem solve

Controlling: controlling other people or oneself to gain the power to solve the problem

Manipulative: using a variety of manipulative styles to solve the crisis

Pathological Coping Styles

Deceptive/antisocial: being dishonest, lying, cheating, or stealing to solve a crisis

Suicidal: using the threat of suicide to coerce someone or to solve a problem

Violent: using the threat of or actual violence to establish control and problem solve

Impulsive: using unpredictable or impulsive responses without anticipation of possible outcomes

Random/chaotic: employing an unproductive and extreme form of trial and error and impulsive style, often seen in prolonged psychotic states steps with the patient several times, handling several crises, before encouraging the patient to attempt these steps as a self-help strategy. This approach has 14 steps.

1. Teach the patient to recognize early warning signs of a crisis, e.g., anxiety, occasional panic, regular feelings of being overwhelmed, a persistent sense of urgency, confusion, disorganization, and suicidal or homicidal feelings, thoughts, or actions.
2. Talk over the crisis or problem with the primary care physician or a trusted friend. The trusted person should not be directly involved in the crisis. For prevention of the next crisis, the physician can develop with each patient a list of available friends and practitioners, with their phone numbers, who may be reached as needed.
3. Crisis resolution begins by discussing the most painful feelings and emotions. The physician can suggest to a patient that discussing the areas of greatest pain has the potential for giving the most relief.
4. Identify the specific area of the patient's life that is most affected by the crisis. Is the primary crisis located at work or at home; or is it an interpersonal, economic, or other crisis in the patient's life?
5. Identify the acute specific precipitants and other stressors over the past 6 weeks that are currently contributing to the crisis. These elements can be identified by developing a timeline with the patient. It is most likely that the acute precipitant occurred on the day of the office visit or within the last week. For example, one patient recognized from his timeline that he always had a crisis each time his wife left him to go on a business trip. He discovered the following repetitive pattern to his crises: separation from his wife led to his feeling lonely, scared, and abandoned. He dealt with these feelings by drinking and driving recklessly and by getting into frequent brawls at the local bars. His timeline led the physician to suggest to this patient that during a separation he should call his wife regularly, not drink, but instead, make arrangements to spend time with a trusted friend.
6. Teach patients to evaluate their own support system by drawing a support network map. Using this map, patients can be assisted in discovering who can help, who they are not calling on, and who may make things worse.
7. Obtain additional information that may help in crisis formulation and resolution.

Table 17.2 Crisis Resolution Strategy

Crisis Resolution Strategy
1. Recognize the early warning signs of a crisis.
2. Talk over the problem with a crisis practitioner or trusted friend.
3. Discuss painful feelings and emotions.
4. Identify the specific area of one's life most effected by the crisis.
5. Identify the stressors over the past 6 weeks. Develop a timeline.
6. Decide who from the support system can help and hurt. Draw a support network map.
7. Formulate the crisis. Use wheel-and-spoke.
8. Obtain necessary information that will help in crisis resolution.
9. Learn about coping style and suggest the use of a new or additional one that might help.
10. Make a specific plan based on new information, newly discovered feelings, and choose a new coping style.
11. Implement the plan for resolution of one of the causes of the crisis.
12. Assess the results. If positive, go to step 13; if negative, go to step 14.
13. Tackle another cause of the crisis, and so on.
14. Try again, get help, then consult with a psychiatrist, if necessary.

8. The most difficult part of the crisis treatment, for both the physician and the patient, is developing the crisis formulation and problems list, setting the priorities of the treatment, and developing treatment options for each problem. Use of the wheel-and-spoke format can be helpful in this regard. With this approach, the crisis is at the center of the metaphorical wheel, and the spokes represent the variety of factors that are causing or contributing to the symptoms. Treatment may be suggested for each problem identified.
9. Learn about the patient's current coping style and why it may not be working. Encourage the patient to use other coping styles that he or she may have forgotten to use, and help the patient develop a new coping style.

10. Based on the new information, newly discovered feelings, and the crisis formulation, choose an effective coping style. The physician and patient should make a specific plan with a specific sequence of actions that will help the patient cope with and resolve the crisis.
11. The patient should implement the plan. Initially, it may be less overwhelming if he or she tries to resolve one cause of the crisis at a time and is faithful to the plan.
12. Assess the results. Is the problem resolved?
13. If the answer to step 12 is yes, then tackle the next problem, and so on.
14. If the answer to step 12 is no, then try again. Go back to step 8 and try to reformulate the crisis, or get additional psychiatric or other professional help.

REFERENCES

Caplan, G. (1961). *An approach to community mental health.* New York: Grune & Stratton.

———. (1964). *Principles of preventative psychiatry*. New York: Basic Books.

Erikson, E. H. (1959). *Identity and the life cycle.* New York: International Universities.

Feinstein, R. E. (1992). Emotional crises. In Morris, L. B. (ED.), *The Columbia University College of Physicians and Surgeons complete home guide to mental health* (pp. 364–373). New York: Henry Holt.

Holmes, T. H., & Rahe, R. H. (1967). The Social readjustment rating scale. *Journal of Psychosomatic Research 2,* 213–218.

Lindemann, E. (1944). Symptomatology and management of acute grief. *American Journal of Psychiatry, 101,* 141–148.

Salmon, T. (1917). War neurosis (shell shock). *Military Surgery, 41,* 674–693.

CHAPTER 18

Family Counseling

Anne A. Brewer and Charlotte Creech

The role of families in family practice is often neglected in the clinical office setting, despite the title of the specialty. This may reflect, in part, the split between biological ("hard") and psychosocial ("soft") sciences within the discipline, with families being relegated to the psychosocial realm. Only when medical care is compromised or if there is severe family dysfunction is attention paid to the role of the family. At that point, many practitioners throw up their hands, conclude that the family and patient are "crazy," and attempt a referral to a mental health specialist. If the referral is refused or unsuccessful, the practitioner is frustrated and the patient and family may remain in an unsatisfactory or dangerous situation. Two cases illustrate this dilemma.

> A 14-year-old boy with insulin-dependent diabetes and multiple admissions was admitted for diabetic ketoacidosis. All the house staff and his attending physician were frustrated with his frequent admissions and poor adherence to his medical regimen. When asked why he "forgot" to take his insulin or binged on sweets, he replied, "I don't know." It became apparent that his family situation might be playing a role in his inability to manage his illness. An interview with his mother revealed that she was divorced from an alcoholic, was struggling to survive financially, had no support network, and had a very conflicted relationship with her son. When these difficulties were addressed through family counseling and the family was helped to access services, the young man's admissions decreased markedly and physician satisfaction improved.

A 42-year-old woman with anemia and weight loss was admitted to the hospital for active tuberculosis. She appeared quite depressed. Further history revealed that she was a recent immigrant from Guatemala. Earlier that same year, her son had been incarcerated for 6 months for a drug-related offense. After her son's imprisonment, she became depressed and stopped eating. Because she had no medical insurance, she did not seek medical attention until she could no longer work. This current hospitalization lasted 6 weeks because her sputum was very slow to become negative for acid-fast bacilli. Perhaps if she had been able to obtain medical care earlier or had social support to help prevent depression, she would not have developed impaired immunity, which prolonged the course of the disease.

These cases illustrate the complex interplay between medical illness and family dynamics. Most primary care physicians have had similar cases and have experienced the frustration of caring for these difficult situations. This chapter will provide an overview of working with families in a primary care office practice.

CLINICAL WORK WITH FAMILIES

There are many clinical situations in which assessment of family function and intervention may improve outcomes or prevent problems (see Table 18.1). It is especially important to consider involving families in the primary care treatment approach during times of transition for families, chronic illness, emergencies, terminal illness, need for making lifestyle changes, nonadherence to medical recommendations, substance abuse, and chronic psychiatric illness.

Families in Transition

There are normal developmental phases in the life cycle of all families. These phases include formation of the family (through marriage or establishment of a partnership); pregnancy and birth; the raising of children; the family with young children; the family with adolescent children; when children leave home (the empty nest); the family with unmarried, then married adult children; families becoming grandparents; and the physical decline of family members; leading to eventual death and perhaps the dissolution of the family.

Table 18.1 Families in Primary Care

Family Involvement Mandatory

- Pediatric and adolescent care
- Emergency medical care
- Child abuse
- Domestic violence
- Elder abuse
- Threats of violence
- Suicidal threats
- Incompetent patient
- Infectious diseases
- HIV spouse notification

Family Involvement Helpful

- Families in transition
- For patients with chronic illness
- For patients with terminal illness
- Lifestyle change
- To foster medical adherence
- Substance abuse
- For patients with chronic psychiatric illness
- Adolescent medical care
- Elderly medical care
- Obstetrical care
- Prevention-oriented care
- Sexually transmitted diseases
- Advance directives
- Choice of health care proxy
- To determine code status
- For wills or estate planning
- When long-term care is required

In addition to normal developmental changes for the family, many families also must adapt to other stresses, including an illness or death of a child, sibling, spouse, or parent; care for ill or aging parents; divorce; job loss; and financial difficulty.

All of the stages of a family's life cycle and stresses require members to cope with change and adapt to new life circumstances. Transition times, while providing an opportunity for growth, are also vulnerable periods for families (e.g., when a chronic illness produces distress or illness in family members). At these transitions, assessment of family function and anticipatory guidance will help families adapt to change. If a family is experiencing difficulty in a time of transition, brief office-based counseling or referral to a mental health professional will aid the family.

For example, the birth of a child is a major transition for families. It requires parents to change their primary focus from each other to caring for a new and helpless member of the family. New parents must cope with fatigue, interrupted sleep, recovery from childbirth, the difficulties of caring for a newborn, and new financial responsibilities. At the same time, the parents need to find ways to nurture their own relationship. The family physician can address these adjustments during prenatal and well-child visits, providing guidance and detecting families who are having difficulty coping. Physicians can also screen for postpartum disorders (see chapter 14, Women's Health Through the Reproductive Cycle). This may prevent disruption of the relationship between parents or failure of attachment to the baby.

Familial Effects From Chronic Illness

Living with chronic illness presents many challenges to families. These include adjusting to the need for frequent medical visits, coping with side effects of medical treatment, adapting to necessary lifestyle changes, dealing with additional financial burdens due to medical expenses, coping with the fear of loss of independence or death, understanding the changing roles of family members, and coping with interpersonal stresses within the family.

If the chronically ill person is a spouse or partner, the other partner is usually the primary caregiver. If the family system is intact, there may be additional assistance from adult children; if not, the ill person may need to call on friends and/or community agencies. The primary caregiver may need to assume additional roles of overseeing and managing medical care and increased child care duties, or the person may need to perform additional household management tasks. Financial worries may loom large, especially if the ill patient is the major financial provider. Caregivers often experience guilt, anger, or excessive fatigue leading to burnout or illness. If marital or family strife existed before the illness, that conflict may be exacerbated by the strains of chronic illness. If the caregiver also has health problems, the family can be easily overwhelmed, leading to placement of the chronically ill patient in a long-term care facility. This can be devastating to the entire family system.

If the chronically ill person is a parent, the family is faced with especially difficult challenges. Commonly, the older children may reenact conflicts of sibling rivalry in which the children vie to fulfill the missing parental roles. Confusion and battles over the new emotional climate of the family, new roles of authority and discipline of the younger children, and dysfunctional family problem solving are common. Reorganization of the entire family life is a necessary and often difficult adaptation.

When a child is chronically ill, the parents face particular challenges. The ill child needs increased attention, which may leave other children feeling short-changed and exacerbate sibling rivalry. Family routines (meals, schedules, and vacations) may be disrupted. The family may become oriented primarily around physician visits or hospitalizations. One parent may devote much time and energy to the ill child, while the other focuses most of his or her life on work as an escape from the pressures of the ill child. Parents typically confront the fear that their child may not survive or may not have a normal life. Guilt may trouble parents, particularly if the child suffers from a genetic disease like cystic fibrosis or an illness caused by prenatal influences, such as fetal alcohol syndrome. Parents frequently overprotect and overcontrol ill children in an effort to control the disease or protect the child from exacerbations. For example, parents may keep a child with asthma home from school in an effort to prevent deterioration from upper respiratory infections. Family cohesiveness may be severely strained by a child's illness; divorce or parental abandonment is frequent. However, the family unit may be strengthened by confronting difficulties together and coping with them successfully.

When adult children care for chronically ill parents, they face role reversal, becoming caregivers for parents who may have difficulty accepting their loss of independence and need for help. Previous parent-child or sibling conflicts may resurface as ill parents become more dependent. Caretaker stress and burnout may occur.

Emergency or Acute Situations

Many emergency situations in family practice warrant assessment of family function and possible intervention. Common emergencies in which families either must or should be involved are reviewed in Table 18.1. A new diagnosis of a serious illness (e.g., chronic obstructive pulmonary disorder, [COPD], myocardial infarction, diabetes, cancer, or renal failure) creates stress for the affected individual and the family. Assessment of the family's level of function, education about the disease process, referral to support services, and referral for family counseling, if indicated, may be done in a family meeting. A sudden change in a person's health status (e.g., pneumonia in a person with COPD or a hip fracture in a previously independent elderly woman) may require a change in family roles and responsibilities. A family meeting can facilitate that change.

Terminal Illness

When a person who has been chronically ill enters the terminal phase of illness, death becomes inevitable and dominates the life of the entire family (see chapter 15, Death and Dying). The dying person must deal with denial, unfinished business, grief and anger over dying, and letting go. The family must face separation, grief, loss, and reconstruction of family life after the death. The family may also face difficult medical decisions on behalf of the ill person. Family meetings to discuss the patient's long-term prognosis and plans for the dying process (especially death without pain) are invariably helpful. Families often need to discuss advance directives, health care proxies, emergency code status, wills and life-end estate planning, and financial issues. A physician-initiated family meeting can often calm and educate a scared support network. The physician can help to resolve some familial conflicts (or refer to a mental health specialist) or prevent conflicting directives from different family members during the death and dying process.

Prevention-Oriented Primary Care and Lifestyle Changes

Prevention of disease is a major goal for primary care physicians. Prevention often works best when explained and implemented in the entire family system.

Changes in lifestyles are important factors in prevention and treatment of many diseases. Lifestyle changes that can be fostered in a family system include family smoking cessation, healthy nutrition, weight maintenance, exercise, and stress management. Lifestyle changes are often difficult for patients to implement and sustain. For example, success rates in individual efforts at smoking cessation are lower than 10% in many studies. The chances of smoking cessation are greatly reduced if the spouse or partner continues to smoke or is critical of the smoker (Mermelstein, Lichtenstein, & McIntyre, 1983). Support from the spouse or partner or family smoking cessation can improve the chances of the entire family living in a smoke-free environment. Family involvement and support are also beneficial in implementing dietary changes leading to healthy family nutrition. Involvement of the entire family in grocery shopping and cooking obviously is crucial for family nutritional change. Without family involvement, family members may undermine efforts to make and sustain dietary changes, which can negatively affect successful change.

Nonadherence to Medical Recommendations

A frequent occurrence in medical practice is nonadherence to treatment (see chapter 19, Behavioral Counseling and Medical Adherence, for a detailed review). Estimates of nonadherence suggest that 50% or more of medications are taken improperly or inconsistently. With complicated medical regimens for chronic illness, this figure is higher. Nonadherence to medical recommendations may be caused by overly complicated medical regimens, side effects of medication, inadequate understanding of medications, illiteracy, cognitive impairment, mental illness, family disorganization, and nonsupport for treatment. Nonadherence can have grave consequences in poor treatment outcomes, drug interactions, and under- and overdosage of medications. Family intervention can improve adherence to treatment regimens. The family can be educated about the importance of adherence, then enlisted to support and monitor treatment and to organize and supervise medications.

Substance Abuse

Substance abuse exacts a terrible toll on patients and families alike. Approximately 10% of adults in the United States abuse alcohol and/or prescription and nonprescription drugs. Because denial is the hallmark of the disease, information from family members is often crucial to making a diagnosis of substance abuse and planning an intervention to reduce harm. Substance abuse in families often surfaces because of distress in other family members, such as depression, chronic somatic symptoms, and acting out or school failure in children. Research with families affected by substance abuse has shown that the substance and substance-related behaviors often become an organizing principle for family behaviors and routines (Steinglass, 1989). (See chapter 4, Substance Abuse, for a detailed discussion of substance abuse diagnosis and treatment.)

Diagnosis and treatment of substance abuse are more successful if families are involved. When a patient is denying substance abuse, it is often much more effective to convene a family meeting than to confront the patient. Confrontation of a patient in denial of substance abuse can lead to a deteriorating physician-patient relationship. A major alternative is to bring in the entire family and utilize them to make substance abuse overt. This can reframe the substance abuse as a problem that requires family support and intervention. This family approach puts the physician in a helping position for the entire family rather than in the role of judge, jury, and sentencer.

Family involvement can include education about substance abuse and its effects on families and about relapse prevention. It can involve family counseling and family support groups like Al-Anon, Alateen, Adult Children of Alcoholics, and Nar-Anon. Support groups can dissipate some of the accumulated anger and resentment experienced by families who live with substance abuse. Family intervention can also help families reorganize their lives around priorities other than substance abuse.

Chronic Psychiatric Illness

Chronic psychiatric illness, particularly schizophrenia, bipolar disorder, depression, panic disorder, obsessive-compulsive disorder, and somatization disorders, have a far-reaching effect on families as well as upon the individuals suffering from these disorders. With a system-wide shift away from institutional care, families have borne increasing responsibilities for mentally ill persons. As with other forms of caregiving, these responsibilities often cause stress in family members.

Intervention with families of patients with chronic mental illness can involve education about psychiatric emergencies (suicidal or violence potential), oversight of ongoing psychiatric treatment and medication adherence (important in relapse prevention), referral to family support groups or family counseling, and stress management for caregivers. Counseling includes offering ways to prevent the chronic mental illness from consuming an inordinate amount of family resources and energy. It may help families to avoid overprotection and overfunctioning (doing for the ill person those things of which he or she is capable), which can worsen dependency.

INTERVENING WITH FAMILIES IN PRIMARY CARE

Family meetings are often valuable in the treatment of patients, yet they are rarely used by physicians in primary care practices. The usual model of care in family practice is still the individual patient visit to a physician or clinician. The individual physician-patient relationship is sacrosanct, and many physicians understandably feel apprehensive about moving into a different mode of data gathering and treatment. In the past, few residencies have offered training in family work, although that pattern is changing. As physicians in training gain experience with working with families as well as individuals, they may move toward greater attention to families in their own practices.

Obstacles to Utilizing Family Treatment in Primary Care

Busy primary care physicians often perceive that they do not have the time and/or the skills to conduct family meetings and are often concerned that these meetings may be lengthy. However, in many situations, a few well-timed family meetings can provide information and a treatment plan that might otherwise require many office visits. Family meetings foster trust and communication with the patient's entire support network. In addition, a family meeting can help to avoid numerous emergency room visits, extra phone calls to the patient or family members, excessive prescription changes, and excessive diagnostic testing, and generally will improve adherence to medical recommendations. A family meeting can also provide a new primary care physician with an opportunity to recruit additional family members as patients if there is a positive physician-family interaction. Family meetings can make the physicians' future encounters with the family more efficient and thus in the long run save time.

Primary care physicians, who often care for several members of a family, are in a unique position to conduct family meetings. They may already have a sense of the family's communication patterns and coping style.

They also may have treated family members for stress-related conditions or may have seen signs of caregiver stress or family difficulties.

Indications for a Family Meeting

Table 18.1 lists many situations in which a family meeting may be valuable. These situations all pose challenges to a family's functioning and represent threats to patients' health and well-being. Physicians need not be skilled family therapists to conduct diagnostic and educational family meetings. A family meeting for information, education, and support can reduce anxiety, enhance family adjustment, and improve adherence.

The Goal of the Family Meeting

Family meetings should be conducted with the goal of assessing family functioning, especially as it relates to the health care of its members. A number of instruments have been developed to assess family functioning. These range from research tools to questionnaires designed for use in a primary care office setting. One instrument that is widely accepted in primary care settings is the Family APGAR (Smilkstein, 1978); (see Table 18.2). This scale estimates family function in the areas of adaptability, partnership, growth, affection, and resolve (sharing of time, space, and money). Another scale, developed by the *DSM-IV* (1994), is the Global Assessment of Relational Functioning GARF scale (see Table 18.3). GARF, which is not yet widely used in primary care settings, may be easier to use than the Family APGAR. This scale rates family functioning in three areas: problem-solving, organization, and emotional climate. If the interviewer prefers not to use the Family APGAR or GARF, he or she can obtain information on family function through a series of open-ended questions (see Table 18.4).

Convening the Family

Once the determination has been made that a family meeting is indicated, physicians should invite all members of a household. In some circumstances (e.g., domestic abuse) it may be appropriate to exclude very young children (infants and toddlers). Extended family members who live nearby or who are a major part of a family's support system should be included as well. A genogram or support network map (see chapter 17, Crisis Intervention in Office Practice) may prove helpful in determining which

Table 18.2 Family APGAR Questionaire

	Almost always	Some of the time	Hardly ever
I am satisfied with the help that I receive from my family* when something is troubling me.	____	____	____
I am satisfied with the way my family* discusses items of common interest and shares problem solving with me.	____	____	____
I find that my family* accepts my wishes to take on new activities or make changes in my lifestyle.	____	____	____
I am satisfied with the way my family* expresses affection and responds to my feelings such as anger, sorrow, and love.	____	____	____
I am satisfied with the amount of time my family* and I spend together.	____	____	____

Scoring: The patient checks one of three choices, which are scored as follows: "almost always" (2 points), "some of the time" (1), or "hardly ever" (0). The scores for each of the five questions are then totaled. A score of 7 to 10 suggests a highly functioning family. A score of 4 to 6 suggests a moderately dysfunctional family. A score of 0 to 3 suggests a severely dysfunctional family.

* According to which family member is being interviewed, the physician may substitute for the word *family* either *spouse*, *significant other*, *parents*, or *children*.

G. Smilkstein: The Family APGAR: A Proposal for a Family Function Test and Its Use by Physicians. *The Journal of Family Practice, 6*:6, 1231–1239, 1978. Reprinted by permission of Appleton & Lange, Inc.

members of the extended or distant family should be included. It can provide important information about events in a family's history that may have bearing on a particular patient's situation and may suggest new supports for help with an intervention strategy. In general, the identified patient should participate in the meeting. If the identified patient is a young child or is severely mentally ill, cognitively impaired, or otherwise

Table 18.3 Global Assessment of Relational Functioning (GARF) Scale

1. Problem solving: Negotiating goals, rules, routines, adaptability to stress, communication skills, and the ability to resolve conflicts
2. Organization: Maintenance of interpersonal roles, subsystem boundaries (boundaries between parents and children), hierarchical functioning (who is in charge of what), coalitions, and distribution of power, control, and responsibility
3. Emotional climate: Tone and range of feelings; quality of caring, empathy, involvement, and attachment/commitment; sharing of values; mutual affective responsiveness, respect, and regard; quality of sexual functioning

Scoring

81–100 overall: Relational unit is functioning satisfactorily from self-report of participants and from the perspective of observers.

61–80 overall: Functioning of relationship unit is somewhat unsatisfactory. Over a period of time, many but not all difficulties are resolved without complaints.

41–60 overall: Relational unit has occasional times of satisfying and competent functioning together, but is clearly dysfunctional; unsatisfactory relationships tend to predominate.

21–40 overall: Relational unit is obviously and seriously dysfunctional; forms and time periods of satisfactory relating are rare.

1–20 overall: Relational unit has become too dysfunctional to retain continuity of contact and attachment.

Modified version of *DSM-IV GARF Scale*.

Reprinted with permission from the *Diagnostic and Statistical Manual of Mental Disorders*, Fourth Edition. Copyright 1994 American Psychiatric Association.

incapable of participating, the meeting may take place without the patient. Families often attempt to protect an ill family member by excluding him or her from meetings. However, this exclusion can lead to isolation and suspicion on the part of the patient.

The physician's ability to recruit the entire family for a family meeting is fostered when the physician or a member of the office staff extends a

Table 18.4 Open-Ended Request for Family Function Information

Component relevant open-ended questions	
Adaptation	How have family members aided each other in time of need? In what way have family members received help or assistance from friends and community agencies?
Partnership	How do family members communicate with each other about such matters as vacation, finances, medical care, large purchases, and personal problems?
Growth	How have family members changed during the past years? How has this change been accepted by family members? In what way have family members aided each other in growing or developing independent lifestyles? How have family members reacted to your desires to change?
Affection	How have members of your family responded to emotional expressions such as affection, love, sorrow, and anger?
Resolve	How do members of your family share time, space, and money?

G. Smilkstein: The family APGAR: A Proposal for a Family Function Test and Its Use by Physicians. *The Journal of Family Practice, 6*:6, 1231–1239, 1978. Reprinted by permission of Appleton & Lange, Inc.

personal request for attendance of each family member. Asking the patient to bring in the family can save time, but there are many circumstances in which this approach will prevent a family meeting from happening. For example, substance-abusing patients may try to exclude family members because they are in denial, wish to avoid conflict, or seek to conceal drug abuse. A physician should determine the whereabouts of all family members before suggesting a family meeting. This will make it more difficult for a patient to make his or her own support network unavailable for help.

Once information about the family has been obtained, the patient can be approached with the idea of a family meeting. The physician's direct contact with family members is often the best way to recruit the entire family for the meeting.

The wishes of patients who refuse to have their families involved should be respected as long as this decision does not put the patient in a life-threatening situation or compromise his or her health. In life-threatening emergencies (a medical emergency, violence, or suicide risk), the physician can contact the family against the patient's wishes. In these circumstances, it is vital that the physician document carefully the reason for this action.

Conducting a Family Meeting

Conducting family meetings is a skill that requires development like other cognitive or performance skills (Doherty & Baird, 1983). Anderson and Holder (1989) provide detailed suggestions for leading family meetings. The following guidelines for conducting a family meeting may be helpful.

Treatment Setting

A family meetings can be conducted in one of the physician's consulting rooms if the group is small. It can also take place in a waiting room before or after regular office hours or in a hospital conference room. Privacy, sufficient seating, and reasonable comfort are the only requirements.

Seating Arrangements

Matching the correct number of chairs to the number of expected family members can give important clues to family structure and organization. In general, arrange the chairs in a circle and let all family members choose their seating freely before the physician or other health care practitioners are seated. This approach allows a potential view of the family structure and/or potential problems. For example, an isolated father who is hurting the family by his substance abuse may sit on one side of the circle while the rest of the family sits huddled together far away from him. Alternatively, a sick child may wind up sitting between the parents while an adolescent who is acting out may choose to sit in the corner. Marital discord may be signaled when the husband and wife sit far apart within the circle. This kind of family process information, although not conclusive, helps the physician formulate possible issues in the family, which can then be discussed and explored as the family meeting proceeds.

Beginning the Family Meeting

When conducting a family meeting, the physician should open with a statement of the purpose of the meeting, expressing concerns about the patient and recognizing and inquiring about the family's concern. The physician can begin the meeting by eliciting patient and family views of the situation, their priorities, and the family's values. The family members' views of the problem may differ radically from the physician's initial view.

It is important to make sure that each family member has an opportunity to express his or her view of the problem and of what is needed. At the beginning of the meeting, the physician should observe who speaks first, who tries to control the meeting, and who is in charge of specific family functions. For example, it is important to know who in the family makes health care decisions, who decides about finances, who decides what is best for the children, and so forth. One or two verbal family members should not be allowed to dominate a discussion. Other, less verbal family members or children have valuable information to impart, and involving them in the discussion helps them engage and commit to the treatment plan.

It is important during the family meeting to avoid criticism and avoid assuming that there are pathological behavior patterns in the family, as this usually provokes family anxiety, defensiveness, and hostility. The physician needs to focus on the family's problems and strengths, rather than highlighting weaknesses. Focusing on family abilities may also allow a family to build on those strengths, to modify behavior, and to change the emotional climate. Provoking defensiveness leads to resistance to change. In some families, however, hostility, ill will, family mood, or threats of violence can make meetings futile or counterproductive. The physician can exclude from such meetings particular family members who are disruptive or dangerous.

Gathering and Giving Information

The physician should gather additional data about family history, family functioning, sources of support, and signs of stress. The relevant information can be used later, if necessary, to assess the family and plan interventions. During the meeting the physician can impart information about the patient's condition, possible complications, and probable course and prognosis. Eliciting the family's concerns and priorities and allowing time for discussion and questions are essential.

The Family Assessment

After learning about the family, the physician is in a good position to determine if members are interested, available, and competent to help the patient. In general, the physician should assume that family members want to help the patient and are trying their best to do so. The family assessment can follow a GARF or Family APGAR format (see Tables 18.2 and 18.3).

The simple number rating that GARF provides is an easy way for the physician to assess family function. Each family is rated according to problem solving, organization, and emotional climate. Problem solving is the family's skills in "negotiating goals, rules, routines, adaptability to stress, communication skills, and the ability to resolve conflicts (*DSM-IV*, p. 758). Organization refers to "maintenance of interpersonal roles, subsystem boundaries (boundaries between parents and children), hierarchical functioning (who is in charge of what), coalitions and distribution of power (which family members are aligned together or oppose each other), control, and responsibility" (*DSM-IV*, p. 758). The emotional climate is the "tone and range of feelings; quality of caring, empathy, involvement, and attachment/commitment; sharing of values, mutual affective responsiveness, respect, and regard; [and] quality of sexual functioning" (*DSM-IV*, p. 758)

Repeat scoring, at subsequent office visits, is an easy way to record the progression or deterioration in family functioning over time. The GARF method of assessing family function is used as part of the critical pathways described throughout this book (see chapters 3, 4, and 13 for demonstrations and application of the use of GARF rating scales).

The assessment should alert the physician to signs of distress in the family. Withdrawal from family or social activities, school failure, somatic symptoms, depression, and poor self-care may be indicators of family dysfunction or caretaker distress. Based on the assessment, the physician should attempt to develop shared priorities and a treatment plan that the family understands and can implement.

Developing a Shared View of the Family Problem

Developing a shared view of the problem and priorities over the course of the family meeting will enhance the alliance between family and physician and will ensure that the patient and the family feel heard and respected by the physician. This may require discussion and negotiation. (See chapter 13, A Model for Office-based Cardiovascular Risk Reduction and Behavioral Change, for a discussion of the process of informed shared decision making.) Once a shared view of the family's problems is accomplished, this should be articulated with the family. For example, the family and the physician might agree that the problem is the need for new medical treatment, more support or home-based resources, additional help from other family members, better cooperation, and less stress.

Family Treatment Plan

The family treatment plan should focus on (1) family activities that can improve the health of the identified patient (e.g., organizing family help with cooking, lifestyle change, medication monitoring, and medical supervision), (2) bolstering the health of other family members (e.g., recognizing burnout in the family member who is the primary caregiver and providing additional medical or psychiatric care for family members in trouble), (3) discovering barriers to medical adherence (see chapters 12 and 19) and negotiating ways to overcoming these problems, (4) helping families locate and access resources from within the extended family (e.g., getting child care assistance from grandparents or asking for transportation assistance from siblings), and (5) helping families access community resources such as support groups, disease-specific education or rehabilitation, social services, home care, hospice, Medicare/Medicaid or other health insurance, or mental health or substance abuse services.

Family Referrals

The physician should recognize signs of severe family dysfunction that warrant referral to a family therapist or other mental health professional. These include severe depression, loss of ability to function in daily activities, severe problems in communication, disorganized family roles, substance abuse, severe conflict, family violence, and child abuse. If a physician identifies family dysfunction or other problems that warrant referral, the initial family meeting can lay the groundwork for a referral, which is often difficult for patients and families to accept. The physician will need tact and patience to gain acceptance of a referral.

The physician should be familiar with referral resources within the community. He or she can facilitate a referral by making the initial contact with a family therapist or mental health specialist or by discussing the case with a psychiatric consultant. It is important to present the referral as a means to help the family access the most appropriate care. The physician should avoid labeling the family as "crazy" or "dysfunctional."

> William was a 42-year-old man who had a history of multiple admissions for hepatic encephalopathy. He had cirrhosis resulting from a chronic hepatitis C infection acquired from intravenous drug abuse. He also had a history of alco-

hol abuse. He lived with his mother, and it was noted that two brothers lived in the area. His hospital admissions were triggered by dietary indiscretions. Numerous conversations with the patient about his diet and medication adherence did not prevent his rehospitalizations. On his last admission, a family meeting was requested to discuss his worsening health, his placement after the hospitalization, and his prognosis. Until this meeting, the patient and his family had always insisted that he would go home and that he was to be treated aggressively in the hospital, including intubation and surgery. Extensive discussion with the family took place. They were able to recognize the dangers of his repeated exacerbations and the long-term prognosis. They agreed to consider placement in a rehabilitation facility. During this hospitalization, William suffered another respiratory arrest and required pressors to maintain his blood pressure. This time, his family was able to make the decision to withhold further aggressive treatment, and the patient died peacefully. Although his family grieved, they felt comfortable with the physicians' care and the decisions that they made on behalf of their family member.

Retrospective analysis of this case suggests that earlier family meetings might have been helpful to discover the reasons for this patient's nonadherence. Earlier family intervention might have prevented the rapid deterioration that ultimately caused his death. His family might have found additional support in dealing with this difficult and very ill man, and the medical staff might have experienced less frustration in caring for him.

Primary care physicians who understand the medical, social, and family contexts of their patients' lives have the opportunity to bring these often disconnected realms together. The benefits to patients are clear: improved adherence to therapy, lessening of isolation, better quality of life, and, perhaps, better outcomes. The benefits to families are decreased caregiver stress and improved communication among family members. Physicians may reduce their frustration in caring for patients and experience the satisfaction of improving quality of life and helping patients to live longer. They also have a unique opportunity to humanize the technological face of medicine, which is experienced by many as impersonal and uncaring. Finally, primary care physicians can participate in understanding the interactions among biological, psychological, and social factors in the pathogenesis of disease and in caring for patients and their families.

REFERENCES

American Psychiatric Association. (1994). *Diagnostic and statistical manual of mental disorders* (4th ed.). Washington, DC: Author.

Anderson, C. M., & Holder, D. P. (1989). Family systems and behavioral disorders: Schizophrenia, depression, and alcoholism. In C. Ramsey (Ed.), *Family systems in medicine,* (pp. 487–502). New York: Guilford Press.

Doherty, W. S., & Baird, M. (1983). *Family therapy and family medicine*. New York: Guilford Press.

Mermelstein R., Lichtenstein, E., & McIntyre, K. (1983). Partner support and relapses in smoking cessation programs. *Journal of Counseling and Clinical Psychologies, 51*, 465–466.

Smilkstein, G. (1978). The family APGAR: A proposal for a family function test and its use by physicians. *Journal of Family Practice, 6,* 1231–1239.

Steinglass, P. (1989). Alcohol and the family system. In: C. Ramsey (Ed.), *Family systems in medicine* (pp. 519–535). New York: Guilford Press.

CHAPTER ***19***

Behavioral Counseling and Medical Adherence

Robert E. Feinstein, Joseph S. Pachman, and Roberta Stiel

Most physicians have not been trained to use techniques for maximizing behavioral change (Thompson, Taplin, McAfee, Mandelson, & Smith, 1995). However, encouraging patients to make health-related behavioral changes is an important role of the clinician, and promoting such changes may be as important as accurate diagnosis and the prescription of appropriate treatments. The skills needed to aid patients in fostering healthy lifestyle change can be learned and incorporated into daily office practice.

This chapter describes a behavioral change model and reviews a method that can be used by clinicians to improve patients' adherence to medical treatment. The use of a cognitive behavioral diary in office-based treatment is described.

STAGES OF CHANGE MODEL

Much research has been done on the structure and process of health-related behavior change in adults. The "stages of change" model described by Prochaska and DiClemente (1983, 1985, 1986, 1992) is arguably the most important new theory to emerge in the field of health promotion in the past decade. According to this model, the five stages of behavioral change are precontemplation, contemplation, preparation, action, and maintenance (Prochaska & DiClemente, 1992). See Table 19.1 for an overview of this model, which encompasses the stage of change, presentation of the patient, common clinician mistakes, and clinician interventions that promote behavioral change.

Precontemplation

A patient in the precontemplation phase of behavioral change either has no awareness of the need to change or has no intention of changing within the next 6 months. The hallmark of the precontemplation stage (Prochaska & DiClemente, 1992) is the patient's resistance to recognizing or modifying a health-related problem. For example, a patient in the precontemplation phase does not recognize a connection between a drinking problem and gastric ulcers, or acknowledges the connection but has no wish to discontinue drinking. Patients in the precontemplation stage often have significant others who are aware of the problem (e.g., the spouse of an alcoholic who clearly sees the relationship between the drinking problem and the patient's stomach pains). Individuals in this stage may eventually demonstrate change; however, making the change usually requires education about the problem, understanding their denial of the problem, and coercion from significant others. For a review of this clinical stage and suggested interventions, see Table 19.1.

Contemplation

A patient in the contemplation phase of behavioral change is aware that a health problem exists and hopes to change behavior within the next 6 months. Although the patient is thinking about change, he or she may not yet be committed to taking the actions necessary for such change. For some patients, moving from this point to the point of actually changing behavior may take years. Patients in the contemplation phase may weigh the pros and cons of the problem and its possible solutions. For example, an adolescent woman who smokes may contemplate smoking cessation but does not take any action at the present time because of her fear of weight gain or ostracism by peers who smoke.

Preparation

Patients in the preparation phase of behavioral change are preparing to make a change within the next month and often report having made partial changes in the past year. For example, a patient is planning to lower his cholesterol level and has tried to do so in the past by changing his diet. In preparation for another attempt to decrease his intake of saturated fats, he plans to read food labels carefully, to buy healthier foods, and to change the way in which his meals are prepared, perhaps with the help of his wife.

Action

During the action phase, patients have begun to demonstrate overt intentions, behaviors, and actions for change, and they continue to do so over the next 6 months. For example, a patient has begun smoking fewer cigarettes and soon will convert to the targeted behavior, abstinence from smoking. By definition, the action phase begins with a change in behavior. This phase is often the busiest one for the patient, because the lifestyle change must be integrated into daily life. For instance, a patient who recently has quit smoking has to deal with friends who smoke; smoking cues that may trigger the desire to smoke again (e.g., being at a bar); and compensatory urges, such as the urge to eat instead of smoke.

Maintenance

During the maintenance phase, patients work to maintain the desired behavior changes. This stage is fundamentally a continuation of the changed behavior. It begins 6 months after the action stage and continues until the change process is no longer a problem for the patient. The maintenance phase is more easily sustained if the patient acknowledges the need for ongoing support. A sign of successful maintenance is that the patient continues to implement the action plan and shows adaptive cognitions and relapse-prevention behaviors. Refusing help or denying the need for ongoing support can lead to relapse, which occurs commonly during this phase. Some patients make several attempts before finally changing their unhealthy behaviors. For example, many patients can lose weight, but maintaining a stable weight requires a consistent behavioral change that typically includes improving nutrition and eating habits, exercising, and managing side effects such as anxiety and depressed mood.

Table 19.1 Implementation of Stage of Change

Stage of Change	Presentation of the Patient	Common Clinician Mistakes	Clinician Interventions
Precontemplation	• Patient unaware of problem behavior (denial) and has no awareness of need to change within next 6 months, or has no intention of changing in the near future. • Family expresses concern about maladaptive health behavior.	• Clinician colludes with patient's denial. • Clinician doesn't ask about problem. • Clinician educates in a didactic manner.	• Ask about the problem each visit. • Assess medical need for change. • Attempt to help the patient see a problem that needs change. • Provide patient education. • Utilize the family. Encourage family health discussions. • Use counseling techniques PRN.
Contemplation	• Patient aware of problem and hopeful about changing his or her behavior within the next 6 months. Patient "wishes" to change.	• Clinician annoyed about absence of change. • Clinician may use scare tactics. • Clinician may avoid discussion of the problem.	• Reflective listening • Ask: "What can you do to change your wish into reality? • Educate: benefits of change. • Have the patient write the pros and cons of behavioral change. • Ask: "What will motivate you to change?"
Preparation planning	• Patient expresses desire to change and is preparing to make a change within next month. Patient demonstrates intent and preparatory action toward change.	• Clinician expects change without a detailed plan for change. • Clinician has excessive expectations for rapid change. • Clinician underestimates the patient's need for support.	• Educate: benefits of change. • Identify/analyze the behavior. • Stimulus trigger: who, what where, when? • Stimulus control: avoid (-) or reinforce (+) stimuli. • Self-monitoring: daily/weekly logs and/or cognitive diaries. • Contract for change. • Set action date and goals. • Discuss barriers to change.

Stage of Change	Presentation of the Patient	Common Clinician Mistakes	Clinician Interventions
Action	• Intentions, behaviors, and actions for change have begun and are ongoing over the next 6 months. • Relapses to old behaviors common.	• Clinician disappointed with relapses. • Clinician expects change to be permanent and the patient to be self-reliant.	• Challenge the patient's plan: "That sounds too hard." • Encourage and affirm change. • Review contract for change. • Begin realistic behavioral goals (e.g., walk up stairs daily). • Identify/plan for high-relapse situations; avoid high-risk triggers. • Discuss barriers to maintaining change. • Utilize a support group. • Stress management. • Discuss target goals, behavioral strategies, and outcome measures. • Make a follow-up plan.
Maintenance and relapse prevention	• Maintains the desired change behaviors that are evident. • Patient acknowledges the need for ongoing support, continues the plan, adaptive cognitions, and relapse prevention behaviors. • Denial of help can lead to relapse. • Relapse is common.	• Clinician minimizes the risk of relapse. • Clinician sees patient's relapse as a failure.	• Continues action plan above. • Emphasize the specific benefits of sustained change. • Praise health behavior. • Be positive, if a relapse occurs, and have the patient try again. • Discuss new barriers to change. • Redo the action plan PRN.

The cycles by which individuals change, then relapse, are characterized by a spiral pattern or nonlinear progression (Prochaska & DiClemente, 1992). After a failed attempt at change, patients usually do not regress to where they began. Ordinarily, the more action taken, the better the prognosis. Certain types of individuals, situations, and problems can benefit from repeated attempts or "recycling" efforts at change, but for others recycling is more like spinning one's wheels. For example, an alcoholic may need to recycle many times before achieving sobriety, whereas "yo-yo" dieting, which is associated with major health risks, rarely results in long-term change.

Different persons will spend different amounts of time in each phase. However, the tasks performed within each phase generally do not vary from individual to individual. The degree of change is a function of the pretreatment stage of change (i.e., the status of the behavior before the patient attempts to modify it). The farther away from action an individual starts out, the longer it will take for him or her to move to action. For example, a patient who has not considered smoking cessation at all will take longer to move to smoking cessation than a patient who has considered quitting. Movement between stages during treatment is highly predictive of success. The stage of change at which the patient begins seeing the clinician is a better predictor of successful outcome or improved adherence than are age, socioeconomic status, problem severity or duration, and social support. Given what is known about stages of change, treating adult patients as if they were all in the same stage of change is a waste of medical resources and time.

When using the stages of change model, the clinician should first determine the patient's current status on the continuum of change. (See chapter 13, A Model for Office-based Cardiovascular Risk Reduction and Behavioral Change, for an expanded application of the stage of change model.) For example, when planning an approach to smoking cessation, the clinician should assess whether the patient has been thinking about quitting (contemplation stage) or has not seriously considered quitting (precontemplation stage). After determining the patient's current stage of change, the clinician should guide the patient from one stage to the next instead of using scare tactics to force the patient to quit smoking.

Change is influenced by both patient and intervention variables. Patient variables that negatively influence treatment efficacy include inadequate motivation, resistance to treatment, defensiveness, and inability to relate to the physician or to those involved with the delivery of treatment.

Intervention variables that affect the chances of change include the relationship skills of the clinician, a mismatch between the clinician's personality and that of the patient (see chapter 8, Personality Disorders in Office Practice), and a clinician's lack of appreciation of the underlying theory of change. The clinician's role as an agent of change should not be underestimated. Many patients will be unable to make health-related changes without input and encouragement from their clinicians. Review Table 19.1 for clinician interventions that can foster the patient's efforts to move from one stage to the next.

MEDICAL ADHERENCE

Medical adherence is the extent to which a patient carries out the recommendations of his or her physician. For example, a drug with demonstrated efficacy will be effective only if the patient takes it in the prescribed manner. Other examples of medical adherence include following a prescribed diet or exercise plan; following through with scheduled immunizations or required laboratory testing; and keeping scheduled appointments, a medical log, or a medical diary. Adherence can be measured using the patient's self-report of compliance, with collateral reports from family or friends that confirm adherence, or with objective indicators of adherence, such as successful control of blood pressure or weight loss (Damrosh, 1995). The number of patients who fail to follow their physicians' instructions ranges from 20% to 80%, while 38% to 95% of patients fail to adhere to their recommended medication schedules (Damrosh, 1995). Patients are most likely to adhere to physician recommendations if they understand the nature and severity of their medical problems, they believe that their probability of getting the disorder is high, they have self-efficacy (i.e., a belief that they can accomplish the necessary tasks), they are confident that the treatment will help, and they intend to adhere (Damrosh, 1995).

The following are general principles about adherence:

- The degree of adherence will decrease over time, especially among patients with chronic diseases. For example, 46% of patients with hypertension are nonadherent with their medication because they think they have been cured, while another 25% think their doctor advised them to stop (Bittar, 1995).

- The more complex the medical treatment, the poorer the adherence. For example, patients on twice-daily medication dosing schedules are less adherent to their regimens compared with patients on once-daily dosing schedules.
- Asymptomatic patients have more problems with adherence than do symptomatic patients. For example, once per day aspirin prophylaxis for stroke may be discontinued by patients with no daily symptoms associated with the need for drug maintenance.

An understanding of the following principles may help the physician enhance patients' medical adherence:

1. The doctor-patient relationship has a major influence on medical adherence. Adherence improves when the physician can assess the patient's needs and adjust the kind and content of the doctor-patient interaction to suit the patient's needs. Patient adherence increases when clinicians listen to their patients, remain empathetic, and use physician-patient interactive interviewing techniques that are tailored to meet the needs of each patient. For example, patients who prefer to follow an expert's opinion may do best with a biomedical approach. Some patients may need a biopsychosocial (collaborative) or psychosocial (less medical focus) approach, whereas others prefer an informational (consumerist) approach (Roter et al., 1997). (See chapter 13, A Model for Office-based Cardiovascular Risk Reduction and Behavioral Change, for a detailed discussion of these approaches.)
2. Consider the impact of the illness and treatment from the patient's point of view. Consider what the illness means to the patient, his or her potential fears about the illness, the necessary changes and the impact of these changes on the patient's lifestyle, and the medication side effects that are likely to be important to the patient. For example, if the patient considers himself or herself to be overweight, avoid using medications that might have the side effect of weight gain.
3. Adherence is promoted by educating the patient about his or her illness, any diagnostic tests required, the prognosis, treatment options, and by encouraging all efforts by the patient at self-care and prevention.

4. Before expecting or asking for adherence by the patient, determine his or her current stage of change for each problem, and use specific interventions based on the patient's stage (see Table 19.1).
5. Patients' cognitive distortions about their medical illnesses often affect adherence to medical care. For example, a sober alcoholic may have an antimedication bias that prevents him or her from taking necessary medications for hypertension. The clinician's use of a cognitive behavioral approach (described below) helps some patients understand and fight their own tendencies toward cognitive distortions (negative thoughts, incorrect or inadequate information processing) that are interfering with medical care.
6. Identify all sources of conflicts that may be affecting adherence. For example, when a patient is angry with the physician (the physician may not be aware of this), medical adherence deteriorates. A patient's cooperation may be adversely affected if a family member with the same illness has had a poor outcome. Conflicts with family members brought on by required health changes can also reduce adherence. For example, smoking cessation may be very difficult for a husband whose wife continues to smoke.
7. Identify other barriers to change, such as insufficient financial resources, difficulty with access to medical services, and lack of insurance, that may be affecting patient compliance, and address each one specifically. Such barriers are reviewed in chapter 12, Cardiovascular and Psychosocial Risk Factors Reduction: Office-based Interventions.
8. Identify and treat moods that are affecting the patient's capacity to adhere to medical treatment. For example, a depressed mood may make smoking cessation very difficult.
9. Help patients in their problem-solving efforts. Table 19.2 summarizes a sample patient's behavioral health change and coping document that can be completed by patients to assist them in problem solving. Individual, crisis, family, and cognitive behavioral approaches offer different problem-solving methods for different patients. These approaches are reviewed in chapters 16, 17, 18, and 19, respectively.

Table 19.2 Health Change and Coping

1. Describe a health problem you want to change.
   - Lower my blood pressure
2. Describe your current stage of change.
   a. Precontemplation: I don't want to change right now.
   b. Contemplation: I am thinking about making the change.
   c. Preparation: I am getting ready to make the change.
   d. Action: I have changed/am changing my behavior.
   e. Maintenance: I have made the change and want to continue.
   - Contemplation: I want to lower my blood pressure.
3. Is the change you want to make (choose one)
   a. Under your control?
   b. Partially under your control?
   c. Under someone else's control?
   - Partially under my control.
4. What is your style of coping with change?
   (describe; or see Coping Styles in Table 17.1, chapter 17)
   - Emotional style
5. Is there a better style you can use? Which?
   (describe; or see Coping Styles in Table 17.1, chapter 17)
   - Informational
6. Describe any barriers to making change.
   (See chapter 12, Barriers to Lifestyle Change)
   - I forget to take my medication.
7. What can you do to overcome a barrier to change?
   - Leave a message for myself on the bathroom mirror.
8. Describe a healthier approach to change.
   - Thoughts: I can keep a cognitive diary.
   - Emotionally: I can check out my feeling with others.
   - Physically: I can begin to exercise.
   - Behavior: I can keep a blood pressure log and decrease salt and alcohol intake.

10. Develop a plan of action. Outline with the patient the details of how medical care should proceed; specify what help the patient can expect from the physician and what is expected of the patient in the future.
11. Consider using a patient contract. Some patients may benefit from a simple contract for adherence that formalizes what both the patient and the clinician can do to promote compliance and improve health. This contract may include an agreement for patient self-monitoring, target dates for action (setting a smoking quit date), and an agreed-upon follow-up schedule. A more sophisticated version of a patient contract is a behavioral contingency contract. This contract with a patient states that an increasing amount of care will be required if adherence decreases. For example, a bulimic/anorexic patient may benefit from a contingency contract stating that if his or her weight is 110 pounds or greater, outpatient treatment is appropriate, but if his or her weight drops to 100 pounds, partial psychiatric hospitalization will be required; if the patient's weight falls below 90 pounds, medical and psychiatric hospitalization will be mandatory. A behavioral contingency contract is more complicated than a patient contract and can specify multiple target goals, self-monitoring, agreement in advance for a treatment change if failure occurs, rewards, and punishments.
12. Examine a daily log kept by the patient before suggesting an intervention, so that it is very clear exactly what the patient is or is not doing. Specify the changes required, and follow up with ongoing daily logs. A log that records the patient's daily, weekly, or monthly patterns can be used to monitor food intake, smoking, exercise, mood, and anxiety.
13. Use stimulus control techniques, which help the patient alter his or her environment to make it convenient and likely that a desired change can occur. This may mean asking the patient to avoid other smokers, to avoid bars, or to resist bringing fattening food into the house. It may also mean asking a patient to set up a comfortable exercise room or to change usual routines to avoid triggers for poor adherence. For example, a patient who used to smoke heavily during a work break should be counseled to avoid the coffee break room, thereby avoiding a behavioral stimulus for smoking.
14. Use stress management techniques that can help manage urges, reduce symptoms, and foster health-related changes. For example,

the clinician can teach the relaxation response as a tool to reduce a craving to smoke or suggest yoga or tai chi class to help a reluctant patient begin to move and exercise.

15. Use a support group. Patients who are suffering with a specific disease can benefit greatly from support from other patients. Alcoholics Anonymous, breast cancer support groups, transplant support groups, cardiovascular support groups, and Alzheimer's support groups are some of the many options available to patients and clinicians to improve adherence to medical treatment and coping with illness.

COGNITIVE BEHAVIORAL TREATMENT IN PRIMARY CARE

Cognitive behavioral therapy has proven to be very effective in dealing with a wide range of psychiatric conditions. This approach can also help promote health-related changes when used in conjunction with a stages of change model. In 1976, Aaron Beck proposed a cognitive-behavioral treatment based on an educational model. Cognitive therapists believe that automatic thoughts are a reflexive, rigid style of distorted or negative thinking, such as exaggerating information out of proportion and presenting a problem as a catastrophe when it is actually manageable. For example, a patient who had asked for a blood test may assume this means he or she has cancer. Automatic thoughts are activated by a stimulus, which causes a mood change such as depression, anger, or anxiety, which then leads to some characteristic misperception, distorted thought, or incorrect interpretation of the meaning of the events.

Cognitive misperceptions can lead to maladaptive health behaviors or inhibitions. This process can be conceptualized as a circle with feedback loops (see Figure 19.1). A cognitive therapist encourages a patient to first recognize the distorted thought process, notes how thoughts change the patient's moods, then corrects the problem by testing the veracity of these automatic thoughts against reality. The clinician can encourage patients to correct these thoughts by repeatedly testing their perception against reality (see Table 19.3 and 19.4). A cognitive diary (see Figure 19.2) can be used by a patient to help him or her identify, test, and change his or her rigid thinking processes. The change in cognitive mind-set creates a change in mood that can subsequently permit a change in health-related

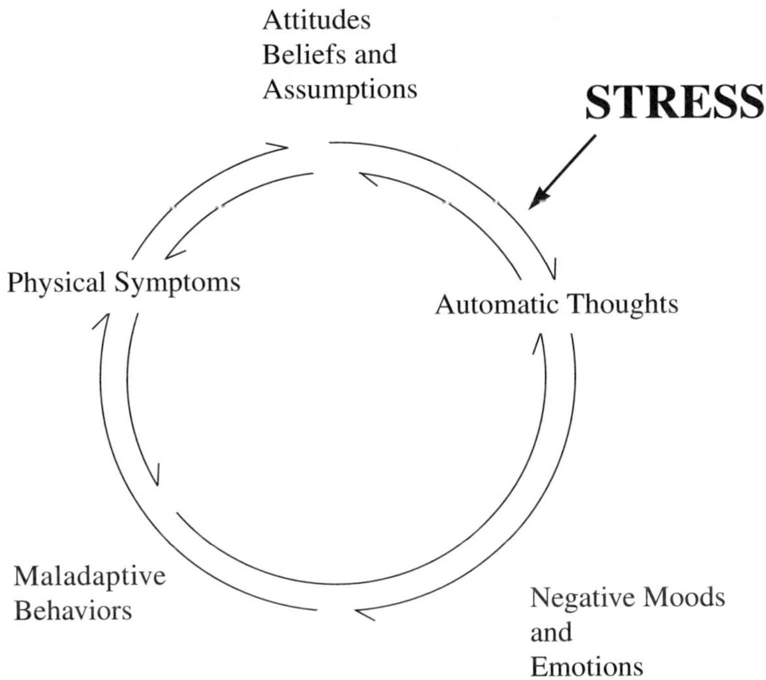

Source: Benson, H. and Stuart, E. M. (1993). *The wellness book*, p. 195. New York: Fireside-Simon & Shuster.

Figure 19.1 Cognitive-Behavioral Therapy.

behavior. The patient gains a broader perspective about what is happening or can happen in a given situation. Identifying cognitive distortions gives the patient the freedom to choose different behavioral responses.

> A stroke victim believed he was useless to his family because of his disability, and he remained in bed all day. His negative view of himself, his defeatist attitude, and his sense of hopelessness were part of his negative thought process. As a focus of treatment, he was encouraged to use a cognitive behavioral diary. In this diary he recorded the results of testing his family to find out if they really saw him as useless and if others blamed him or viewed him as bad. He was also encouraged to test his physical capacities (with the assistance of a physical therapist) to see if he was truly incapable or as hopeless as he felt. Based on the review of his diaries, his cognitive distortions began to change

Table 19.3 Illogical Styles of Thinking

1. EXAGGERATING THE NEGATIVE OR POSITIVE
   Emphasizing negative thoughts and invalidating positive ones.
   Example: "I ate pizza; it ruined a whole week of healthy eating."
   Emphasizing the positive and ignoring the negative.
   Example: "If I eat healthy foods tonight, it discounts all the junk food I ate all week."
2. SELF REFERENCE
   Taking things personally, when they have no reference to you.
   Example: "The doctor is mad . . . I did something wrong."
3. NEGATIVE SELF TALK
   Insulting oneself, name calling, or predicting personal failure.
   Example: "I am an idiot." or "I will never be able to do that."
4. EITHER/OR THINKING.
   Thinking in extremes or opposites. Thoughts that people or things are all good or all bad.
   Example: "People are either caring or they are cruel."
5. DETAILED OR OBSESSIVE THINKING
   Emphasizing details and facts; omitting emotions and impressions; preventing a broader perspective.
   Example: "I can't see the forest for the trees."
6. MOANS
   M = Must O = Ought A = Always N = Never S = Should
   Example: "I must exercise daily." "I should lose 50 pounds."
7. PERFECTIONISTIC THINKING
   Thinking there can be no mistakes. All must be perfect.
   Example: "Everything must be perfect, or it is no good."
8. AFFECTIVE & IMPRESSIONISTIC THINKING
   Thinking based on emotions or impressions, not facts/evidence.
   Example: "I feel it is bad . . . it must be bad."
9. FUTURE THINKING
   Believing one can predict the future.
   Example: "I am sure I will die young."
10. NEGATIVE PAST THINKING
    Thinking a troubled past predetermines a future of failure.
    Example: "I had a bad childhood . . . I won't amount to anything."
11. IMPULSIVE THINKING
    Making quick decisions without gathering facts or evidence; being unaware of potential negative consequences.
    Example: "I felt angry . . . yelled at my boss . . . got fired."
12. THOUGHT READING
    Thinking others know your thoughts and think badly of you.
    Example: "Without facts, I know my doctor doesn't like me."
13. SUSPICIOUS THINKING
    Always thinking that others are out to hurt or exploit you.
    Example: "I am sure they are out to get me."

Table 19.4 Combating Illogical Thinking

1. EXAGGERATING THE NEGATIVE OR POSITIVE
   What is the good news that I am not considering?
   What is the bad news that I am not considering?
2. SELF REFERENCE
   Is this really me, or is it the other person?
3. NEGATIVE SELF TALK
   Use positive self talk, and encourage yourself.
4. EITHER/OR THINKING
   If thinking all is good, ask, "What can be bad?" Find a balance.
   If thinking all is bad, ask, "What can be good?" Find a balance.
5. DETAILED OR OBSESSIVE THINKING
   These are the facts and evidence . . . but what do I feel? What is my overall impression? What is the big picture?
6. MOANS
   Do I have to be so extreme? Must I? Why ought I? Is it always or never, with nothing in between? Why should I?
7. PERFECTIONISTIC THINKING
   Is it really that important if it/I am not perfect? What is good enough?
8. AFFECTIVE AND IMPRESSIONISTIC THINKING
   This is how I feel or this is my impression . . . but what are the facts and evidence, and what do I think? Describe the logic.
9. FUTURE THINKING
   Can I really predict the future outcome, or am I just fulfilling a negative self prophecy?
10. NEGATIVE PAST THINKING
    Why can't the future be free of a troubled past?
11. IMPULSIVE THINKING
    Slow down, wait, think things over, and examine the possible future consequences.
12. THOUGHT READING
    How can anyone know what I am thinking if I don't tell them? Tell them, and give others a chance to respond.
13. SUSPICIOUS THINKING
    Are they out to get me, or am I mad or angry?

and his mood state improved, he felt less self-critical and had a more hopeful attitude, with realistic optimism. This treatment helped increase his motivation to get out of bed and return to physical rehabilitation and improved his chances to optimize his functioning.

Cognitive behavioral therapy is based on several principles and techniques:

1. Cognitive therapy is brief and time-oriented. In a busy primary care practice, it may be used as a tool by the physician to assist the patient in initiating a specific health-related behavior such as smoking cessation, weight reduction, exercise, or abstinence from substance abuse.
2. A sound therapeutic relationship between the clinician and the patient is necessary for successful treatment.
3. Treatment is a collaborative effort between the clinician and the patient. The patient is invited to be an active participant in treatment, to negotiate a behavioral contract with the clinician, to keep daily logs, and to use a cognitive behavioral diary. This approach, like all counseling approaches, may require some additional clinician time in the office setting to review cognitive diaries and counsel the patient.
4. Cognitive therapy using a cognitive behavioral diary is structured and directive.
5. Cognitive therapy is problem-focused. When using a diary, the clinician should focus on one priority health-related issue at a time. For example, a patient's diary should focus on only one health-related issue at a time, such as smoking cessation, exercise, weight, anxiety, or depressed mood.
6. Homework is a central feature of cognitive therapy; that is, having the patient keep a cognitive behavioral diary is the focus of the clinician's office-based treatment effort.

The Cognitive Behavioral Diary

A cognitive behavioral diary has the following elements: triggering situation, mood/feelings, physical symptoms, automatic thoughts (Beck, 1976) or "hot thoughts" (Greenberger & Padesky, 1995), pros (information that supports the belief), cons (information that does not support the belief), a realistic view based on the pros and cons assessment, and a new mood rating. A typical diary that can be given to patients is illustrated in Figure 19.2.

Triggers/Situation

In the first column, the patient describes the situation that he or she is trying to change. This means describe the four *W*s: what, where, when, who. What situation causes the problem? *Example:* "I smoke a lot after each meal or on a relaxation break." Where does this occur? *Example:* "It is worse at work." When does it occur? *Example:* "After one of my five meals or snacks and during two coffee breaks." Who do you smoke with?

Triggers of Distress	**Mood or Feeling**	**Physical Symptoms**	**Disturbing Thought**	**Pros of Thought**	**Cons of Thought**	**Revised Thought**	**Anxiety or Fear**
Who? What? When? Where? Why?	What is your mood (e.g., sad, depressed, anxious, irritable)? Rate the severity: 1 = minimal 5 = severe	List physical symptoms (e.g., pain, headache, palpitations).	Write down one of your most anxious or fearful thoughts.	Write down the evidence that supports your thinking.	Write down the evidence that does not support your thinking.	Write down a more realistic thought about your troubled thought.	Is your mood or physical symptom improved? Rate the severity: 1 = minimal 5 = severe

Figure 19.2 Cognitive Diary.

Example: "I smoke with work friends, never at home, because I don't want my wife and kids to see this." In addition, the patient describes common triggers for the behavior. *Example:* "My smoking is triggered after meals, often after coffee or sex, and is worse when I am on a break from work."

Moods/Feelings

In the second column, the patient describes his or her mood or feeling associated with the behavior and rates the severity of each mood from 1 (minimal/not a problem) to 5 (severe/major problem). *Example:* Describe how you feel after you smoke. A patient may say, "I feel guilty every time I smoke." The patient can record guilt as one mood associated with a smoking behavior. A typical mood list associated with unpleasant mood or feelings might include depressed, lonely, sad, panicked, anxious, worried, annoyed, irritated, angry, impatient, urgent, guilty, embarrassed, humiliated, devalued, frightened, disappointed, frustrated, and hurt. A typical mood list associated with pleasant feelings might include at peace, pleasant, happy, fulfilled, proud, excited, hopeful, optimistic, cheerful, loving, and secure. In addition to naming the mood or feeling state associated with the situation, the patient rates the mood at the beginning of the diary and again at the end. For example, at the beginning the patient notes, "I feel 4 [moderately severe guilt] when I smoke, and my anxiety level is 3 [moderate]." At the end, he writes, "I feel 2 [mild guilt] and 2 [mild anxiety]."

Physical Symptoms

In the third column, the patient lists all physical symptoms associated with the behavior. If no symptoms exist, he or she lists none. For example, during a smoking cessation effort, a patient might write, "I feel jumpy . . . my heart is racing, my hands are trembling slightly." Physical symptoms can stimulate negative thinking, which, in turn, can exacerbate emotional or physical symptoms. For instance, symptoms of nicotine withdrawal can trigger the thought "I can never stop smoking. . . . I can't stand this," which creates a feeling of hopelessness, defeat, and more physical discomfort.

Disturbing Thoughts/Negative Thoughts

Disturbing or negative thoughts are critical factors in failure to change. Negative thinking is often an outgrowth of our long-held attitudes, beliefs, and assumptions about the world (see Figure 19.1). Negative thoughts and a belief system are related but are not the same. Automatic thoughts are generally event-specific and are an immediate response to a given situation: Something happens, and negative thinking occurs. For example, a patient reaches for a cigarette and thinks, "I'll never stop smoking." Beliefs, on the other hand, are more fundamental, generalizable, and serve as the underlying schema through which events are interpreted and the world is perceived. For example, "My father and mother both died of cancer, so I will too. So what difference does it make if I smoke?" The core belief here is "I will die of cancer no matter what I do." Belief systems are much harder to change compared with negative thinking but can be modified with ongoing psychological treatment. For a more detailed approach to refuting irrational beliefs, refer to Eshelman and McKay (1995).

Negative thoughts related to health behaviors (that are not heavily influenced by powerfully negative belief systems) often can be modified using a cognitive diary. In the column headed "Disturbing Thought," the patient records all negative thoughts about the behavioral change in the specific situation in which it occurs. For example, the negative thought during a brief smoking relapse could be "I will never stop smoking . . . here is the proof. . . . I am doing it again." It takes time for a patient to become aware of his own self-defeating thoughts. Having the patient keep a diary gives the patient and the clinician access to negative thinking that is interfering with change.

Pros and Cons

Once a negative thought is identified, the patient records in each column all the pros that support the negative thinking and all the cons against it. For example, "I will never stop smoking." The pros, or evidence supporting this negative thought, are "I am still smoking" and "I have failed to stop many times in the past." The cons, or evidence that does not support this negative view, are "Just because I am smoking now does not mean I have to smoke in the future" and "Change is possible. I have lowered my blood pressure by taking medication. In fact, I can put my cigarette out now, before I have completed smoking it. Maybe I can use a nicotine patch."

Revised Thoughts and New Mood Rating

Weighing the pros and cons can lead to revised thinking that is much less negative or is more positive and realistic. An example of a revised thought is "I probably can stop smoking. It will be hard. I may fail several times before I actually succeed. Keep trying, and get the nicotine patch to help."

After recording the revised thought, the patient rates his or her mood or feeling again to see whether it has improved. For example, "When I was smoking I felt 4 [moderately severe guilt] for smoking, and my anxiety level was 3 [moderate]. After recording my revised thinking, I now feel 2 [mild guilt] and 2 [mild anxiety]." The patient can be asked to keep a daily thought diary. The clinician can review one or several diaries with the patient during an office visit.

Encouraging a patient's health-related behavioral changes and medical adherence can be a goal of every office visit. By understanding the stage of change model, using stage-specific interventions, and promoting adherence to medical recommendations, the clinician can be an agent of change who can actively help patients improve their health-related behaviors and lifestyles. Daily logs, behavioral contracting, and cognitive behavioral diaries are tools that can be useful in fostering health-related changes.

REFERENCES

Beck, A. T. (1976). *Cognitive therapy and the emotional disorders.* New York: Plenum Press.

Bittar, N.(1995). Maintaining long-term control of blood pressure: The role of improved compliance. *Clinical Cardiology, 18*(Suppl. III), III-12–III-16.

Damrosh, S. (1995). Facilitating adherence to preventive and treatment regimens. In D. Wedding (Ed.), *Behavior and medicine* (2nd ed., pp. 379–388). St. Louis: Mosby.

Eshelman, D., & McKay, M. (1995). *Refuting irrational ideas: The relaxation and stress handbook* (4th ed.). Oakland, CA: New Harbinger Publications.

Prochaska, J. O., & DiClemente, C. C. (1983). Stages and processes of self-change in smoking: Toward an integrative model of change. *Journal of Consulting and Clinical Psychology, 51,* 390–395.

———. (1985). Common processes of change in smoking, weight control, and psychological distress. In S. Shiffman, & T. Wills (Eds.), *Coping and substance use* (pp. 345–363). San Diego: Academic Press.

———. (1986). Toward a comprehensive model of change. In W. R. Miller & N. Heather (Eds.), *Treating addictive behaviors: Processes of change* (pp. 3–27). New York: Plenum Press.

———. (1992). Stages of change in the modification of problem behaviors. In M. Hersen, R. M. Eisler, & P. M. Miller (Eds.), *Progress in behavior modification* (pp. 184–218). Newbury Park, CA: Sage.

Roter, D. L., Stewart, M., Putnam, S. M., Lipkin, M., Jr., Stiles, W., & Inui, T. S. (1997). Communication patterns of primary care physicians. *Journal of the American Medical Association, 277,* 350–356.

Thompson, R. S., Taplin, S. H., McAfee, T. A., Mandelson, M. T., & Smith, A. E. (1995). Primary and secondary prevention services in clinical practice. *Journal of the American Medical Association, 273,* 1130–1135.

Index

('i' indicates an illustration; 't' indicates a table)